BOOK OF

Proven Home Remedies and Natural Healing Secrets

Thousands of Proven
Home Healing Tips
You Can Use Without Doctors,
Drugs or Surgery

by the editors of FC&A

BOOK OF

Proven Home Remedies and Natural Healing Secrets

Notice:

This book is for information only. It does not constitute medical advice and should not be construed as such. We cannot guarantee the safety or effectiveness of any drug, treatment or advice mentioned. Some of these tips may not be effective for everyone.

A good doctor is the best judge of what medical treatment may be needed for certain conditions and diseases. We recommend in all cases that you contact your personal doctor or health care provider before taking or discontinuing any medications, or before treating yourself in any way.

Pleasant words are like a honeycomb,
Sweetness to the soul and health to the body.

— **Proverbs 16:24**

For I will restore health to you, and your wounds
I will heal, says the Lord...

— **Jeremiah 30:17a**

FC&A Publishing
103 Clover Green
Peachtree City, GA 30269

Fourteenth printing July 2000

ISBN 0-915099-51-9

Contents

Breathing and Lung Health 83

Caffeine 86

Cancer 88

Cholesterol 107

Weight Loss 350

Concluding Remarks 361

Introduction

Do you ever feel like Groucho Marx running around with a cigar hanging out of the corner of your mouth shouting, "Is there a doctor in the house?! Is there a doctor in the house?!"

Unfortunately, the answer to our plea for medical wisdom is almost always a resounding, "NO!" There's no doctor in the house to tell us what to do when little Cindy's ear gets red and puffy after a day at the beach. There's no doctor we can call for a bit of advice about how to prevent husband Kevin's allergies.

There's no one to ask about that funny reaction you seem to be having to your glaucoma medicine. And there sure isn't anyone around to tell you why you may be depressed or what you should eat to minimize your cancer risk.

If you went to see your doctor every time you had a health question, you'd be broke!

And don't envy those people who do have a doctor in the family, either. Take it from someone who has a sister who's a pharmacist and a mother who's a nurse. After a while, you get too embarrassed to ask all the health questions you'd like answered. You're sure they're thinking, "Man, she doesn't know *anything*!"

Well, compared to the doctors, pharmacists and nurses, we lay people may be ignorant, but obviously you do know one thing. You know where to go for the answers to your health questions.

You have in your hands the most handy, economical "doctor's visit" you've ever made. The *Book of Proven Home Remedies and Natural Healing Secrets* will tell you how to combat your insomnia, ease the pain of your arthritis, lower your high blood pressure and cholesterol naturally, avoid hemorrhoids, and prevent cataracts from developing.

We give you practical advice on how to lose weight, what kind of bottled water you should buy, how to use and store your medicines, and how to buy the best walking shoes. We even tell you how to pick out a pet and care for it so your pet won't make you and your family sick.

How do you know you can trust the information we're bringing you? It's a good question — conflicting news about health issues appears in the newspapers and on the radio every day. We thought we'd never hear the end of the debate over which is better for you — butter or margarine!

You can trust our information because it comes from the most reliable sources out there. To write a book, we spend months researching the latest, most up-to-date medical journals where doctors and scientists report their ground-breaking medical findings and their tried-and-true methods of healing.

In this book, you have at your fingertips the health wisdom of the ages and the medical data from the scientific laboratories of the 1990s. And it's all in language you don't have to be a scientific genius to understand.

Notice that buying this book doesn't mean you'll never have to see a doctor again, as nice as that may sound. Although we have included plenty of home remedies to help you treat yourself and your family, there are many diseases which require a doctor and prescription medicines to treat properly.

You'll notice we were very careful to add "See your doctor" at the end of many of the articles about diabetes, cancer, heart problems or liver disease. Although "home remedies" can't cure these diseases, this book will give you natural healing methods that will help you prevent some diseases and will help give you the knowledge you need to make better choices about your health.

We think you'll agree that you're holding a wonderful collection of home remedies and healing secrets. Please enjoy reading it, and enjoy your trip along the road to better health.

God bless you!

Aging and Health

What is 'normal' aging?

Although "old age" may be a state of mind, you can expect certain physiological changes to occur in your body as you age.

A report in *Postgraduate Medicine* (85,2:213) lists changes you may experience as you get older and that you should consider "normal." (Please note that not everyone experiences these changes.)

❏ **Heart**—The heart's ability to work efficiently generally decreases by about one percent each year between ages 30 and 80, although regular exercise may lessen the decline. That means that normal aging will cut your heart's efficiency in half by age 80, the report indicates. "By age 80, renal [kidney] blood flow is 50 percent less and cerebral [brain] blood flow is 20 percent less than in the same person at age 30," say doctors P. E. Perlman and William Adams.

❏ **Lungs** — Lungs function less efficiently due to a loss of muscle tone. Smoking also reduces lung efficiency.

❏ **Kidneys** — The kidneys become less efficient at flushing wastes, so certain drugs may be poisonous to the kidneys. Because the kidneys become less efficient at regulating thirst, older people are also susceptible to dehydration and hypernatremia (excess sodium in the blood).

❏ **Digestion** — Older people have constipation more often than younger people because the digestive tract doesn't move food as well and the stomach secretes less acid. The ability to absorb drugs through the intestines is unchanged, though. Older people also find it harder to swallow food because their esophagus is less efficient at moving things along.

❏ **Nervous system** — Impaired or confused thinking is caused by disease, not aging. But, it's natural that the brain functions more slowly, causing reflexes to slow down.

❏ **Immune system** — Older people are more susceptible to infections. Vaccines have less of a beneficial effect on older folks, mainly because their immune systems have slowed down. Vaccines work by stimulating the immune system.

❐ **Metabolism** — Metabolism is the process by which cells release energy for maintaining the body's vital functions, such as pumping blood and regulating body temperature. Older people have more difficulty perceiving cold and are susceptible to hypothermia (body temperature dangerously below normal). Skin is less elastic and more prone to pressure sores (bedsores).

❐ **Thyroid gland** — The thyroid gland is located at the base of the neck and produces hormones that affect the nervous system and the digestive system. Older people are prone to hypothyroidism (decreased activity of the thyroid gland). Doctors often identify the symptoms of hypothyroidism as "failure to thrive."

'Failure to thrive' in the elderly

"Failure to thrive" is a murky term used by doctors to describe age-related illness in older patients. The symptoms of failure to thrive include fatigue, weakness and loss of appetite, says Dr. Richard E. Waltman. Older people may fail to thrive for a number of reasons, such as poor nutrition and stress, according to the doctor in *Senior Patient* (1,4:30).

Depression — Retirement, grief, financial problems or moving to a new home can cause depression, masked by pain, fatigue, weakness and loss of sleep and appetite — in other words, failure to thrive.

Doctors have difficulty helping older patients with depression because they are less likely to talk about what's bothering them than younger patients, Dr. Waltman said.

The good news, however, is that once you talk to your doctor, he probably will be able to help you.

An active social life and regular exercise will give you more energy and a happier outlook on life. Talk to your doctor about starting an exercise routine.

He will advise you based on any physical limitations you might have.

Lack of exercise — Lack of exercise may contribute to decreased heart efficiency, muscle tone and mobility. Ironically, older people who complain of feeling tired may be told to slow down or to take it easy. That may be the worst possible advice.

"The more they rest, the more they will slow down and the worse they will feel," Dr. Waltman says. Joining an exercise group is a great way to meet new people.

The activities recommended most often for older people are walking, swimming and stationary bicycling.

Always check with your doctor before beginning any exercise program.

Poor nutrition — A proper diet is essential for good health and "many older people simply do not eat well, especially those who live alone," Dr. Waltman said. A report in *Geriatrics* (44,8:61) points out two essential nutrients that many older people neglect.

The first is fiber, which has been shown to help prevent colon cancer by ridding the body of toxins more quickly and cleansing abnormal cells from intestinal walls.

If your diet is deficient in fiber, gradually add more. A sudden increase may cause bloating and cramps.

High-fiber foods include kidney and pinto beans, acorn squash, raspberries and prunes.

The second is calcium, which is essential in preventing osteoporosis (brittle bone disease). Doctors recommend that you get 1,000 to 1,500 milligrams of calcium every day.

Dairy products are the best source. An eight-ounce glass of whole milk contains 291 milligrams of calcium.

Medication problems — If you feel poorly, and you take a number of medications prescribed by different doctors, this may be your problem, according to Dr. Waltman.

"Many older [people] take as many as 12 different medications a day. … In addition to causing side effects severe enough to justify hospital admission, medications may cause more vague symptoms of fatigue, weakness and failure to thrive," the doctor says.

Alcohol problems — This is not a subject many people like to talk about. But alcohol abuse does exist among older people. Too much drinking can aggravate other problems, especially those involving the liver, brain, pancreas and digestive tract.

Excessive drinking also can lead to depletion of vitamin B12, itself a serious problem. And people who consume a lot of alcohol tend to neglect their nutritional needs, leading to a kind of starvation.

Cut down on your drinking if it has been a problem, says Dr. Waltman. Get help from your doctor, your local mental health association or from Alcoholics Anonymous.

Always speak your mind! If you feel something is wrong, by all means, tell your physician.

Don't wait for him to ask you about specific symptoms or stress-causing events. Says Dr. Waltman, "I have been impressed by the fact that when older patients feel something is wrong, if even vaguely, they are frequently right."

Loss of appetite and weight loss in the elderly

Loss of appetite and weight loss can lead to deteriorating health in the elderly, but doctors and families are often frustrated when they try to help.

However, a recent article in *Postgraduate Medicine* (85,3:140) says that loss of appetite, known as anorexia, can usually be traced to physical or social problems and can often be alleviated.

What can trigger anorexia in the elderly? Stomach problems, prescription drugs, heart and lung diseases, dietary restrictions, isolation or even something as simple as poor-fitting dentures or a sore tooth can cause the lack of appetite and eventual weight loss, according to the study. Doctors Cynthia Olsen-Noll and Michael Bosworth of Wright State University School of Medicine co-authored the study.

Once weight loss or loss of appetite has been identified, a thorough physical exam should be given to see if a medical problem is the cause, the doctors recommend.

Some of the medical problems that the study linked to loss of appetite include the following:

- **Stomach problems — peptic ulcer disease, intestinal obstruction, gallstones, stomach reflux, stomach cancer, delayed emptying of the esophagus or spasms of the esophagus.**

- **Dental problems — "Absence of teeth and poor-fitting dentures can result in the avoidance of solid foods," the researchers explain. A toothache, sensitive teeth or poor dental hygiene can also affect the appetite and the amount of food an elderly person will eat.**

- **Heart and lung diseases — emphysema, heart failure, and chronic bronchitis.**

- **Other problems — hyperthyroidism, hypothyroidism, uremia, neoplasms (unusual new tissue growth which could be cancerous) or liver problems.**

Prescription and over-the-counter drugs can also affect the appetite. Levodopa (brand names Dopar and Larodopa) and digitalis (digoxin or Lanoxin) are "two drugs especially implicated in appetite suppression," the authors warn.

"Oversedation by psychotropics, abuse of over-the-counter laxatives or appetite suppressants, ... thiazide diuretics," antibiotics, sedatives, narcotics and some other drugs are implicated as well.

Nutritional problems and education should not be overlooked. "Often, physicians prescribe dietary restrictions [like low-salt, high-fiber, low-fat diet] without adequately evaluating the patient's ability to understand and prepare the diet or find suitable substitutions for favorite foods," the study says. "Older patients are more likely than younger ones to have incorrect knowledge and hold myths concerning nutrition."

Social problems can lead to appetite loss, according to the report. Since "the elderly more commonly eat for social reasons than for satisfaction," the setting and presentation of meals becomes very important.

If a person lives alone, he is less likely to prepare and eat a full meal for himself. Someone with a hearing loss may lose the enjoyment of meals because she finds it difficult to talk to her companions.

If the senses of taste, smell or sight are impaired, the body's natural appetite stimulants are suppressed, and people may not feel hungry or may not enjoy the food as much as they used to.

In an institution, a limited choice of food can cause problems. "Free choice of foods and improved socialization at mealtime improve the elderly person's overall functioning," Bosworth says.

Depression, loneliness, isolation, undiagnosed alcoholism, loss of memory, drug abuse or anxiety can also contribute to a loss of appetite.

To overcome these problems, Olsen-Noll and Bosworth recommend a physical exam for the elderly person, reviewing and eliminating all unnecessary prescription and nonprescription drugs, improving dental care and providing better education.

They also suggest that the elderly get help in preparing special foods and allow plenty of time to eat in a comfortable social setting.

The doctors also recommend an increase in physical activity when possible (such as an afternoon walk) for the elderly patient suffering from poor appetite or excessive weight loss.

Can vitamins help slow the aging process?

Can vitamin supplements actually help improve the immune system and delay the aging process? Scientists now think it may be possible.

Vitamin supplements may help strengthen the immune system in elderly people, suggests a study in *The Journal of the American College of Nutrition* (9,4:363).

Maintaining a proper balance of vitamins is crucial in helping the body ward off illnesses quickly and effectively. However, the study shows that most elderly people frequently have low levels of important vitamins in their bodies.

This shortage of important vitamins often results in a sluggish immune system that has great trouble fighting off sicknesses.

So, many elderly people suffer needlessly from common illnesses simply because their immune systems have slowed down.

Many elderly people who eat very well-balanced meals still suffer from vitamin deficiencies. They may be taking medications that can "block" the vitamins in the food from being absorbed and used in the body.

So, scientists are suggesting that elderly people talk to their physicians about vitamin supplementation.

The vitamin supplement will help bring the level of vitamins in the body up to the proper level and help the immune system function as effectively as possible.

RDA for those over 50

The following tables give the official Recommended Dietary Allowances for vitamins and minerals in amounts considered necessary for people over age 50.

The tables contain two measurement categories —

❒ those vitamins and minerals that are needed in milligram amounts

❒ those needed in much smaller microgram amounts.

A milligram is one-thousandth of a gram. A microgram is one-thousandth of a milligram, or one-millionth of a gram.

Vitamins	Males	Females
Vitamin A	1000 micrograms	800 micrograms
Vitamin D	5 micrograms	5 micrograms
Vitamin C	60 milligrams	60 milligrams
Folic acid	200 micrograms	180 micrograms
Niacin	15 milligrams	13 milligrams
Riboflavin	1.4 milligrams	1.2 milligrams
Thiamine	1.2 milligrams	1 milligram
Vitamin B6	2 milligrams	1.6 milligrams
Vitamin B12	2 micrograms	2 micrograms
Vitamin E	10 milligrams	8 milligrams
Vitamin K	80 micrograms	65 micrograms

Vitamins	Males	Females
Calcium	800 milligrams	800 milligrams
Phosphorous	800 milligrams	800 milligrams
Iodine	150 micrograms	150 micrograms
Iron	10 milligrams	10 milligrams
Magnesium	350 milligrams	280 milligrams
Selenium	70 micrograms	55 micrograms
Zinc	15 milligrams	12 milligrams

People on medications or on special, restricted diets should check with their doctors before using the information above. Certain nutrients — like selenium — are dangerous in amounts only slightly above the recommended range.

Check with your doctor before taking any vitamin or mineral supplements.

Vitamin A: Too little or too much can be dangerous, especially for the elderly

Vitamin A is essential for your health, but if you get too little or too much, it can be very dangerous.

Night blindness or loss of vision in near darkness is the earliest symptom of a vitamin A deficiency. A severe deficiency of vitamin A may cause xerophthalmia (dry eyes) and can lead to permanent blindness if the eye tissue becomes ulcerated, two researchers explain.

Other symptoms of vitamin A deficiency are dry, brittle hair; cracked, dry or blemished skin; reduced hormone production; poor growth; and difficulty in fighting infections, says *Vitamin and Mineral Encyclopedia* (FC&A Publishing). The digestive system and the urinary or reproductive systems may also deteriorate.

Natural sources of vitamin A or carotene are liver, cod liver oil, eggs, milk and dairy products, broccoli, spinach and other green, leafy vegetables, carrots, turnips and other yellow vegetables, apricots and cantaloupe.

Meats naturally contain vitamin A, while plants contain beta carotene, a "pre-vitamin" form that the body converts into vitamin A.

A recent study in the *Journal of Food Science* (52,4:1022) has shown that "the carotene content of wet vegetables, either fresh or cooked, was always significantly greater than that of dried ones." Fresh vegetables have more carotene than dried beans, potatoes or rice.

The best part about carotene is that it's usually not converted into vitamin A unless the body really needs more of the vitamin. It's just burned as food energy or passes on through the body.

Therefore, you can eat a lot of carotene and not suffer from the bad effect you would from eating too much vitamin A. Your body would get all the benefits of vitamin A without the dangers.

Overdoses of vitamin A can be caused by eating too much animal liver over a period of several weeks. But usually overdoses are the result of high doses of vitamin supplements, Bendich and Langseth report in *The American Journal of Clinical Nutrition* (49,2:358) — in other words, taking too many vitamin pills.

A study from the Human Nutrition Research Center on Aging shows that "elderly people who take vitamin A supplements may be at increased risk for vitamin A overload."

Adults taking repeated high daily doses have complained of harmful side effects like buildup of pressure within the skull, vomiting, irritability, peeling of skin, loss of hair and dry, itching skin, reports *Vitamin and Mineral Encyclopedia* (FC&A Publishing). Megadoses can cause a toxic reaction or even, in rare cases, death.

Vitamin A is fat-soluble. That means it dissolves in body fat. Because of that, it can be stored in the body for a long time, unlike water-soluble vitamins that are quickly flushed out of the body by the kidneys.

The liver can store up to a two years' supply of vitamin A, so the amount of vitamin A in the body can become extremely high over many years, researchers at Tufts University report in *The American Journal of Clinical Nutrition* (49,1:112).

"Our study suggests that elderly people should limit their intake of supplemental vitamin A, particularly over the long term," warns Stephen Krasinski, who headed the research team. "Our data may also indirectly support a lowering of the RDA for vitamin A."

The good news about vitamin A overdose is that most bad symptoms will go away when the high doses are stopped. In some cases permanent damage does occur, but usually if the overdose can be diagnosed, and the additional vitamin A eliminated, the recovery will be quite rapid.

Here are some ways to avoid vitamin A overdoses:

❐ If you take a vitamin supplement, check the fine print on the bottle. Be sure that you never take more than the RDA for vitamin A unless your doctor specifically says it's okay.

❐ Do not take vitamin A supplements if you are taking cod liver oil or fish oil supplements. Both contain high levels of vitamin A. Cod liver oil or other fish oil should be used with caution, and under your doctor's supervision, because of the risk of vitamin A overdose.

❐ If you want to supplement your body's store of vitamin A, take carotene supplements instead of vitamin A supplements.

❐ Do not take vitamin A supplements if you are taking isotretinoin (brand name Accutane) or etretinate (brand name Tegison). Both are prescription drugs that are made from vitamin A.

❐ Do not take vitamin A supplements if you are on birth control pills, unless you're under a doctor's supervision. Women taking birth control pills usually show an increase in levels of vitamin A in their blood of 30 to 80 percent, says *Vitamin and Mineral Encyclopedia*.

❐ Always remember to report your vitamin and mineral supplements to your doctor and, in the case of a medical emergency, the hospital staff.

Take 'the best anti-aging vitamin' in existence — water

Water, water, everywhere, but not enough drink it.

Older folks simply don't drink enough water, especially with their medicines, says a pharmacist specializing in problems of over-age-50 patients. Maybe doctors should write prescriptions for water to make sure their older patients get enough liquid, suggests Madeline Feinberg in *Senior Patient* (1,4:26).

"All medications, including liquids, need to be taken with a half to a full glass of water," she says. "This will help the medication dissolve more quickly in the stomach and be more readily absorbed. It will also reduce any stomach irritation from the drug."

Most elderly people have to guard against drinking too little water, the article says. Older people don't get as thirsty as younger folks. Some elderly patients even try to drink less water, thinking they are "helping" their medicines. "Some people think that if pills are supposed to get rid of excess fluid, then decreasing fluid intake will be that much better!" the pharmacist writes.

Other older people try to control loss of bladder control (incontinence) by drinking less water. Drinking less water is nearly always harmful, the article indicates, except for the few seniors who are on doctor's orders to reduce their fluid intake.

Water has these benefits:

- **Holds down urinary tract infections by keeping the bladder well-flushed.**

- **Makes the best and cheapest diet drink available. Drinking water makes you feel full with zero calories.**

- **Smooths out skin and prevents tiny wrinkles from forming. "In fact, water is probably the best 'anti-aging vitamin' we have for skin," the article says.**

But water means water, not other beverages like coffee, tea, soft drinks or even fruit juices, the pharmacist says. "These (other) beverages may contain caffeine, may be high in sugar and calories, or may interfere with drug action," the article concludes.

Positive outlook on life helps you age 'gracefully'

The old saying "pretty is as pretty does" may have more truth than we know. Doctors think that a person's standards of personal cleanliness, grooming and dress actually may tell a lot about her health condition.

Researchers now realize that signs of self-neglect in elderly people are often the first warning signs of hidden illnesses, according to *Senior Patient* (2,9:45).

In other words, a sudden decline in a person's personal care and hygiene may be a warning sign of a health problem or disorder.

For 25 years, the British Red Cross has provided basic "beauty care" to people in hospitals and nursing homes, *Senior Patient* reports. Red Cross workers provide hair, skin and nail care for elderly people. They even help the patients put on fresh makeup and clean clothes.

Such assistance improves patients' self-esteem, fosters a positive outlook on life, and possibly even helps reduce the time it takes for recovery.

Many people may think of the idea as frivolous and too time-consuming. But a little makeup and a fresh hairstyle may actually shorten a person's recovery time in the hospital.

It seems that elderly people who keep a positive outlook on life and continue to keep themselves well-groomed and as youthful-looking as possible are more likely to age "gracefully" than those who neglect their personal care and hygiene.

Elderly people who try to maintain an attractive appearance through their later years may actually be nurturing their own self-esteem, sense of well-being, social interaction and zest for life.

Change in lifestyle can create a longer life span

Middle-aged men who adopt healthy lifestyle changes can greatly reduce their risk of dying from a heart attack a decade later.

High blood pressure, high cholesterol and smoking are known risk factors for heart disease, but they don't have to end your life. Beginning a program of intervention aimed at halting the consequences of heart disease may just help save your life!

The Multiple Risk Factor Intervention Trial (MRFIT) was set up to determine the effects of lifestyle changes in men who fit the high risk category of coronary heart disease.

According to *The Journal of the American Medical Association* (263,13:1795), researchers at the University of Minnesota in Minneapolis conducted a ten-year study to determine the benefits derived from an intervention program designed to overturn the negative effects of lifestyles that promote heart disease.

The MRFIT program consisted of over 12,000 men, aged 35 to 57, all fitting the high risk requirements. These men were divided into two categories — those in the intervention program and those using only their private medical care (no extra intervention).

The intervention program, with a total of 6,428 men, involved diet changes to lower cholesterol levels, counseling to stop smoking, and any necessary treatment to control high blood pressure. The 6,438 remaining men received no special instructions, but used their normal sources of health care.

During the decade following the onset of the program, the value of intervention became obvious. The cardiovascular disease mortality rate was 8.3 percent lower in the group that received special instructions.

In narrowing the analysis to fatal heart attacks, the researchers found a 24 percent drop in deaths among the intervention group compared to the usual-care group.

Change can be difficult, but when the benefits include a longer and more productive life, the effort seems worthwhile.

Ask your doctor if a diet lower in saturated fats and cholesterol, medication or exercise to lower your blood pressure and a program to stop smoking would take you out of the "high risk" category.

Weight lifting helps reverse the weakness of old age

Does getting old automatically mean becoming weak, frail and subject to life-threatening falls?

No! says a new study at Tufts University in Boston reported in *The Journal of the American Medical Association* (263,22:3029).

The secret to staying young — Lift weights to strengthen weakened leg muscles. Ten nursing home residents, ranging in age from 86 to 96, volunteered to pump iron with their legs for eight weeks.

Eight of them had a history of falls, and seven used a cane or other appliance to help them walk. In addition, seven had osteoarthritis, six had heart disease and previous broken bones from osteoporosis (brittle bone disease), and four had high blood pressure.

In other words, most had diseases or disabilities common to the very old.

Each started with about 17 pounds of weight for each leg and progressed to more than 45 pounds on each leg after eight weeks. They exercised three times a week.

During each session, they did three sets of eight repetitions each, with a one- or two-minute rest period between sets.

One repetition means raising and lowering one leg one time. A set is a sequence of repetitions without a rest break.

Despite their frailty, "the average strength gain at eight weeks was 174 percent in the right legs and 180 percent in the left legs," the report says.

Their strength never got stuck on a plateau; it was still on the rise when the weight-lifting sessions ended.

"It is likely that at the end of the training these subjects were stronger than they had been many years previously," says Dr. Maria A. Fiatarone, study director.

Not one experienced any falls during or after the weight training, the study says. Only one of the four men dropped out, and that was because he strained an old hernia repair.

But the point of the weight training showed up in improved mobility.

Half of the volunteers were able to walk faster confidently — as much as one-and-one-half times faster than before the leg-weight sessions, the study reports.

Two who had used canes before the weight lifting put their canes away and walked without assistance.

And one of three people who, before the exercise sessions, couldn't rise from a chair without pushing with the arms were able to rise just using the strength in the more muscular legs.

Unfortunately, when the volunteers went back to their old ways of no exercise and sedentary habits, they lost a third of their new-found leg strength within four weeks. Exercising needs to be continued indefinitely to maintain the benefits.

The weight training caused no problems for those with heart disease or arthritis, the report says.

Although weight rooms may not become widespread in nursing homes and senior citizen centers, aging experts predict that stretching and movement exercises to strengthen muscles and improve the sense of balance will become common for people even into their 90s.

Since this was an experimental study conducted under strict medical supervision, you should not try similar exercises without checking with your doctor first.

Appendicitis in the elderly may not be obvious: a telltale sign

Appendicitis in the elderly can be difficult to diagnose because older people may not show the more common symptoms and signs of the illness, warns *Geriatrics* (44,4:113).

Two elderly patients at Duke University Medical Center had symptoms indicating problems in the nervous system. The nervous system symptoms included seizures, dizziness, disorientation and confusion.

Those nervous system symptoms "masked" or hid the real cause of their illness. Each of them had a severe infection of the appendix, commonly known as appendicitis. Appendicitis is a common, life-threatening condition. It usually requires hospitalization and surgical removal of the infected appendix.

Even though both patients had unexplained high fever, a classic symptom of appendicitis, it took seven days for one of the patients to be accurately diagnosed.

The journal suggests that "acute appendicitis in the elderly is often difficult to diagnose" because:

- **The elderly patients may also be experiencing chronic diseases.**

- **They are reluctant to seek medical help.**

- **Their signs and symptoms are often very different from appendicitis in a younger person.**

According to the Duke doctors, the two signs of appendicitis to look for in the elderly are unexplained high fever and nervous system symptoms. If those two signs are present, the doctors suggest that appendicitis should be considered.

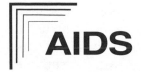

AIDS

AIDS: a growing threat to the elderly

There may be as many as 27,000 cases of AIDS in people over 50, and 1,100 AIDS cases in people over 70 years of age, according to Dr. Philip G. Weiler, director for Aging and Health at the University of California, Davis.

Weiler is worried that AIDS in the elderly is "largely an unrecognized problem" because AIDS in older people often mimics the problems of senility or Alzheimer's disease, *Geriatrics* (44,7:81) reports.

Older AIDS patients often experience loss of memory and personality changes which could easily be misdiagnosed. But Weiler points out that severe weight loss, tiredness and weakness often will accompany the mental problems in older AIDS patients and separate them from senility patients.

"AIDS has become a diagnostic imitator. It could manifest as a psychiatric illness — for example a psychosis or depression — or simply as generalized fatigue and weight loss, perhaps mimicking cancer," says Dr. Weiler.

Why are so many elderly affected by AIDS although they haven't been considered a high-risk group? "One-fourth of all blood transfusions are in those ages 50 to 60, and you can add another 15 percent for people over age 60," he explains. "I think there is still a risk from blood transfusions that predated screening of blood donors for AIDS, which began in 1985."

AIDS typically may take many years to develop into a full-blown disease. While the diagnosis may not help the elderly person with AIDS, an accurate diagnosis will allow loved ones and others who give care to the victim to take appropriate precautions — precautions that might be ignored in the absence of an AIDS diagnosis.

Before finalizing a "dementia" diagnosis, doctors should check the patient's history of blood transfusions and the spouse's blood transfusion record, according to Weiler.

"The possibility of infection via sexual contact should not be ruled out," says Dr. Robert Butler, in a *Geriatrics* (44,7:21) editorial. "Physicians should not ignore or underestimate the extent of sexual involvement of people in their 50s, 60s, and older," Dr. Butler says.

"According to most estimates, 10 percent of AIDS cases are found in the over-55 population. Since this age group received more blood transfusions than any other age group, and since it may take longer to notice overt symptoms of AIDS in older persons than in younger ones, we may eventually see more cases of AIDS in the older population," says Dr. Butler.

AIDS through blood transfusions: how to be 100% safe

If you have surgery and need a blood transfusion, how can you be sure the donated blood is free of the deadly AIDS virus? That's a question many are asking since it was discovered that the fatal disease can be transmitted through blood transfusions.

Although every pint now undergoes strict testing to eliminate tainted blood, a small danger remains. Since March 1985, blood donated in the United States has been screened for the HIV virus, which leads to AIDS.

Hepatitis B, syphilis, and another rare form of hepatitis also are screened out. But even with screening, the U.S. Surgeon General estimates that at least one pint in every 100,000 donations carries the AIDS infection and slips through to an unsuspecting recipient.

One sure way to avoid AIDS through transfusions is to donate your own blood and have it saved until you need it. A second sure way works like this: During surgery, the doctors collect blood seeping from your wounds, recycle it, and put it back in your body.

These techniques are called autologous transfusion. "Autotransfusion" is another term for the same thing. This means that you give your own blood back to yourself.

Because of the AIDS crisis, many doctors are more reluctant to give blood transfusions. The National Institutes of Health (NIH) have asked that all transfusions "be kept to a minimum." They definitely should be given when absolutely needed. But in some cases, the doctor will monitor the patient during the first stages of recovery and prescribe iron supplements to avoid a transfusion.

"With every [regular donated blood] unit you get, the risk incrementally increases; therefore, the fewer the better," said Tibor J. Greenwalt of the University of Cincinnati in a report in *Science News* (134,3:41). Dr. Greenwalt was chairman of a recent conference on transfusions at the NIH.

Still, situations may arise when you need blood, and transfusion is a medical necessity. Following are some ways you can help ensure the safety of the blood you receive.

Autotransfusion during surgery — Some hospitals are now capable of "recycling" blood lost during surgery, reducing the need for transfusions. Blood that was previously drained out of the body and thrown away is now being filtered, cleaned, treated and returned to the patient. This is known as autotransfusion, because the blood is actually from the same patient.

First, the blood is suctioned out of the wound. Next, the blood is filtered to remove dangerous blood clots and any foreign materials. Blood thinners may be added.

In some systems, the blood is separated in a centrifuge, and only the red cells are kept. Finally, the blood may pass through a sterile solution before it is returned to the patient.

Approved in 1988, the Solocotrans autotransfusion system is used to help collect and recycle blood during orthopedic operations. Other systems have been in limited use for several years, but the AIDS crisis and improvements in the systems have increased their use.

The Cell Saver System can be used in several types of surgery where there is usually a great loss of blood — open heart surgery, ruptured liver or spleen, ectopic (outside the uterus) pregnancy or orthopedic operations.

Autotransfusions can be quick and cost-effective (and are usually covered by insurance companies). It takes less time to set up the equipment than it does to test for blood type and then cross-match potential blood donors from a blood bank.

But some additional blood may still be needed. Doctors estimate that only one-third of the patients who use autotransfusions will not require additional blood. Two-thirds of such patients still will need donated blood.

If you are planning open heart or other surgery, find out if your hospital has a machine for autotransfusions. If you need emergency surgery, you won't have much time to make autotransfusion arrangements. To be on the safe side, check your local hospitals ahead of time.

Pre-donating your own blood — If you are planning elective surgery, many hospitals or blood banks will allow you to donate your own blood in advance. This blood can be stored and given back to you if it's needed during surgery.

There is a time limit. Fresh blood can be stored for only about 35 days, and you can only give a limited amount just before planned surgery.

Blood can be donated, frozen for up to three years and thawed for transfusion, but this can be extremely expensive. One pint of blood can cost $150 for freezing and $250 for thawing, not including the storage time, some officials estimate.

Storage space is also limited, which often adds to the high cost per pint. Some hospitals, like Central General on Long Island, N.Y., have started hospital blood banks where patients can donate their own blood for future use.

People over age 50 or those with low blood counts may not want to give their own blood because it could weaken them and slow their recovery from surgery. Also, in cases of repeated surgery, a patient may not have enough time for recovery to pre-donate blood before the next operation.

Pre-arranging safe donors — Learn the blood types of yourself, your immediate family, close relatives and best friends. Agree with each other that, in case of an emergency, each would donate blood to anyone in the group with a compatible blood type.

Keep a list of the people with your blood type, along with their telephone numbers, with you at all times.

If you are in an accident or require emergency surgery, those people can be alerted. Or, if you are planning surgery, your family or friends can give a "recipient-specific" donation. The blood is tagged and kept for your use.

However, be aware that even people you know may themselves be at high risk for AIDS, but may feel pressured into giving blood for you. In that case, your safety factor would vanish.

Make sure that none of these people have engaged in what the U.S. Surgeon General calls "risky behavior." This means homosexuality, injecting illegal drugs, sexual promiscuity or intimate contact with people who have done such things.

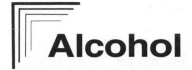

Alcohol

Alcohol robs your body of a vital nutrient

If you must drink, you'd better stop at two beers, a major new heart study suggests. More than that amount of alcohol daily may spike your blood pressure and may drain a vital nutrient, calcium, from your body, says a report by the American Heart Association. That harmful effect shows up even if you take extra calcium supplements, the study indicates.

"Our study suggests that for the average person, at more than two drinks a day, some bad things start happening physiologically," says Dr. Michael H. Criqui, co-author of the study published in *Circulation* (80,3:609). "Your blood pressure goes up, and you begin to lose the benefits of the calcium in your diet," Dr. Criqui says.

Criqui and co-workers studied 7,011 men of Japanese descent who participated in the Honolulu Heart Study. The study shows that nondrinkers and light drinkers who had higher calcium intakes also had correspondingly lower blood pressures, the AHA report says.

But, the study warns, those who averaged more than two alcoholic drinks a day suffered at least two bad effects:

- **The alcohol seemed to raise their blood pressure.**
- **The drinking also seemed to prevent the blood-pressure-lowering effects of calcium.**

Previous studies show that drinking alcohol apparently leads to poor absorption of calcium in the intestines, the report says. In addition, a heavy drinker passes a lot of calcium through the kidneys in urine, draining the body's stores of calcium.

Heavy drinkers sometimes have bones that appear to be "washed out" in x-rays, because they lack calcium, the researcher says. That's added bad news for people at risk from osteoporosis, a bone-loss disease that strikes many women and some men over the age of 50.

You can't get around the bad effect of alcohol on blood pressure simply by taking more calcium every day, Dr. Criqui says. "We found that regardless of the level of calcium or potassium in the diet, alcohol still had an independent (bad) effect," says the researcher. "Alcohol seemed to be a much more powerful influence on blood pressure than either calcium or potassium."

The researcher recommends that you eliminate alcohol from your diet. Short of that, he says, you should average two or fewer alcoholic drinks a day.

Alcohol and the immune system

Heavy drinkers may be ruining more than just their liver. Excessive alcohol intake may severely damage the body's whole immune system, making it more susceptible to serious, even life-threatening infections like pneumonia, according to an editorial in the *British Medical Journal* (298,6673:543).

Heavy drinking over a period of several years may drastically decrease the number of natural "killer cells," the body's powerful defense against invading bacteria and viruses, said the report.

Heavy drinkers have much higher rates of lung infections, including tuberculosis, than other people.

The drinking habit also greatly weakens the liver so that "alcoholic subjects may be at increased risk of both hepatitis and HIV [AIDS] infection," the journal said.

Undernutrition — caused by lowered intake of proteins, vitamins and sources of energy — also lowers resistance to infections among heavy drinkers. Many have severe vitamin deficiencies.

Vitamin C helps beat drinking problems, boosts recovery rate

People with an alcohol problem might help their short-term recovery by taking two grams of vitamin C a day, suggests a study reported in *The Journal of the American College of Nutrition* (9,3:185).

Studies about alcohol detoxification — "drying out" — show that taking large doses of vitamin C really helps in clearing alcohol out of a person's system quickly.

In an experiment with 111 New York City alcoholics, three out of four of those who completed a year-long program centered around taking extra vitamins and minerals stayed sober. Regular non-nutritional therapy produces much lower success rates, reports *Men's Health* newsletter (6,8:12).

A Special Amino Acid and Vitamin Enteral (SAAVE) supplement seemed to help keep twice as many alcohol abusers in a sobriety program in

California, says the manufacturer, Matrix Technologies, Inc. The findings were reported in the *Journal of Psychoactive Drugs* (22,3:173).

The studies are adding up: Special medically supervised diets that emphasize balanced nutrition dramatically improve chances for long-term recovery from heavy drinking.

The Recommended Dietary Allowance for vitamin C is 60 milligrams a day for people over 50. Check with your doctor before taking supplements.

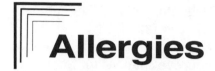

Allergies

Achoo! Yes, it's pollen season again

For most of us, spring fever means a hammock and a lazy "I'll worry about it tomorrow" attitude.

For millions of people with pollen allergies, however, spring fever means just one thing: Kleenex.

According to *Health After 50* (2,2:4), pollen allergies are more common in the fall but often last longer in the spring.

In fact, what you may think of as a spring cold may be an allergy. Other allergic symptoms include headache, fatigue, irritability and sore throat.

An allergy is a supersensitivity to "substances that don't bother most people," according to *The Allergy Self-Help Book* (Rodale Press, Emmaus, Penn.). Substances that cause allergic reactions are called allergens.

When you come into contact with any allergen — by touching, tasting or inhaling it — your body's natural defenses spring into action.

The immune system releases a flush of histamine to ward off the intruder. The immune system doesn't break down often. But if it goes haywire and mistakenly targets a harmless substance (such as strawberries or dust), the body releases too much histamine. And it's too much histamine that causes those annoying allergic symptoms.

Generally, allergies develop over time, although you could have an immediate reaction.

Often, your body resists the first few encounters with an allergen and then "gives in" to it. (Many people reach their 50s or 60s and wonder why they've "suddenly" developed an allergy to something they've eaten all their lives.)

Although pollen is a notorious allergen (more than 15 million Americans have hay fever), you could be allergic to just about anything. Common allergens include food (such as eggs and wheat), drugs, wool, smoke, dust, pet hair, mold and mildew.

Interestingly, if your parents had allergies, chances are you do, too, but not necessarily the same ones. For some reason, many people choose to "live with" their allergies rather than treat them. You do have to know what you're allergic to before you can treat the allergy.

Skin testing is the most common way to test for allergies. Your doctor will inject an allergen just under the surface of your skin, and if a welt appears, you are allergic to that substance.

Skin testing works well in tracking down pollen allergies, but is less successful for food allergies and just about useless for drug allergies (with a few exceptions).

Radioallergosorbent testing is a better allergy detective. RAST is a simple blood test, measuring the amount of antibodies in the blood, which tells your doctor whether your body is trying to fight off an allergen.

Natural ways to control allergies

Knowing you have a pollen allergy doesn't make it much easier to control. Although drugs can help relieve annoying symptoms, specialists agree the best way to control a pollen allergy is to prevent an outbreak in the first place.

Here are some tips from the *Johns Hopkins Medical Letter* (2,2:4):

❒ Pollen levels are highest between 5 a.m. and 10 a.m., so stay indoors during those hours.

❒ Keep windows in your home and car closed.

❒ Keep your home 10 degrees cooler than the outside temperature. A too-cold house can aggravate allergies. Keep your air conditioners and vents clean to prevent dust particles from circulating.

❒ Keep your lawn mowed short to prevent grass from blooming. Blooming releases pollen into the air.

❒ Wear sunglasses outdoors to protect your eyes from pollen.

❒ Don't dry clothes on a clothesline outdoors.

❒ If you think you've been exposed to pollen, shower as soon as you return home.

❒ And finally, if you can, take a break from pollen season in your area of the country. A cruise is the ideal choice!

House dust — an army of allergens

If that ball of fuzz under your bed makes you sneeze or wheeze, you may already know that you're allergic ... but what exactly are you allergic to?

House dust is made up of lots of different things, and two of the worst offenders are so tiny you can't even see them!

Molds are microscopic plants that live on decaying plant and animal matter in and outside your home. These funguses thrive in warm, moist air.

If you are allergic to funguses, breathing in their airborne spores will cause you to have an allergic reaction. Spores are the "seeds" of the tiny plants.

You can control molds in your environment by following these simple procedures suggested by *Pharmacy Times* (56,5:113):

> • **Kill mold in your bathrooms and basement by applying a solution of equal parts water and household bleach.**
>
> • **If you must rake leaves and cut grass, use a face mask when you do these chores.**
>
> • **Buy an artificial Christmas tree rather than a real one.**
>
> • **Store firewood outside instead of inside.**

A tougher problem may be getting rid of dust mites.

These tiny relatives of spiders and ticks hide in your upholstered furniture, bedding, curtains and carpets. And they feed on flakes of human skin that you shed every day.

It's not the dust mites themselves that cause your nose to tickle. The trouble comes from the waste products given off by the tiny creatures.

Dust mites' waste products lodge in your furniture or bedding or float through the air in your house, causing some people to have runny noses, asthma or even eczema, a skin problem.

You can control dust mites and molds by keeping the humidity between 30 and 50 percent in your home. It will also help to remove carpeting and to cover mattresses, box springs and pillows with dust-proof cases.

You can control dust mites

There are a few special precautions you can take to control dust mites in your home:

> • **Choose washable bedding, not wool or down blankets.**
>
> • **Wash all bedding weekly in hot water.**
>
> • **Take down heavy curtains and Venetian blinds.**
>
> • **Remove carpet.**
>
> • **Ask your doctor about Acarosan — a new product that kills dust mites in carpets, beds and upholstered furniture.**

Keep the cat, not the allergies

Are you tired of the runny eyes, stuffy nose and wheezing caused by an allergic reaction to your house cat?

Don't throw out the cat yet! There may be another solution, says a report in *Science News* (138,7:109). Researchers have developed a spray that contains tannic acid, a compound found in oak bark, coffee and tea.

Apparently, the tannic acid can chemically alter house dust, pollen and dust-mite debris so that they no longer cause allergic reactions.

Spraying the tannic acid in carpeted rooms also helps reduce the amount of cat dander in the carpet. The cat dander may be the culprit behind your allergic reactions.

Even if the cat has been gone for a while, the bits of cat fur and skin that remain in the carpet may take several months to die down to tolerable, nonallergic levels. Spraying tannic acid can reduce the dander level to a tenth of its former power. Tannic acid sprays may be found in pet stores.

A bit of advice: Test the spray on a small section of carpet before spraying the whole room to make sure the tannic acid doesn't discolor your carpet.

Sudden unexplained coughing?
Check your gloves

Asthmatic reaction triggered by your gloves? Sounds strange, but it could be true if you wear latex gloves while you work.

Several cases of people developing asthma in response to their latex gloves have been reported in *The Lancet* (336,8718:808).

Apparently, the powder on the gloves can trigger an allergic asthmatic reaction. The chemicals in the glove itself might also cause the coughing and wheezing that accompany asthma.

Many health care workers and food preparation workers commonly wear latex gloves for sanitary purposes. And many people wear latex gloves around the house when cleaning.

If you are coughing and wheezing for no apparent reason, ask your doctor about the possibility of being allergic to your gloves.

Photocopy blues

If you've been suffering from hay-fever symptoms, but none of your hay-fever remedies have worked, you may be reacting to the copy machine in your office building or local drug store.

A recent report in *The New England Journal of Medicine* (322,18:1323) states that nasal stuffiness, headaches and other common allergy-like reactions may be caused by laser printers and photocopying machines.

Apparently, the machines give off emissions which contain some volatile organic compounds. These compounds have been associated with allergic reactions.

Inadequate air circulation inside the buildings that house laser printers and photocopying machines leads to "stale" air. Stale air contains emissions and results in headaches, sore throats and runny noses, often referred to as "sick building syndrome."

If you suspect you're suffering from "sick building syndrome," you may consider spending as little time around these culprit machines as possible.

Occasional breaths of fresh air away from the machines may be all you need to clear up your symptoms. Be sure to check with your doctor if you have questions about this condition.

Delayed allergic reaction to insect stings

You think you're starting to have an allergic reaction but don't understand why. It has been two weeks since you encountered that wasp, and his sting didn't cause much of a problem then.

Most reactions to insect stings are immediate — within minutes.

However, a recent study reported in *Emergency Medicine* (22,7:99) found that some individuals may experience an allergic reaction to a sting several hours or even days later.

Some New York doctors found that a group of their patients suffered typical allergic reactions up to fourteen days after being stung by insects.

Reactions varied but included some of the following symptoms:

- **localized swelling at the site of the sting**

- **itching, generalized skin rash**

- **difficulty in breathing**

- **painful swollen joints**

Many people in the delayed-reaction group had been stung several times at once. Therefore, many researchers think that a larger amount of insect venom might be a factor in a delayed reaction.

Some patients had allergic reactions at the time they were stung and also experienced a second reaction several days later.

A very severe allergic reaction is called anaphylaxis. This means the body overreacts when it tries to protect itself from an allergen (something that causes an allergic reaction).

Symptoms of anaphylaxis include:

- **rash**

- **itching**

- **swelling in the throat to the extent that the airway is obstructed**

- **circulatory difficulties**

If you think you're experiencing an allergic reaction that could be the result of an insect sting within the past couple of weeks, report this to your doctor immediately. Your doctor might need to test you for hypersensitivity to insect venom.

If you are hypersensitive (or allergic) to insect stings, you will need to take proper precautions to avoid future stings and reactions.

Mild reactions serve as a warning that the next insect sting could be more serious, possibly even deadly.

Alzheimer's Disease

Recent research on Alzheimer's disease

Alzheimer's is a disease — always fatal — in which portions of the brain responsible for thinking, memory and routine physical functions are destroyed over a period of a few months to five years.

It mainly strikes elderly people, and women get the disease more often than men.

Experimental drug — Researchers in a 12-city study are looking for additional evidence that the experimental drug THA improves the ability to think and remember in patients suffering from Alzheimer's disease.

Recent research suggests that THA (tetrahydroaminoacridine) slows down the abnormal loss of acetylcholine, an essential "memory" chemical made by the brain.

Some researchers believe that Alzheimer's symptoms — memory loss, inability to think clearly, irrational behavior and dementia — may be caused by the decline in acetylcholine.

A second phase of the study is comparing the effectiveness of THA when taking it with and without lecithin, a natural fatty substance found in egg yolks, soybeans, corn and animal tissues.

Smoking — Meanwhile, studies in recent years have shown that smokers are four times as likely as nonsmokers to develop Alzheimer's disease. An obvious way to lower your risk of getting the fatal disease is to stop smoking, researchers say.

Aluminum — Suspicions are growing about the link between Alzheimer's and aluminum in our diet. Some doctors are warning that aluminum in large amounts can be leached from metal utensils during cooking.

Science News (131,5:73) reports that experiments in Sri Lanka suggest that cooking in aluminum cookware with water containing fluorides increases the aluminum concentration by up to 1,000 times more than cooking with water without fluorides.

Most Americans routinely drink fluoridated water and use it in cooking, and many use aluminum cookware. New evidence suggests the combination may be unwise.

Alzheimer's disease from your home tap water?

Drinking water may be harmful to your health, a new research report suggests. Aluminum levels in tap water may be linked to deadly Alzheimer's disease, one of the leading causes of senility in people from age 40 to 60, according to researchers in England.

As aluminum concentrations in ordinary drinking water increased, the rates of Alzheimer's disease among persons using that water also increased, said the report in *The Lancet* (1,8629:59). In some cases, the rates increased by as much as 50 percent.

The greatest risk, they found, occurred in areas where the aluminum concentrations were greater than 0.11 milligrams (the same as 110 micrograms, or four-millionths of one ounce) per liter of water. (One liter is equal to a little more than a quart.)

Below 0.01 milligrams (10 micrograms) aluminum per liter, the researchers found, there seemed to be no added risks of getting Alzheimer's disease.

Aluminum sulfate, or alum, is commonly used by water systems during the treatment process, the report said. The chemical is added at the water plant as a coagulant to make suspended solids settle out of the liquid.

The amount of aluminum added varies from plant to plant, within certain limits, depending on the amount of solid materials in the raw water being treated.

In many cases, increased amounts of aluminum added to the raw water means that technicians have to use less chlorine to purify the water later in the treatment process.

While much of the added aluminum is removed before the water is pumped to homes and schools, some aluminum remains dissolved in the treated water and is consumed by water users, the report said.

Higher levels of aluminum in untreated water also occur naturally in some geographic locations because of mineral deposits in the ground.

For comparison, a recent chemical analysis of water treated by the Atlanta, Ga., water system showed that the after-treatment aluminum level was 0.06 milligrams (60 micrograms) per liter. The British study indicated that, at that level, Alzheimer's disease rates increased by about 40 percent in the areas studied in England and Wales.

Aluminum is not among the "toxic" chemicals for which many U.S. water systems routinely test their water supplies and for which maximum limits are set.

For example, there are no current standards or limits on aluminum concentration for Georgia water systems.

The 12-nation European Economic Community currently permits water aluminum concentrations up to 0.2 milligrams (200 micrograms) per liter, according to an editorial in the same issue of *The Lancet*.

The researchers were concerned that the water treatment process may add to the already high levels of aluminum consumption in most Western countries.

In Britain, for example, they estimated that an adult consumes an average of five to 10 milligrams of aluminum each day, occurring naturally in food. But, researchers say, only a small portion of that is actually absorbed by the body internally.

Aluminum-based preservatives in food may add another 50 milligrams (50,000 micrograms) daily.

An adult American may get that much or more of the chemical, especially since many people regularly take aluminum-based antacids for heartburn and upset stomach.

While much of that aluminum passes through the body without being absorbed, the British researchers were concerned that water aluminum is much more "bioavailable."

That means it is more easily absorbed during its passage through the digestive system.

They recommended that water plants use as little aluminum as possible during the treatment process to cut down on the long-term accumulation of the chemical in humans.

Although aluminum is considered a "trace element" (*Taber's Cyclopedic Medical Dictionary*, 16th edition) and is found in minute quantities in food, water and living tissues, the body does not require aluminum for any metabolic processes. In fact, aluminum is increasingly under suspicion as a potent brain poison.

Autopsies have revealed abnormally high amounts of aluminum in characteristic "tangles" of diseased tissue in brains of persons who died with Alzheimer's disease.

More suspicions were raised in the mid-1970s when young patients undergoing dialysis treatment for kidney disease developed symptoms of senility.

Doctors found that aluminum in the water used in the treatment caused the rapidly developing senility.

When they lowered the aluminum below 0.03 milligrams (30 micrograms) per liter, the senility symptoms were quickly reversed, and the patients returned to normal mental states.

Residents of the island of Guam, where the water is high in aluminum and low in calcium and magnesium, have more cases of amyotrophic lateral sclerosis, also known as Lou Gehrig's disease.

Lou Gehrig's disease also causes senility and leads to death. It is very similar to Alzheimer's disease, especially in the abnormally high amounts of aluminum found in the brain tissue at autopsy.

The British researchers indicated that they are convinced of a strong relationship between long-term aluminum consumption and increased risks of getting Alzheimer's disease.

"This survey, conducted in 88 county districts within England and Wales, shows that rates of Alzheimer's disease in people under the age of 70 are related to the average aluminum concentrations present in drinking water supplies over the previous decade," the report said.

"A positive relation between rates of Alzheimer's disease and water aluminum concentrations was present whichever way the data were analyzed."

Readers may want to call their local water system to find out the concentration of aluminum in drinking water. If it is above 0.01 milligrams (10 micrograms) per liter, some home filtering system may be warranted.

In addition, water treatment plants might be encouraged to use less aluminum in the treatment process, pending further scientific study of the potential threat of long-term aluminum ingestion.

New hope for a cure for Alzheimer's disease

A cure for Alzheimer's disease, a brain disorder that affects the elderly, may be just a few years away, researchers report in *Science* (247,4941:408).

The hope comes in the form of nerve growth factor (NGF for short), a naturally occurring protein that helps keep certain kinds of nerve cells healthy.

Dying nerve cells cause memory loss, one of the first signs of Alzheimer's. Scientists don't know why brain cells begin to die.

Although NGF can't restore memory and brain function that has already been lost, researchers believe it will help stop further memory loss and brain damage.

They are now reproducing the protein in the laboratory to use in animal studies.

NGF treatment is experimental and hasn't even been tested in humans yet, but researchers say its potential is "very exciting." They also hope to find other proteins as useful as NGF.

Researchers admit there is a risk in trying any new treatment on humans, but the hopelessness of Alzheimer's may outweigh the risk.

As many as four million people in the United States have the disease, they say.

Ask your doctor about aspirin therapy for Alzheimer's disease

If you take an aspirin every other day to ward off stroke and heart disease, you may be getting another unexpected benefit as well.

U.S. Pharmacist (15,5:62) reports that some Alzheimer's experts believe that aspirin and the other drugs commonly given for rheumatoid arthritis can prevent Alzheimer's disease.

This theory is only in the testing phase right now. Be sure to check with your doctor before you start taking aspirin regularly.

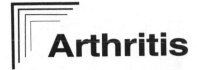

Arthritis

Weapons for fighting arthritis

Arthritis, in one of its more than 100 forms, afflicts millions of Americans. A lot of sufferers want answers about what's causing the pain and what can be done to treat it.

Here are a few questions and answers:

Q. Arthritis — what is it?

A. The term means "inflammation of a joint." There are more than 100 different diseases that are considered forms of arthritis. All of them attack joints and connective tissues in the body. But each form has different symptoms, and each must be treated differently.

The most common form is osteoarthritis, affecting 16 million Americans. This type happens when the elastic surfaces at the end of bones — called cartilage — begin deteriorating. Osteoarthritis usually strikes people over 60, affecting mostly joints in the feet, fingers, hips and knees. It usually hits only a few joints at any one time.

Next most common is rheumatoid arthritis. In this disease, the film-like membrane surrounding a joint becomes inflamed, eventually leading to destruction of the joint itself.

Rheumatoid arthritis strikes people of various ages and can affect many joints at once. It can even cause problems with other organs like the eyes, lungs, blood vessels and skin.

Other forms include spinal arthritis (known medically as ankylosing spondylitis), lupus, gout, scleroderma and juvenile arthritis, according to *Arthritis Today* (3,3:22).

Q. What causes arthritis?

A. Although exact causes are still uncertain, scientists are beginning to think that some people may inherit the tendency to get arthritis, especially the rheumatoid variety, according to the Arthritis Foundation.

Several forms also seem to be triggered by infections. For example, some kinds of diseases caused by tick bites can lead to arthritis-like inflammations in the joints.

Q. *What can be done to treat arthritis?*

A. There is no known cure. However, crippling pain of arthritis usually can be controlled, especially if the disease is caught early. Control measures include medicines, diet, exercise, rest, protection of the affected joints and, sometimes, surgery. A surgeon can replace whole joints with artificial materials.

Many people seem to believe that arthritis is a natural result of growing old and think that arthritis isn't harmful, so they treat themselves rather than going to a doctor. However, since there are several different types of arthritis, and because of the high death-rate in rheumatoid arthritis, a doctor should always be consulted. Early and aggressive treatment of rheumatoid arthritis is very important. British researchers have found that waiting too long to treat rheumatoid arthritis can be fatal.

According to a 25-year study by the Royal National Hospital for Rheumatic Diseases in Bath, England, one-third of people with rheumatoid arthritis died because of arthritis-related problems. "People really do die from arthritis," cautions Dr. Theodore Pincus of Vanderbilt University in Nashville.

Furthermore, medical treatment within the first six months of rheumatoid arthritis also can prevent irreversible damage to the joints and cartilage, as well as lowering the death rate, the researchers concluded. Treatment varies, depending on the patient and the specific type of arthritis.

Q. *What medicines are used to treat arthritis?*

A. There are three categories of drugs used to control arthritis.

(1) The main type fights inflammation, the major source of arthritis pain. Among these are the nonsteroidal anti-inflammatory drugs (known as NSAIDs) and the corticosteroids. Aspirin is the best-known of the NSAIDs and probably is used more than any other single medicine to treat arthritis, says *Arthritis Today*.

(2) Another category of drugs acts to slow down the disease process, which, untreated, leads to destruction of the affected joint. This

second class of drugs includes gold compounds, penicillamine, methotrexate and anti-malarial drugs. All these are very powerful and have some serious side effects.

(3) The drugs of last resort are extremely powerful immunosuppressives. That means they put a damper on the body's own self-defense system. They may halt the disease's progress, but the potential side effects are severe.

Q. *What are some other treatments?*

A. The Arthritis Foundation says sufferers get some relief from both heat and cold therapies. "Cold temporarily deadens nerves that carry pain and also reduces swelling and inflammation," according to the report in *Arthritis Today.* "We really don't know why heat works. It does increase circulation in the affected area. ... One popular technique for pain relief is a contrast bath ... alternating use of heat and cold."

Q. *What about diet and other natural means?*

A. Aerobic exercise is recommended for people who have mild or moderate forms of arthritis. Studies have shown that low-intensity exercise like fast walking or golfing actually can reduce joint pain in patients with rheumatoid arthritis and osteoarthritis, according to the medical journal *The Physician and Sportsmedicine* (17,2:128). In gouty arthritis, diet may play a major role in prevention of the painful attacks.

If rheumatoid arthritis is suspected, fish oil may reduce the painful symptoms, says Dr. Edward Harris, chairman of medicine at Stanford University. This is especially effective if treatment with the oil is supplemented with daily aspirin. Doctors recommend getting the essential ingredients in fish oil — the omega-3 fatty acids — by eating cold-water fish rather than by taking fish oil capsules. High levels of these beneficial oils are found naturally in all cold-water fish. Increase your intake of trout, salmon, mackerel, or cod.

Packaged fish oil supplements, available at the store, could cause other problems, such as reducing the ability of your blood to clot. For that reason, most doctors believe the supplements should be used with caution.

Arthritis, a sleep-robber?

Eight out of 10 people with rheumatoid arthritis report that they often feel very tired during the day. Doctors usually say that daytime fatigue is just part of the suffering that rheumatoid arthritis patients have to learn to put up with.

Many doctors just think the arthritis itself and the drugs used to fight it cause the tiredness.

But a new study in *Arthritis and Rheumatism* (32,8:974) suggests that many cases of fatigue may be due to sleep disturbances, rather than to the disease itself.

Doctors at the Minnesota Regional Sleep Disorders Center studied 16 patients with chronic, active rheumatoid arthritis, but who were otherwise healthy. The youngest was 54; the oldest, 71. They found no "sleep deprivation" as such.

The doctors were surprised, however, to find that all 16 rheumatoid arthritis patients thrashed their arms and legs much more than "normal" sleepers.

Perhaps more significantly, all 16 awoke frequently throughout the night, many times more than nonarthritic patients, the report indicates.

Based on brain-wave readings, the rheumatoid arthritis patients averaged waking up and dozing off an amazing 46 times per hour, "which permitted only 1.3-minute sleep periods," the report says.

More than 10 of those awakening periods lasted more than a minute each, the study says. That's two to three times the sleep-arousal rate of a group of nonarthritic 75-year-olds in another study.

Perhaps even more amazing, none of the 16 realized the next day how badly he had slept. All remembered waking up only about half the times they actually did, as measured objectively by the researchers on their instruments.

Interestingly, not one of the 16 blamed waking up on joint pain.

The doctors did not try to control the effects of medicines on the tests. They reasoned that rheumatoid arthritis patients generally take medicines, and that must be factored in. Nine of the patients were taking prednisone, but the seven who were not taking that medicine had the same sleep problems.

None was taking any kind of sleeping pill. One was taking amitriptyline, and one was on imipramine, both only occasional, low doses.

"These striking abnormalities of sleep" may cause excessive daytime sleepiness in rheumatoid arthritis patients, the researchers conclude, "and may play a role in early-onset fatigue." The implication from this study is that this rheumatoid arthritis "symptom" may be a separate illness.

Until now, doctors have treated the arthritis but generally have not tried to fight the "accompanying" fatigue. Now, they may want to start treating the tiredness itself, separate from the arthritis.

Commonsense relief from arthritis pain

You can take the initiative in battling that relentless enemy, osteoarthritis, researchers say.

Rest — The first and best weapon against arthritis is a good balance between rest and exercise, says a report in *Senior Patient* (2,1:55).

Getting a good night's sleep, plus morning and afternoon rest periods, helps take pressure off weight-bearing joints and rests tired muscles.

Gentle Exercise — But balance your rest with gentle exercise, experts suggest. One of the best forms of exercise for arthritis patients is swimming in a mildly heated pool. Even if you can't swim, you can still enjoy gentle exercise in the shallow part of a pool, researchers suggest.

Heat — Use heat to relieve the pain that comes with osteoarthritis. Try soaking in a warm tub or using a heating pad or hot pack to help ease pain in sensitive joints.

Elderly patients should avoid hot tubs and whirlpools, however, because the water is often too hot.

Massage — Gentle massages can also help relieve those stiff, aching muscles. Using heat and massage regularly provides great relief from arthritis pain without the extra cost of professional therapy.

Walkers and Canes — One of the best methods of relieving arthritis pain is simply reducing the stress on sensitive joints. Walkers and properly fitted canes can help improve balance, relieve over-tired muscles and provide stability.

But the cane or walker must "fit" the patient.

Many patients use canes that are too long. Or they may have the correct size cane, but don't know how to use it properly, according to another report in *Senior Patient* (1,2:93).

It's very easy to determine if a cane is the right length. Wear shoes and stand up straight, with your arms hanging loosely at your side. Have someone measure the distance from the crease in your wrist to the ground. This measurement is the best height for the cane, the report says.

Flat, contoured handles at right angles to the cane are better than curved handles (the ones shaped like a shepherd's staff). Flat handles are more comfortable for longer periods of time.

Use flat-bottomed rubber tips for the end of the cane. Rounded rubber tips don't grip the ground as well as tips with flat bottoms. Remember that rubber tips wear out with regular use just like tires and shoes.

They should be replaced occasionally. You can find replacement rubber tips at most drugstores.

And, make sure you hold the cane the correct way — on the side away from the painful body part. For example, if your *left* knee pains you, hold your cane in your *right* hand, the report recommends.

Home Safety — Simple devices in the home can also help ease stress on arthritic joints and improve safety.

To get around better, consider using raised chairs and toilet seats, shower chairs, grab bars in bathrooms and nonslippery rugs and bathmats.

Take away the need to stretch by installing lowered closet shelves and bars. And replace buttons and zippers with Velcro to ease stress on arthritic hands and arms.

All of these commonsense tips are easy and inexpensive. They're good ways to help relieve osteoarthritis pain and promote more independence in everyday activities.

For more information, contact the Arthritis Foundation, 1314 Spring Street N.W., Atlanta, Ga. 30309. Ask for their free booklets, "Arthritis: Basic Facts," "Taking Care: Protecting Your Joints" and "Coping With Pain."

Arthritis patients said to benefit from moderate aerobic exercise

Aerobic exercise can actually decrease joint pain while improving muscle strength and aerobic capacity in people with arthritis, according to two separate reports in *The Physician and Sportsmedicine* (17,2:128 and 18,1:123).

Studies show that aerobic exercise helps produce better heart and lung health.

And that helps make a person more self-sufficient, decreases pain and stiffness and leads to improved overall fitness.

It has always been difficult for arthritis patients and doctors to balance the need for exercise with the joints' need for rest.

However, three doctors at the University of Michigan say that patients with rheumatoid arthritis or osteoarthritis can "participate in low-intensity aerobic exercise programs" without aggravating their disease. Low intensity exercise includes things like fast walking and golfing.

"Findings from studies of patients with either rheumatoid arthritis or osteoarthritis who participated in an aerobic exercise program show that the subjects made significant gains, in aerobic capacity, functional status, muscle strength and other aspects of performance," according to the doctors who conducted the study.

The patients also improved in areas "that might have a positive impact on quality of life, including pain tolerance, joint pain, mood, and social activity," say the researchers.

"Despite increasing evidence that regular aerobic exercise yields many benefits for patients with arthritis," the report says, "patients often are advised to curtail physical activity." But the doctors warn that an inactive approach is not good for most patients because it "may contribute to fatigue, weakness and poor functional performance."

Unfortunately, many people with arthritis give up on exercise just because of pain or stiffness in one or two joints. This results in deterioration of the whole body. People with arthritis should realize that muscle strength actually helps protect weakened joints, researchers say.

In an evaluation after five years of regular exercise, another researcher found that the arthritis symptoms had not developed as quickly in patients who exercised as in patients who did not. The people who exercised had also taken less sick time and sick pension from their employers.

Try exercises that use "smooth, repetitive motions such as walking, ice skating, cross-country skiing, and bicycling," recommends Dr. Richard Kyle, chief of the orthopedics department and staff physician for the Arthritis Care Program at Metropolitan-Mount Sinai Medical Center in Minneapolis.

When the weather is bad, go to indoor jogging or cycling machines. "Swimming, cycling, golf, dancing, gymnastics, fast walking, and jogging ... may be good exercise alternatives," the doctors conclude.

Experts emphasize that some activities should be avoided. Sports that involve jumping up and coming down hard (basketball, volleyball) may aggravate sensitive joints.

Avoid the risk of joint damage. Proper jogging or walking shoes, for example, are very shock-absorbent and can help cushion arthritic joints.

Help your joints by shedding a few pounds. Losing weight reduces the extra stress on the joints.

A warning: If you've led a sluggish life-style for a while, be careful not to gear up too quickly and thus over-exercise, suggest researchers.

Instead, observe the "two-hour rule." This simple rule says that if you feel pain for two hours after stopping an exercise, you're probably overdoing it. If this happens, just temporarily scale down the level of exercise, or modify the exercise or equipment in some way.

Be sure to warm up and cool down properly, doctors say. They suggest that you apply light massage and heat or ice as a pain-control measure.

When you exercise also is important. People with rheumatoid arthritis may need to exercise later in the day due to morning stiffness. However, people with osteoarthritis who feel worse at the end of the day may need to exercise in the morning.

Be alert to warning signs from your body, experts suggest. If you experience dizziness, faintness, chest pain, nausea, extreme joint pain or pain enduring long after finishing the exercises, tell your doctor right away.

If you just dread the thought of exercise, you may find it more enjoyable to exercise with music. Exercising with a friend or with groups of other arthritis patients also makes the experience more fun.

Regular exercise is important, but the sessions don't have to be long. "As little as 15 minutes of exercise three times per week is sufficient to improve aerobic capacity in arthritis patients with severe limitations," reports T.H. Harkcom in *Arthritis and Rheumatology* (28,1:32).

If you're interested in an exercise program, ask your doctor before beginning. Your doctor can help plan a program designed especially to meet your needs and abilities.

How to exercise safely when arthritis cramps your style

The Physician and Sportsmedicine (17,2:128) gives some guidelines to aerobic exercise for people with arthritis.

❑ Only people with mild or moderate arthritis, who can take care of themselves, should be considered for aerobic exercise.

❑ People who want to take an active role in their own health care will get the best results. You need to be motivated to exercise and be willing to work with your doctor's supervision.

❑ All patients should have an exercise tolerance test, a complete physical and laboratory studies before they start an exercise program.

❑ The first six weeks of an exercise program should be supervised by a doctor or physical therapist. Regular check-ups should continue — improvements may change the need for medication.

❑ Warm-up and cool-down exercises should be learned and faithfully observed.

❏ You should strive to attain 70 percent of your maximal heart rate during your exercise session.

❏ Proper footwear, with cushioned support to prevent shock to your joints, should be worn.

❏ Ice treatments can be used on aching joints before and after exercise.

❏ Choose the best time of day for you to exercise. Some people have more joint problems in the morning and others experience more discomfort later in the day.

❏ Listen to your body and try to learn the difference between pain normally generated by exercise and pain related to the arthritis. "Joint pain that lasts longer than one hour after exercise ... should be recognized as a reason to curtail ... activity until the pain subsides."

Walk your way to stronger bones and easier joints

You know your heart benefits every time you "take a hike." But did you know that your bones and joints are strengthened as well?

According to *Arthritis Today* (4,3:19), even a moderate walking program can do wonders in reducing joint and muscle stiffness, while actually making bones stronger, denser and less subject to bone-thinning osteoporosis.

Although most people don't realize it, walking is a good aerobic exercise. Dr. James M. Rippe, cardiologist and director of the exercise physiology and nutrition laboratory at the University of Massachusetts Medical School, says that walking, when done properly, is just as beneficial as running or jogging — it just takes longer.

"You don't have to have sweat pouring down your brow to get benefits from aerobic exercise," says Dr. Rippe. "Consistency is more important than intensity."

But don't take that to mean you should "stop and stroll." Try to set a pace that allows you to reach your target heart rate (see article on finding your target rate in the Exercise and Fitness chapter), then maintain it for at least 20 minutes.

People with arthritis often fear exercise will intensify painful flare-ups. The truth is, inactivity causes joints to become stiff and muscles to become smaller and weaker. Walking breaks the cycle of pain and the resulting inactivity.

> • **To loosen stiff joints before walking, try soaking your feet in warm water.**
>
> • **Wiggle your toes back and forth as far as they will comfortably move.**
>
> • **Dry your feet, dress properly and go for a walk. When you return, soak your feet again, but this time in cool water for about five minutes.**

As with any exercise, a warm-up period will increase blood circulation in your muscles, making them more flexible and less likely to suffer from strains, pulls and soreness.

Five minutes of walking slowly should be sufficient. Then pick up your pace, but keep it comfortable, for 10 to 20 minutes.

Do this at least four times a week for a month. Gradually increase your speed, distance and time until you can walk briskly, and continuously, for 30 minutes without feeling fatigued.

Be sure to breathe deeply, in through the nose and out of the mouth. Keep track of your pulse to make sure you stay within your target heart range.

At this point, you are receiving a good aerobic workout. Just remember — if you can't carry on a conversation while you're walking, or you find yourself huffing and puffing, you're pushing too hard.

During the time of an arthritis flare-up, it would be wise to check with your doctor to determine exactly how much exercise is right for you.

But even when the walking is somewhat awkward, or you feel limited to shorter walks due to mild pain, the rewards are still definitely worth the effort.

People with arthritis report feeling less stressed and having a better outlook on life due to their daily walks. Walking gives them added flexibility that carries over into other activities and is credited with increasing their life span. Not a bad return on a 30-minute investment!

Natural relief for arthritis pain

Ginger — You may be able to reach into your kitchen spice cabinet for relief from the pain and inflammation of rheumatoid arthritis. People with arthritis reported "significant relief" from pain after taking less than a tablespoonful of ginger every day for three months, reports Dr. Krishna C. Srivastava of the Institute of Odense in Denmark. Long known as a folk remedy for various ailments, ginger now is being studied in medical trials to determine its usefulness as an arthritis medicine.

The arthritis patients took ginger in two ways: either about five grams a day of fresh ginger root, or from a half-gram to 1.5 grams daily of ginger powder.

All reported that "they were able to move around better and had less swelling and morning stiffness after taking the spice," says *The Medical Tribune* (30,18:16). No side effects were reported.

Chinese herb — Another potential medicine comes from China and has been used there for centuries as a folk remedy. Researchers are planning large-scale trials of an extract from an herb known as Triptery-gium wilfordii hook.

The Chinese extract "achieved a 90 percent reduction in pain and other typical RA [rheumatoid arthritis] symptoms in 30 patients who were treated for 12 weeks," according to the *Tribune* report. Control patients given a placebo (a harmless fake medicine) recorded less than a fourth as much relief. The main side effects were skin rash in half the patients and mild diarrhea in about a fifth.

Indian tree bark — Still another natural source of arthritis help is showing up in bark extracts from an Indian tree known as Dysoxylum binectariferum.

The extract, known as rohitukine, has been shown to reduce inflammation and prevent the body's immune system from turning against itself, according to Dr. A.N. Dohadwalla in Bombay. Even high dosages produced no bad side effects in animal tests, the doctor says.

Polish peat — In addition, possible arthritis help may come from deposits of decaying vegetation. A plant extract tested recently comes from some rich peat bogs in Poland. Peat is a soft forerunner of coal.

The refined product seems to cut down on the autoimmune response that, in rheumatoid arthritis, points the body's anti-disease weapons at the body tissues themselves.

Fish oil supplements provide relief from rheumatoid arthritis

People with active, painful rheumatoid arthritis discovered they had less pain, fewer swollen joints, decreased morning stiffness and improved strength in their hands after taking daily "fish oil" pills for nearly six months.

The daily supplement of omega-3 fatty acids also appeared to halt and even reverse arthritis's invasion of other joints, says a report in *Arthritis and Rheumatism* (33,6:810).

Researchers at the Albany Medical College in New York tried "high" and "low" doses of omega-3 oils on the volunteers. They gave a third group pills containing olive oil, the report says.

The amounts given were linked to a person's weight. For example, the "high" dose was the equivalent of a quarter-ounce of fish oil per day for a man weighing 180 pounds, or less than two ounces per week. Women in the study also got amounts corresponding to their weights.

The "low" dose was half that of the "high."

About one person out of every four of the volunteers experienced fishy after-taste or belching, usual side effects of taking fish oil capsules. The researchers suggest that such side effects are minor compared to side effects of standard drug therapy for arthritis.

Fish oil supplements can also cause increased bleeding times, the report notes.

Those taking the olive oil supplements reported that 24 weeks of olive oil failed to ease joint tenderness, morning stiffness or pain levels. Only the high-dose fish-oil group got significant pain relief, the report says.

The "high-dose" and "low-dose" concepts were defined by the researchers just for the purposes of their clinical trial. However, other studies have used daily doses of omega-3 oils many times higher than that used in this study, but always with close medical supervision.

Always check with your doctor before taking any supplements, natural or otherwise.

Put an end to rheumatoid arthritis?

A protein produced in the laboratory may soon offer relief to rheumatoid arthritis (RA) sufferers by bringing a certain hormone under control, according to the *Johns Hopkins Medical Letter* (2,2:1).

Too much of the hormone, known as interleukin-1, destroys healthy tissues and leads to pain, swelling and deformity. In animal studies, the protein blocked the production of interleukin-1.

The protein did not repair damage already done but did prevent further damage to healthy tissue. Human studies are planned.

Hot flashes and cold tips for relief from aches and pains

Whether you have arthritis or you're a weekend gardener who has overdone a good thing, the correct use of heat or cold therapy can be your ticket to temporary relief from minor aches and pains. *Arthritis Today* (3,3:22) reports that you can gain relief from arthritis pain by using both heat and cold therapy.

Cold therapy temporarily "deadens nerves that carry pain and also reduces swelling and inflammation," states the report. Heat therapy helps relieve stiffness and pain by increasing circulation in the affected area.

Another popular technique used for pain relief is a contrast bath — alternating use of heat and cold.

To get the best results from heat or cold therapy, it's important to use them correctly. Here are a few tips to help you use heat and cold safely and effectively.

Before using heat or cold:

- **Check with your doctor or therapist, especially if you are sensitive to cold or heat.**

- **Avoid using heat or cold on areas where you have poor circulation or vasculitis (inflammation of a blood or lymph vessel).**

- **Make sure your skin is healthy and dry.**

- **Use extra padding between your heat or cold source and areas where the bone is close to the surface (wrap the heating pad or cold pack in a towel, etc.).**

- **Allow your skin to return to normal temperature between treatments.**

During use:

- **Avoid using creams, lotions or heat rubs on your skin with heat or cold packs.**

- **Time yourself. Using heat or cold too long can hurt you. (Ask your doctor about the best length of time for cold or heat therapy.)**

- **Stay awake, and don't lie on top of the heat or cold pack.**

- **Remember that a bath or shower that is too hot may make you tired or dizzy.**

After use:

- **Normal skin will be a uniform pink color. Watch out for warning signs of blisters or dark red or red and white areas.**

- **Check for any new discoloration or swelling.**

Talk to your doctor or therapist about how heat and cold therapy can fit into your overall plan to relieve arthritis aches and pains.

Fibromyalgia: an arthritis-like disease

Fibromyalgia is a condition affecting the muscles that causes intense, widespread pain at various "tender points" throughout the body.

Other symptoms include anxiety, fatigue, headache, disturbed sleep, bowel problems and numbness or tingling sensations. Fibromyalgia affects an estimated five percent of Americans, mostly women, and is often mistaken as an inevitable side effect of arthritis.

The disease, once called fibrositis, is kin to arthritis, and people with arthritis also can suffer from fibromyalgia at the same time.

Doctors still don't know what causes it. They point out that the symptoms are very similar to those of chronic fatigue syndrome. That leads some to speculate that stress, anxiety, depression and emotional upsets may trigger the condition or make it worse.

Researchers are trying to find out whether these emotional factors cause the disease or result from the disease. Other doctors think that the disease may be caused by some kind of virus.

No X-ray or laboratory test yet exists that can identify the condition. Because of that, over the years, people with fibromyalgia have been told by doctors that the pain is "all in their heads."

However, doctors are finally getting a grip on diagnosing this hard-to-pin-down disease.

Recently, rheumatologists have identified several specific tender points to distinguish fibromyalgia from other painful rheumatic conditions like osteoarthritis.

Doctors now can test a patient's pain level just by pressing those areas with their hands. That eliminates the need for expensive blood tests and X-rays.

You can tell whether you have the disease by touch. If you feel pain at 11 out of 18 touch points, you could be suffering from fibromyalgia, the report indicates.

"Tenderness in at least 11 of 18 specified sites on the body, accompanied by widespread pain, identifies the syndrome and distinguishes it from other ... disorders," says Dr. Frederick Wolfe, chairman of the Multicenter Fibromyalgia Criteria Study.

The tender points that you and your doctor can look for are:

❏ **Neck** — four points: one point on each side of the larynx (voice box). Also, on the back of the neck, one spot on either side of the spinal column at about the midway point on the neck.

❏ **Back** — four points: one on the outside of each shoulder blade, and one point near the middle of the shoulders at an outward angle from the shoulder blade.

❏ **Hips** — four points: one at the top of each buttock, and one point on the lower outside of each hip.

❏ **Chest** — two points: one spot on each side of the breastbone at the second rib, just below the collarbone.

❏ **Legs** — two points: one site on the inside of each knee.

❏ **Arms** — two points: one spot on the inside of each elbow.

Though there is still no cure for fibromyalgia, doctors are discovering some treatments for it, according to reports in *Arthritis Today* (3,3:50) and *Medical World News* (30,11:10).

❏ You can put ice packs or heating pads on the painful areas. Sometimes a combination of both these approaches can help.

❏ You can do some aerobic exercises that work on the muscle areas giving you pain.

❏ You can do certain stretching exercises that may provide some relief.

❏ You can stand erect and sit properly. Poor posture is known to aggravate the condition.

❏ You can learn several stress-reducing techniques, such as meditation, reading the Bible, etc.

Check with your doctor first about these and other natural ways you can ease the pain. Your doctor also may want to prescribe sleeping pills and some muscle relaxers. Treatment is tailored to the patient, depending on how badly she hurts and where.

For more information about fibromyalgia and what you can do to fight its painful effects, contact your local Arthritis Foundation chapter.

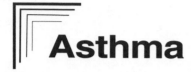

Asthma

New research about asthma and allergies

All asthma is caused by allergies, according to a new study by researchers at the University of Arizona. "These findings challenge the concept that there are basic differences between so-called allergic ("extrinsic") and nonallergic ("intrinsic") forms of asthma," reports Dr. Benjamin Burrows in *The New England Journal of Medicine* (320,5:271).

In the new study, doctors found that the prevalence of asthma was related to the level of the serum immunoglobulin (IgE) in the body. "And no asthma was present in the 177 subjects with the lowest IgE levels for their age and sex," they report.

IgE is the antibody that causes immune system response in the body. When your body has an allergic reaction — in other words, when your immune system overreacts to a stimulus — you get excessive amounts of the antibody IgE in your body.

Researchers studied 2,600 volunteers with asthma or allergic rhinitis and concluded that asthma is almost always associated with some type of IgE-related reaction and therefore has an allergic basis.

Since 1918, doctors have believed that some asthma is caused by allergies to dust, molds, pollens, animal danders and other airborne particles. But if the asthma is triggered by emotional factors, infection or irritants, it is classed as nonallergic.

According to *The Merck Manual*, about 10 to 20 percent of adults have allergic asthma, 30 to 50 percent have nonallergic asthma and some seem to have both allergic and nonallergic responses.

Now, this belief will have to be reevaluated.

Can asthma be caused by dust mites?

New research suggests that some asthma, especially in children, might be caused by exposure to house-dust mites, spider-like creatures too small to be seen with the naked eye.

The mites, which cling to specks of dust in your home, give off a kind of protein called an allergen that triggers allergic responses.

Such exposure possibly could touch off asthma in susceptible people, suggests the study in *The New England Journal of Medicine* (323,8:502).

While the study focused on mites' effect on children with asthma, the information implies that adults also could be affected so long as they come into contact with dust-borne allergens.

"Over the past 30 years, many of the changes we have made in our houses — such as increased temperatures and the use of fitted carpets, tighter insulation, and detergents effective in cool water — have improved the conditions needed for dust mites to grow," says study author Dr. Richard Sporik.

Soybean dust linked to severe asthma attacks

If you suffer from asthma attacks, the villain causing your distress may be as near as your pantry. Epidemics among dockworkers and residents living near the docks in Barcelona and Cartagena, Spain, have led researchers to identify a new asthma trigger: soybean dust, according to reports in *The Lancet* (2,8662:538) and *The New England Journal of Medicine* (320,17:1097).

Soybeans are a member of the legume family, which includes peas and beans. A common U.S. farm crop, soybeans are high in protein and are used in many commercially prepared foods.

Soy products include soy flour and oil, both of which are used in many food products, from margarine to fillers in canned and frozen meat products.

According to the reports, "extracts of the bean can cause an immediate allergic response." During one epidemic, researchers found that 64 of 84 adults were allergic to soybean products.

For some reason, children under age 14 were not affected. In another epidemic, 65 patients were sent to the hospital with acute asthma. One died, and nine others needed a respirator to help them breathe.

Experts have known for some time that air pollution and thunderstorms, which stir up a lot of dust, cause asthma epidemics. But, the reports say, the weather was not a factor in the 13 epidemics in Barcelona. On each asthma epidemic day, however, dockworkers were unloading soybeans. No epidemics were reported on days when soybeans were not unloaded.

Researchers point out that the increasing popularity of soybean products may lead to asthma epidemics in other parts of the world. If you are experiencing unexplained breathing difficulties or allergies, ask your doctor to test you for sensitivity to soy products.

Blood Pressure

The facts about high blood pressure

High blood pressure is the major risk factor for stroke and one of the major risk factors for heart attacks and cardiovascular problems as well as kidney failure. Although high blood pressure may be partly hereditary, several "environmental" factors increase the likelihood you may get it. They include stress, obesity, a sedentary lifestyle, low potassium intake and too much fat, salt and alcohol.

Many Americans take medication to control high blood pressure. Although medication does help, researchers are concerned about the effects of long-term use — especially for people whose blood pressure is just above normal — and are exploring ways to lower blood pressure naturally through diet and exercise.

A plan to prevent high blood pressure naturally

If you are prone to high blood pressure, are you destined to take powerful drugs to fight the disease? The answer is, maybe not. You may have a natural option to prevent high blood pressure from ever developing, say eight researchers at Northwestern University Medical School in Chicago.

"Results indicate that even a moderate reduction in risk factors for hypertension among hypertension-prone individuals contributes to the primary prevention of the disease," the report says. (Hypertension is the scientific name for high blood pressure.)

You may be able to cut your risk of developing high blood pressure by making moderate changes in lifestyle, the scientists indicate in a report in *The Journal of the American Medical Association* (262,13:1801).

The researchers studied 201 men and women who were slightly overweight, ate salty foods, smoked, downed several alcoholic drinks a day and rarely exercised. All of them had blood pressure in the "high-normal" range. That means a diastolic (lower number) pressure of from 80 to 99 mm Hg. But, otherwise, they all were healthy.

These prime candidates for high blood pressure agreed to work on better nutrition and to shoot for four goals:

- **Lose at least 10 pounds.**

- **Reduce daily salt intake to less than one-tenth of an ounce.**

- **Cut back to no more than two alcoholic drinks a day.**

- **Exercise for 30 minutes three times a week.**

Smokers were advised to kick the habit. The researchers encouraged the study participants to stick to a "fat-modified American Heart Association-type diet."

For five years, the participants — ranging in age from 30 to 44 — kept food diaries, visited with the doctors regularly, were given blood and urine tests, and had their blood pressures checked periodically. Three-quarters of them exercised faithfully, mostly walking, jogging and bicycling.

One out of four met the weight-loss goal, but fewer than two in 10 reduced salt intakes. All said they averaged no more than two drinks a day.

They cut their daily calorie intake by an average of 800 calories, a drop of 30 percent. They cut back modestly on saturated fat and cholesterol.

During the same period, doctors kept track of another, similar group that took no special dietary, weight-loss or exercise measures — in other words, just everyday folks who continued to eat, drink and do what they pleased.

After five years, the researchers found that the "do-as-you-please" group had double the rate of high blood pressure as the study group.

The nutritional approach also helped even those in the study group who did develop high blood pressure by delaying its onset for a year or more in most cases. Those who lost the most weight experienced the most benefits, the researchers report. On the negative side, smokers were nearly four times as likely to develop high blood pressure as nonsmokers, the report indicates.

One in five people in the "do-as-you-please" group developed high blood pressure during the five-year trial, compared with one in 11 in the nutrition study group. That proved true even though most in the study group did not reach their original goals. Just the emphasis on nutrition seemed to help a lot.

Such modest changes in lifestyle could slash the risks of heart disease and stroke in 1 million people with high-normal blood pressure over the next five years, the researchers believe. The researchers recommend that doctors start aiming for "primary prevention [of high blood pressure] by safe nutritional-hygenic means" in addition to prescribing drugs to fight the disease.

These findings were confirmed by a new four-year study by the University of Minnesota. The researchers found that even people with mild high blood pressure, who had been taking prescription blood-pressure lowering drugs, could maintain lower blood pressure without drugs by losing weight, reducing salt and reducing alcohol.

"Drugs have saved the lives of many people with high blood pressure," explained Dr. Richard H. Grimm, Jr. who led the study. "But in recent years, the medical community has been more and more concerned about the potential adverse side effects of drugs and the cost of drugs."

In the study, 189 men who had mild high blood pressure (diastolic blood pressure more than 80 mm Hg but less than 90 mm Hg) were divided into three groups.

The first group stopped taking prescription drugs and received nutritional counseling. "They were instructed in weight control, dietary sodium reduction and alcohol reduction," Grimm explained.

The second group discontinued drug therapy but did not receive any nutritional counseling.

Group three continued on their prescription drug regimen.

"Four years after the study began, almost 40 percent of group one participants remained off drugs with normal blood pressures," the researchers reported. But 95 percent of groups two and three had to return to or continue with drug therapy.

The nondrug, nutrition group lost an average of 5 to 10 pounds and kept the weight off during the four years. Their salt intake was reduced by 36 percent, and the amount of alcohol they consumed was also reduced.

However, the other groups gained weight and showed no change in their salt and alcohol intakes.

Group one also had improved levels of cholesterol, potassium and uric acid in the blood, an unexpected but pleasant side effect, the doctors noted.

"The promising nondrug treatments include weight control, dietary sodium reduction, alcohol reduction, and programs to increase physical activity in people with mild high blood pressure," Grimm reported.

Grimm is also heading another study, called the Treatment of Mild Hypertension Study, sponsored by the National Heart, Lung and Blood Institute.

Grimm hopes the study will reveal the following:

- **whether nutrition therapy combined with drug therapy will lower the death rate from high blood pressure**

- **whether lowering mild blood pressure will prevent coronary heart disease**

- **how different blood pressure drugs affect life expectancy**

"Approximately 60 million Americans — about 25 percent of the adult population — have high blood pressure," Grimm reports. "The medical costs of hypertension are estimated about $10 billion annually ... approximately 75 million patient visits to primary-care physicians for high blood pressure treatment each year."

When lowering high blood pressure can be dangerous

Just how much should high blood pressure be lowered? That's the question being asked by doctors at Albert Einstein College of Medicine in Bronx, N.Y., after a study there indicated some dangers associated with both very big and very small drops in blood pressure. The "moderate" declines seemed to be safest, says the report in *The Journal of the American Medical Association* (262,7:920).

Researchers say many more people eventually had severe or fatal heart attacks following blood pressure treatment that resulted in drops of less than six points or more than 18 points. People whose diastolic blood pressure dropped from seven to 17 points had the least amount of heart attacks.

People with very large and very small drops in blood pressure face three to four times the risk of heart attack compared with people with moderate declines, the study says.

Seen in another way, the risks of fatal heart attack were about the same for those whose high blood pressure remained virtually unchanged as for those with a large fall in blood pressure. Why those with big drops in blood pressure should face the same risks as those whose blood pressure remained high is unknown, the *JAMA* report says.

The research indicates that an "ideal" blood pressure figure may be an unrealistic goal and may even be dangerous for many people, according to a *New York Times* report of the study.

One speculation was that a big blood pressure drop may result in poor blood flow through heart arteries, starving the heart muscle and leading to a heart attack.

They downplayed other possible factors like reaction to the medicines, other diseases and behavior like smoking and drinking.

That's because those same factors were present in the ones who had moderate drops in pressure and fewer heart attacks.

The doctors tracked 1,765 patients, three-quarters of them male and with an average age of 52 years.

All patients had blood pressure higher than 160 systolic or 95 diastolic when they entered the study, the report says. Most of them took standard drug treatments, like diuretics, calcium channel blockers or beta-blockers, to lower their blood pressure.

But, "drug type mattered less than the magnitude of blood pressure decline," according to the *Times* report.

The researchers say there was no direct time relationship between the big drop in blood pressure and a subsequent heart attack. Some attacks took place within a few weeks of the treatment; some occurred many months later.

The doctors make two suggestions:

❐ The attending doctor should seek a very specific treatment tailored to each patient that will protect the heart while trying to lower blood pressure, and

❐ "Until this goal is attainable, the cautious physician should seek modest (in the range of seven to 17 mm Hg of diastolic blood pressure) ... reduction for those with mild to moderate hypertension."

Important new risk factor for blood pressure deaths

Measuring a common waste product from your body may be the best early warning sign yet discovered to signal your risk of death from high blood pressure. Researchers have discovered that a blood test frequently performed during routine medical examinations may be a highly accurate predictor of fatality in patients with hypertension.

More than 50 percent of people with a combination of high blood pressure and high levels of a substance called creatinine in the blood will die within eight years, the report says.

Researchers analyzed data from a massive study involving 14 U.S. medical schools. Among the 10,940 high blood pressure patients enrolled in the study, a high level of a substance called creatinine in their blood serum (2.5 milligrams per deciliter or more) was associated with a surprisingly high death rate, according to a report in *Hypertension* (13,1:1).

"These data suggest that in patients with high blood pressure and a serum creatinine level equal to or greater than 2.5, more than 50 percent will die within eight years," says Dr. Neil B. Shulman, a principal investigator in the study.

Beginning at a serum creatinine level of 1.2, there was a noticeable, continuous increase in risk of death at increasing levels of creatinine, Shulman says.

A normal creatinine range is usually considered to be between 0.7 and 1.5 milligrams per deciliter, he adds. It's not that creatinine by itself causes anything bad to happen. High levels of it just serve like a smoke detector's buzzer, warning that something bad is going on in the body.

Creatinine is a waste product of metabolic processes in muscle cells, like smoke from a fire, explains Shulman, associate professor of medicine at Emory University in Atlanta. Normally, the kidneys filter creatinine out of the blood. For that reason, high levels of creatinine in the blood also may indicate kidney problems.

But the patients with high creatinine levels tended to die of heart disease and stroke, not of kidney disease, the scientists found. "We don't know why the hearts and brains of these patients with kidney dysfunction are so vulnerable to heart attacks and stroke," Shulman says.

The new finding is important, he adds, because it might lead to new approaches to preventing the complications of high blood pressure, which include heart attack and stroke.

According to Shulman, the study indicates that high blood levels of creatinine should be recognized as a risk "marker" for stroke and heart attack. An abnormal electrocardiogram (ECG) or an enlarged heart are other risk "markers." Conventional risk factors include cigarette smoking, elevated serum cholesterol and high blood pressure.

"I think our finding will be valuable both to the researchers who are trying to unravel the mysteries of high blood pressure and to the practicing physicians who need to identify which patients deserve special attention," Shulman says.

Patients with high creatinine levels are in such a "risky situation" that physicians should work hard to help them reduce their risk factors for heart attack and stroke, he says.

Studies show the benefits of exercise and weight loss in controlling blood pressure

Two recent medical studies praise the benefits of exercise and weight loss in controlling cases of mild high blood pressure.

At the same time, both studies suggest that adding drugs to the exercise and weight loss programs might be just a waste of money, at least in mild cases.

The two natural ways do the job as well as or better than hypertension medicines, according to reports in *The Journal of the American Medical Association* (263,20:2766) and *Medical World News* (31,10:35).

In the *JAMA* report, doctors at three Maryland clinics studied three groups of men with high blood pressure averaging 145/97 mm Hg. All were sedentary, meaning they didn't exercise much, if at all.

They put one group on a beta-blocker, propranolol hydrochloride. A second group got a calcium channel blocker, diltiazem hydrochloride. A third group received only a placebo, a fake, harmless pill with no medical effect.

All three groups performed the same kinds of exercises.

Three times a week, all 49 men lifted weights for 30 minutes on a 20-station weight-training circuit. Then they performed 20 minutes of aerobic exercises, either stationary bicycling, walking or jogging.

After 10 weeks, average blood pressure had fallen 14 points systolic and 13 points diastolic, to 131/84, the *JAMA* report says. More significantly, the drop occurred whether or not the men were taking blood pressure medicine, the report says. Exercise alone accounted for the improvement, the researchers conclude.

In addition, the men experienced a drop in total cholesterol and LDL ("bad") cholesterol levels. Levels of HDL ("good") cholesterol increased with the calcium channel blocker but actually decreased with the beta-blocker propranolol, the report says.

Added benefits: The men lost a little weight and increased their overall strength by an average of 25 percent. A second study involved nearly 800 overweight people with mild high blood pressure, according to *Medical World News*.

First, researchers divided the big group into two smaller ones. They put one of the groups on a diet to lose weight, but let the second group keep eating normally.

Next, they divided each of the two groups into three smaller groups and gave them either a diuretic (chlorthalidone), a beta-blocker (atenolol) or a placebo.

They found that people on the placebo who dropped 10 pounds or more had an average diastolic reduction of 12 points, about the same as those taking blood pressure drugs, the report says.

The catch is this: To get a blood pressure reduction from weight loss alone, you apparently have to lose at least 10 pounds, says Dr. Herbert Langford, chief of hypertension research at the University of Mississippi at Jackson. Lose less than 10 pounds, and blood pressure remains above normal, the study suggests.

Learning to like a low-salt diet

A low-sodium diet is one of the basic, natural ways to lower high blood pressure, but many people are hesitant because they think that a salt-free diet is bland. However, researchers at the University of Minnesota discovered that your desire for salt and your taste changes when you start a low-salt diet.

"The study was initiated because many participants in earlier studies reported that once they were on a low-sodium diet, many foods that had been acceptable were now 'too salty' or even unpleasant," Dr. Richard Grimm recently announced.

Participants in a low-salt diet compared salted crackers at regular intervals. "The highest sodium content crackers were rated more salty and less pleasant," Grimm said. "The level of sodium preferred also decreased ... these changes in taste occurred early and were evident by the sixth-week visit."

"In questionnaires, men on low-sodium diets reported they were more sensitive to the taste of salt, found many high salt foods to be unpleasant, and stated that the diet was easier to follow the longer they stayed on it," Grimm explained.

This confirms other studies that suggest our craving for salt is a learned behavior — an acquired taste. According to *High Blood Pressure Lowered Naturally* (FC&A Publishing), other studies with twins also show that salt craving is created by a high-salt diet and is not something we're born with.

It will take up to three months to lose the craving for salt completely, according to Mrs. Dash, a manufacturer of no-salt products.

The average American eats five to 10 grams of sodium, or one-third to one-fifth of an ounce of salt per day. This is much more salt than is needed for bodily functions.

Most people only need one-tenth that amount. Many scientific studies show that reducing salt intake, ideally to 500 milligrams per day, will lower blood pressure in most people.

Processed foods, anything that comes in a can, a frozen package or a box, is likely to have salt added as a preservative or flavor enhancer.

Tips to provide flavor without salt

- Use lemon juice on food instead of salt.

- Use one of several salt-free mixtures of herbs and spices now available.

- To spice chicken dishes, add fruit such as mandarin oranges or pineapples.

- Marinate chicken, fish, beef or poultry in orange juice or lemon juice.

- Use homemade mustard or honey to glaze meat dishes.

- Use green pepper, parsley, paprika or red pepper.

- In baking, use extracts instead of salt.

- Learn about the many natural herbs, spices and fruit peels that are available.

Could a low-salt diet send your blood pressure soaring?

For years doctors have been telling you too much salt can send your blood pressure soaring. Apparently, one doctor has changed his mind.

Dr. Brent M. Egan, a blood pressure specialist, told the audience at a recent annual American Heart Association meeting that a low-salt diet may actually be harmful for some people.

He and his colleagues studied 27 men who were put on a very low-salt diet for one week. They then ate their regular diet for two weeks and then repeated the low-salt diet once more.

Many men with normal blood pressure were "salt-resistant," says Dr. Egan, meaning that their blood pressure did not automatically fall when their salt intake was reduced. In fact, blood pressure actually increased by as much as five points in some men who reduced salt intake, he reports.

Studies have shown that insulin, a hormone produced by the pancreas, in some cases contributes to hardening of the arteries by helping the body produce excessive cholesterol. Insulin also encourages the body to retain salt in the kidneys, the report says.

Many men in the study had higher levels of insulin, and Dr. Egan suggests that the body may "adapt" to a low-salt diet by producing more insulin.

The American Heart Association recommends that Americans eat no more than one and a half teaspoons of salt a day. (The AHA has no plans to change that recommendation.)

If you are on a low-salt diet — or if your doctor has recommended one — Dr. Egan suggests that you carefully monitor your blood pressure at home. (You can buy blood pressure monitors at your local drugstore.)

Take your blood pressure every day for one week to establish your baseline measurement before starting the diet. Once on the diet, monitor your blood pressure regularly.If your blood pressure doesn't fall after one to two months on the low-salt diet, talk with your doctor because, Dr. Egan says, the diet "apparently is not helping."

Bran and other fiber lowers blood pressure

Daily fiber supplements help lower high blood pressure, according to a recent study. The systolic pressure of the study participants dropped an average of 10 points, and the diastolic pressure decreased an average of five points in just three months with fiber supplements, Danish researchers revealed in *The Lancet* (2,8559:622). People in the control group of the study who took a placebo experienced no change in their blood pressure levels.

Your fiber intake should be at least 30 grams each day and should include a variety of fiber types, says the National Cancer Institute. Good sources of fiber include wheat bran, oat bran, fruits, vegetables (with skins), whole-grain breads and cereals.

Until modern times, our ancestors ate a high-fiber diet, and many present-day digestive, colon, and bowel problems were rare in those days. Our digestive system is designed to handle a diet that contains bran, the outer fiber of cereal grains. Modern food processing methods remove much fiber from our food, which leads to constipation and other health problems, as well as high blood pressure.

Low-fiber diets have been linked to heart and artery disease, constipation, appendicitis, colon cancer, diverticulosis, cancer of the large bowel, hemorrhoids and obesity.

New role for vitamin C: It may lower high blood pressure

Doctors one day might tell people with borderline high blood pressure, "Take one vitamin C tablet every day to get your blood pressure back to normal."

That's because researchers have discovered that vitamin C might prevent healthy people from developing high blood pressure and might even help lower slightly elevated blood pressure readings to normal levels, according to a report in *Science News* (137,19:292).

Checking 67 healthy men and women ages 20 to 69, researchers at the Medical College of Georgia in Augusta found that those with high levels of vitamin C in the blood averaged a blood pressure reading of 104/65.

Those with one-fifth those blood levels of vitamin C — but still within acceptable, normally healthy levels — averaged blood pressure readings of 111/73, the report says. The "normal" blood pressure reading usually is considered 120/80.

Researchers suggest that the vitamin somehow pushes blood pressure down, keeping levels at or below "normal." That provides a cushion against blood pressure rising beyond healthy levels. Even people with established high blood pressure may benefit from more C, suggest researchers at Tufts University in Boston.

They checked 241 elderly Chinese-Americans and found the same result: the lower the blood levels of vitamin C, the higher the blood pressure.

Another common thread in both studies: Even at the lower ranges of vitamin C measured in the volunteers, none of the people suffered from a vitamin C deficiency. So the question researchers will be asking is this: are current "minimum" recommended levels of vitamin C (60 milligrams daily) large enough to give this apparent protection against high blood pressure? Or should people with a tendency toward high blood pressure increase their daily vitamin C intake to around one gram per day, as suggested by U.S. Department of Agriculture scientist David L. Trout?

Check with your doctor first before taking extra vitamin C. Some studies show that taking more than one gram of vitamin C a day can cause kidney stones, gout, diarrhea, cramping and interference with some blood tests.

In addition, suddenly stopping big doses of vitamin C can cause "rebound" scurvy, a serious vitamin deficiency.

You can get vitamin C naturally by eating citrus fruits and dark-green vegetables like broccoli.

Potatoes and bananas may help lower high blood pressure

A low-potassium diet may contribute to high blood pressure, according to two reports in *American Family Physician* (41,1:318) and *British Medical Journal* (301,6751:521).

In a recent study, 10 healthy men ate either a low-potassium diet or a normal-potassium diet for four to eight weeks.

Those on the low-potassium diet had significantly higher blood pressures after eight weeks than the men on normal-potassium diets.

Researchers suggest that potassium also protects your heart by lowering blood cholesterol levels.You can add potassium to your diet by eating more fruits and vegetables, such as bananas, beans and peas. Potatoes and potato flour are especially high in potassium.

The estimated minimum daily requirement for potassium is somewhere around two grams, or about one-fourteenth of an ounce.

Other experts urge even higher amounts of potassium for its anti-stroke and blood-pressure-reducing benefits — up to 3.5 grams per day, according to the official government recommendation reported in *Recommended Dietary Allowances, 10th Edition* (National Academy Press, Washington, D.C.).

Earlier studies have shown that a low-potassium diet can also lead to stroke, and researchers plan more studies to confirm their results.

The moral of the story — eat more fruits and vegetables to get more potassium.

If you are taking medicines or suffer from an illness or disease, check with your doctor about how much potassium you should take in each day.

Stressed out? Put down that coffee cup

If you have a high-stress job, put down your coffee cup.

University of Oklahoma researchers say more than five cups of coffee a day can send your blood pressure soaring, reports *Modern Medicine* (57,11:22).

Thirty-four men took a simple test. Half of them drank a glass of grapefruit juice containing the amount of caffeine equal to that in two or three cups of coffee, and half drank a regular glass of grapefruit juice. Their blood pressures were measured 15 minutes after finishing the glass.

Before the test, 17 men had been identified as high risk for hypertension, the medical name for high blood pressure. They had mildly high blood pressure (135/85 to 155/95 mm Hg) and a parent with hypertension.

The men who were at high risk for hypertension and who drank the caffeinated grapefruit juice had the highest blood pressure levels 15 minutes later. They were given tasks to measure their reaction time, and while they were working on the tasks, their cortisol levels rose.

A rise in cortisol levels usually means a rise in blood pressure levels. So, if your "tasks" at work already stress you out, caffeine will make you even more stressed.

Although coffee has not been proven to increase the risk of heart disease, another team of researchers recommends that people with heart problems drink decaffeinated coffee or no coffee at all, says another report in *Modern Medicine* (57,11:118).

Fish oil lowers 'mild' high blood pressure

High doses of fish oil lowered blood pressure in men with mild high blood pressure, according to a new study published in *The New England Journal of Medicine* (320,16:1037).

"We found that dietary supplementation with high doses of fish oil given for one month lowered blood pressure in men with mild essential hypertension, whereas a lower dose of fish oil, the same amount of safflower oil, or a mixture of saturated and unsaturated oils produced no significant change," reports Dr. Howard Knapp of Vanderbilt University.

The researchers compared the effect of the fish oil (15 grams daily, or slightly more than one-half ounce) with common prescription blood-pressure reducers. "The magnitude of the effect that we found was similar to that of propranolol or a thiazide diuretic in the Medical Research Council trial," Knapp says.

Although these results are promising, the researchers warn that "the clinical usefulness and safety of fish oil in the treatment of hypertension will require further study."

Licorice lovers alert

Those who like a bit of licorice candy every day may be left with a bad taste in their mouths.

Adults who eat licorice every day run a higher than normal risk of developing high blood pressure and heart disease.

According to a report in *The New England Journal of Medicine* (322,12:849), licorice causes the body to store excess salt, which in turn raises blood pressure and puts a strain on the heart.

Researchers recommend that licorice lovers cut way back on their treat and eat it only on special occasions.

Marriage helps protect against high blood pressure

Married people have an increased chance of surviving cancer.

Married couples also are less likely to have high blood pressure than people who are single, widowed, separated or divorced.

However, the researchers in several different studies are quick to say that they don't know exactly why marriage has such a positive effect on your health.

"It may simply be that married people live healthier lives," suggests Dr. Marjorie A. Speers. In a study by the Yale University Medical School and the University of Texas, where Speers is an assistant professor of preventative medicine, married people were 20 percent less likely to have high blood pressure than singles.

In the Speers study, married people were also more likely to know if they had high blood pressure, more likely to get treatment for it, and more likely to keep their high blood pressure under control.

Unmarried people tend to wait longer to go to a doctor to be diagnosed, so their cancer and other problems are usually more advanced and more difficult to treat, doctors note. Unmarried people are also more likely than married people not to get any treatment at all, reports *The Journal of the American Medical Association* (258,21:3125).

Dr. James Goodwin, who has helped research several cancer studies, believes that marriage provides a support system and better finances for early diagnosis and treatment.

It seems apparent that marriage is good for your health.

Job demands influence blood pressure

If you've ever suspected that your high-pressure job is bad for your health, you may have been correct.

According to a study reported in *The Journal of the American Medical Association* (263,14:1929), men who hold jobs with high demands over which they have little or no control are three times more likely to suffer from high blood pressure than men who don't.

These workers are also more likely to suffer from physical changes to the heart that could lead to heart disease over time.

Researchers report that the risk of job-related hypertension increases with age.

Take a deep breath to protect yourself from high blood pressure

How deeply you can breathe may determine whether you develop high blood pressure, a startling new statistical study suggests.

Researchers say that the smaller the volume of air you can inhale and exhale from your lungs, the higher your risk of high blood pressure, according to a report in *Science News* (137,25:398).

How much air you can take in and breathe out is called "forced vital capacity."

That and levels of a substance in the blood called uric acid have emerged as possibly "two of hypertension's most predictive risk factors," says the report.

Researchers discovered the early warning signs by examining the detailed medical records of 26,429 people who had been members for at least 18 years of the Kaiser Permanente Medical Care Program in Oakland, Calif.

The group at the highest risk for high blood pressure was the shallow breathers.

The one-fifth with the lowest lung capacity were more than four times as likely to develop high blood pressure as the ones in the upper fifth.

People in the upper fifth of uric acid levels were twice as likely to develop high blood pressure by age 55 as the ones in the lowest fifth.

Uric acid is a natural by-product that occurs when the body breaks down old or damaged cells.

Since uric acid can't be further broken down by the body, it must be excreted, usually through the kidneys into the urine.

The uric acid and "forced vital capacity" risk factors stood out even after accounting for the effects of smoking, family history, cholesterol levels and being too fat.

So far, scientists don't know why these two easily measured factors figure so heavily in predicting the risk of high blood pressure.

Before you treat high blood pressure, read this

Blood pressure readings taken at home are more accurate than readings taken at a doctor's office when it comes to predicting heart disease, a new study has discovered. This means that if a doctor only relies on the office readings, many people could be incorrectly treated for mild high blood pressure.

Although doctors have known for almost 50 years that a trip to the physician or the hospital can cause an inflated blood pressure reading — often called "white coat hypertension" — doctors did not know if these people were at higher risk for heart disease than people with normal readings.

Higher office readings are labeled "white coat hypertension" because blood pressure sometimes rises when people feel stressed by a visit to the doctor. According to the study, 10 to 20 percent of all people with mild high blood pressure may suffer from "white coat hypertension."

However, a report just published in *The Journal of the American Medical Association* (261,6:873) showed that people with "white coat hypertension" did not have the heart damage associated with high blood pressure — an enlarged heart and reduced heart function.

Sustained and untreated high blood pressure can damage the heart, arteries, kidneys, brain and eyes. People with uncontrolled high blood pressure have seven times more strokes, four times as much congestive heart failure and three times as much coronary heart disease as people with normal blood pressure.

In the study at the University of Connecticut, people with high office readings but normal readings at home were compared to two groups — one that had high blood pressure and one that had normal blood pressure.

The office and home blood pressure readings of all three groups were recorded. The size and capacity of their hearts were evaluated at rest and during exercise. People with "white coat hypertension" were found to have normal heart function and no physical signs of true high blood pressure.

The researchers suggest that since there is no apparent heart damage, people with "white coat hypertension" do not have high blood pressure.

To avoid unnecessary treatment, people with mild high blood pressure could be monitored at home before any drug treatment is started. Portable units are available to take and record blood pressure at regular intervals.

You wear the monitor throughout the day and keep a record of your physical activities. Later, the doctor compares your blood pressure readings to the corresponding physical activities. Also, many doctors are now encouraging their patients with high blood pressure to monitor their own levels manually. You use your own stethoscopes and cuffs and record your readings at home.

You bring your "blood pressure diary" to each checkup by the doctor. This way, the doctor can evaluate you based on your normal daily blood pressure, rather than on an inflated blood pressure reading taken during an occasional, but stressful, visit to the doctor's office.

Since about 45 million Americans are estimated to have "mild" high blood pressure, and up to 20 percent of those are estimated to suffer from "white coat hypertension," over eight million Americans could be affected by these findings.

Breast Cancer

Natural body rhythms play vital role in combatting deadly cancer cells

The old song, "What a difference a day makes," is especially true in treating breast cancer, new research shows.

In studying chronobiology, scientists are beginning to realize that timing is crucial to the success of breast cancer surgery and chemotherapy, according to a report in the *Journal of the National Cancer Institute* (81,23:1768).

Chronobiologists have discovered that tumor cells have precise schedules for division and growth, different from normal cells. Using that growth cycle information, they have been able to "target" cancerous cells for destruction with chemotherapy while safeguarding normal cells, the journal report says.

Chronobiologists have also found that menstrual cycles in women are closely linked to immune system responses. Because of this link, the cure rate and survival time after breast cancer surgery depends greatly on when during a woman's menstrual cycle the surgery takes place, says a new scientific study reported in *The Lancet* (2,8669:949).

Women who had breast surgery — both lumpectomy and mastectomy — during or around their menstrual periods had more than four times the rate of recurrence and death, the report says.

On the other hand, women who had their breast cancers removed during days 7 to 20 of the menstrual cycle seemed to have much greater protection against developing another breast cancer or a spread of the disease, says the report.

"The time of resection [surgery] in relation to the menstrual cycle is an independent predictor of the likelihood of future metastatic [spread of] disease," writes Dr. William J.M. Hrushesky of Albany (N.Y.) Medical College.

He and three other colleagues studied the five-year records of 44 premenopausal women who underwent surgery to remove breast cancers.

Three women were pregnant at the time of surgery, and all three died. Eight of 19 patients who had surgery near or during their periods developed breast cancer again.

Three patients developed new breast cancers plus cancers that popped up elsewhere in their bodies (metastatic cancers). Those three had surgery during or near their periods.

Not a single patient who had surgery between days 8 and 18 of the menstrual cycle developed new or metastatic cancers.

"Our findings indicate a striking effect of the timing of breast cancer surgery on the incidence and rapidity of disease recurrence and upon disease-free and overall survival," the report says.

The authors speculate that changes in hormone levels in a woman's bloodstream affect the number of natural killer cells in the bloodstream. That in turn has a great effect on whether the cancer will recur or spread, they believe.

On the basis of both animal and human studies, they believe that a woman's immune system is at a low ebb near and during the menstrual period, possibly to help the egg become implanted in the womb. During this time, there are fewer killer cells in a woman's body.

On the other hand, a woman's immune system kicks into high gear between days 7 to 21 of the cycle, peaking in the middle, they believe. A woman has a maximum amount of killer cells flowing in her bloodstream during the mid-cycle, they think. Those armies of killer cells may be more efficient at mid-cycle at hunting down and killing any cancer cells that escape during surgery, the report indicates.

The study breaks new ground in linking surgery timing and cancer spread to the menstrual cycle. But it points out a weakness in medical charting and record-keeping by many U.S. doctors and hospitals.

In fact, the study had trouble getting off the ground because of a lack of accurate records. They discovered that many surgeons and hospitals never chart women's menstrual cycles. "This omission may hinder any attempts to retrospectively study the relation of menstrual cycle to disease and intervention in large numbers of patients," the authors say.

Another implication of this study is that women's menstrual cycles may play a larger than previously suspected role in many disorders, not just breast cancer.

The study cautions that the findings have several limitations, including the small size of the study group. But the authors have some advice: "We urge doctors to note the date of the [patient's] last menstrual period before any major medical or surgical intervention for any serious illness."

The breast cancer study results imply that survival times and cure rates for other kinds of cancers may hinge on coordinating treatments with the body's natural rhythms.

While the coordination of treatments with cell division cycles, the circadian sleep-wake cycle and the menstrual cycle holds much promise for potential benefits, most doctors have ignored the new science. "The medical establishment ... has been rather slow in accepting the discipline, chronobiologists believe," according to the report in *JNCI.*

Radical may not always be better — lumpectomies are just as effective

Radical mastectomy is "out" and lumpectomy is "in" as treatment for early-stage breast cancer, according to reports in the *Journal of the National Cancer Institute* (82,14:1180) and *Medical World News* (31,13:31).

A panel of cancer experts agreed that cutting out just the cancerous tumor is usually just as effective as the more extensive surgery.

Sometimes lumpectomy is even better than taking the entire breast and associated tissues in the chest and armpit, the reports indicate.

Of the 150,000 people who will develop breast cancer this year, about 75 percent of them will have stage one and stage two cancers.

Those are the two kinds for which lumpectomy and follow-up radiation therapy "are as effective as total mastectomy," says the *MWN* report.

Women with ductal cancer of the breast usually choose a total mastectomy, since the cure rate is nearly 100 percent, reports *The Lancet* (335,8688:519). Ductal cancer usually is confined to one breast and normally doesn't spread beyond that breast, unlike other forms.

They might do as well to choose a less radical option that takes only a quarter of the breast in about three out of four cases, the report suggests.

High risk factors for breast cancer

Dense breast tissue increases the risk of breast cancer about fourfold, according to new research from the Centers for Disease Control (CDC) in Atlanta. "Women whose mammograms showed over 65 percent dense tissue developed breast cancer at a rate more than 400 percent higher than women with densities of less than 5 percent," Audrey F. Saftlas of the CDC and John N. Wolfe at the Hutzel Hospital in Detroit report in *Science News* (135,14:213).

Mammograms can be used to identify dense breast tissue. Once women know they are at high risk for breast cancer, they can have mammograms more frequently and possibly catch the cancer at a very early stage, says the *Science News* article.

Dense breast tissue "is at least as important as family history" in determining a woman's risk for breast cancer, Saftlas says. Women with a family history of breast cancer are at highest risk, according to *The Journal of the American Medical Association* (253,13:1908).

In addition to having dense breast tissue, if you fall into one of the other high-risk categories listed below, be sure to get regular mammograms:

> • **If you gave birth to your first child after the age of 30.**
>
> • **If you never gave birth.**
>
> • **If your mother or sister has developed breast cancer.**
>
> • **If you reached sexual maturity very early.**
>
> • **If you have a history of cysts in your breasts.**
>
> • **If you are overweight.**
>
> • **If you are over 40 years of age.**

Despite a family history of breast cancer, women past the age of 60 have about the same risk as women with no such history, says a report in *Archives of Internal Medicine* (150,1:191).

The family history risk apparently affects mostly women of child-bearing age. The longer a woman lives without developing breast cancer, the less likely her heredity will catch up with her, at least in breast cancer risk, the study suggests.

How to detect breast cancer early

Early detection is very important in surviving breast cancer, especially if you are at high risk. Have regular mammograms and examine your breasts every month.

The American Cancer Society recommends that women 50 and over should have a mammogram once every year. Women between 40 and 49 should have a mammogram every second year. The first mammogram should be given when a woman is between 35 and 39 years of age. This will be used as a baseline to detect any irregularities later, the Cancer Society explains. A mammogram is a special x-ray of the breast which enables doctors to detect the earliest and most curable breast cancer.

Since a woman knows her own breasts, it is easier for her to detect changes in her breast tissue than for her doctor. Examining your breasts each month, in addition to your doctor's exam once a year, will help detect changes as early as possible. Besides lumps, watch for other possible signs of cancer including:

❏ Any change in the shape, size or color of the breasts. Do this by comparing them in a mirror each month. Compare them to each other and to how they looked the previous month.

❏ Any unusual discharge should be noted and reported to your doctor.

❏ Scaliness or crustiness on the breasts, especially around the nipple.

❏ Any new dimples in the breasts.

❏ Any lumps or thickening of the breast tissue.

❏ Asymmetry — any difference in the shapes of the breasts.

A dietary secret that may prevent breast cancer

Can you change your diet and prevent breast cancer? Some researchers are saying cautiously that such a dietary prevention plan may be good ammunition against one of the biggest killers of women. The secret — lower the amount of fat you eat, suggest two studies.

Keeps tumors from turning into breast cancer — "Dietary fat is a risk factor for breast cancer," conclude researchers in an Israeli study of 2,300 women. In general, the Israeli study shows that women with high-fat intakes are three times as likely to develop the types of tumors that turn into breast cancer.

Breast cancer develops from benign tumors. A high-fat diet promotes a change from benign (noncancerous) breast disease to cancer, the researchers report in *The American Journal of Clinical Nutrition* (50,3:551). They point out that breast cancer develops in stages over a number of years, and if diet influences the process, women may be able to change their diet to help prevent cancer.

Diet apparently had no effect on two types of benign breast disease. But, among those with the most advanced stage (grade 3) of benign breast disease, they spotted a link between high-fat diets and numbers of women with breast cancer.

"The results suggest that saturated fatty acids, but not the other food groups, are associated with grade 3 disease," says the report. Although the women with grade 3 disease ate more starches, sugars and proteins than other women, their fat intake was the greatest risk factor, the researchers conclude.

In a separate study published in the *Journal of the National Cancer Institute* (81,4:278), Dr. Paolo Toniolo of the Department of Environmental

Medicine at New York University Medical Center studied over 700 Italian women by analyzing their daily diet in 70 food categories.

Most strongly linked to increased rates of breast cancer were dairy products like high-fat cheese and whole milk, he reports. Ranked just under dairy products were animal fats and meat.

Women who ate foods rich in animal fat, such as meat and cured meat, showed a "modest" increase in the risk of breast cancer. "Consumption of fish, eggs, bread, pasta, olive oil, vegetables, and fruit did not reveal any evident relationship with breast cancer," the study says.

To reduce the risk of breast cancer, women need to reduce their consumption of total fat to less than 30 percent of their total daily calorie intake, saturated fat to less than 10 percent, and animal proteins to less than 6 percent, Toniolo suggests. The current typical American diet relies on fats for between 35 and 45 percent of total caloric intake.

Breast-cancer patients in Japan have better outcomes than their counterparts in the United States. One possible reason for the difference is that Japanese women generally eat a relatively low-fat diet. Obesity and low-fiber, low-carbohydrate diets may lead to lower survival rates, researchers speculate.

This is affirmed in a report in *Science News* (134,7:100) that says eating a lot of saturated fats makes active breast cancer grow faster and spread farther, especially among older women. Canadian researchers studied the progress of recently diagnosed breast cancers in 666 women.

Those with diets high in the kind of fats found in butter, cheese and coconut oil developed larger cancers that spread more rapidly to the lymph nodes, indicating a more severe (and less curable) form of the disease. The more cancer involves the lymph nodes, the harder it is to get rid of the disease.

On the other hand, those who ate foods high in polyunsaturated fats — such as corn, safflower, sunflower and cottonseed oils — showed less invasion of the lymph tissues, the report said, indicating a more treatable form of the disease.

Affects recovery rates after surgery — A high-fat diet also may affect the recovery rates of women who undergo breast cancer surgery, according to a related study in *The Journal of the National Cancer Institute* (81,16:1218). Swedish researchers evaluated the diets of 240 women aged 50 to 65 who had breast-cancer surgery between 1983 and 1986, says the *JNCI* report.

They were particularly interested in protein, carbohydrate, fat, alcohol and vitamin intake, but they also considered other factors such as height, weight, smoking and physical activity.

Women with larger tumors reported eating less fiber, carbohydrates and vitamin A but more fat than women with smaller tumors. The high-fat eaters generally had larger tumors that spread farther, the research indicates. Women who drank alcohol also showed an increased risk, researchers said.

Keeps cancer from developing even after it's active — On the positive and preventive side, another study reported in *Journal of the National Cancer Institute* showed that women who ate a "very low-fat diet" for a year developed fewer than half as many breast cancers as those who ate the "typical" diet.

The low-fat diet apparently cut the cancer rate in half. Nearly 40 percent of the calories consumed in the "typical" American diet is in the form of fats, way too high for long-term health, the studies indicate.

According to the *JNCI* report, doctors at two Toronto hospitals put half of a group of 180 women whose mammograms showed unusual breast shadows on a specially formulated low-fat diet. Only about 20 percent of the diet's total calories was in the form of fat, while 56 percent was in carbohydrate form.

The other half of the group stuck to the "typical" diet — 37 percent of its calories in fat and 43 percent in carbohydrates.

After a year, five on the "typical" diet developed breast cancer, but only two on the low-fat diet came down with the disease, the Toronto study showed. A larger, follow-up study is planned.

While many studies have demonstrated higher risks of getting breast cancer because of fat-rich eating habits, the Canadian research is among the first to show that the growth and spread of the cancer is affected by what we eat — after the cancer has become active.

This suggests that a low-fat diet could be an important weapon in fighting breast cancer, even after it has been diagnosed. All the studies put together indicate that a low-fat diet over many months:

- **could lower the risk of getting breast cancer,**

- **could lessen the severity of the disease once it's active,**

- **and could even increase the cure rate after surgery.**

To boost your protection against breast cancer, eat fruits and vegetables, especially those high in vitamin C, instead of fats, says the *Journal of the National Cancer Institute* (82,7:561).

If women in North America were to cut their daily consumption of saturated fats to less than one-tenth of their total calories, the breast cancer rate for women past menopause would drop 10 percent, says a report in *Science News* (137,16:245).

Just by eating enough fruits and vegetables to get 380 milligrams of vitamin C daily might drop the breast cancer rate by another 16 percent for all women over age 20, the report says.

That's more than six times the current officially Recommended Dietary Allowance of 60 milligrams.

Soybeans and breast cancer

Would eating soybeans several times a week slash your risk of getting breast cancer?

Some researchers suspect that a diet loaded with soybeans may be the reason Asian women have one-fifth the number of cases of breast cancer that American women have, says a report in *The Atlanta Journal* (March 27, 1990, B7).

Women of the East eat tofu, or soybean curd, the way we Americans eat eggs and potatoes.

So far, animal tests have raised hopes that soybeans may provide some powerful cancer prevention, but no tests have been made on people.

Soybeans contain isoflavones, substances that may block some cancer-causing chemicals. The big drawback — soybean products like tofu generally don't win any taste tests.

Indulging a sweet tooth may increase your risk of breast cancer

A taste for sweet things might be dangerous for women with diagnosed breast cancer, suggest two recent scientific studies.

Eating and drinking foods with high sugar contents produced faster-growing and more deadly tumors in animal tests, report cancer researchers in *Clinical Nutrition* (9,2:62).

Mice fed diets that were high in sugar were nearly three times more likely to die quickly than mice on low-sugar diets, the report says.

Tumors seemed to thrive on sugary diets and were nearly five times as deadly as the same kind of cancerous tumors in mice on a low-sugar diet, reports the journal article.

The researchers found that adding vitamin E and selenium to the diets helped a little bit. Mice on high-sugar diets that received the two nutrients — known as antioxidants — still developed big, fast-growing tumors, but the tumors were less deadly.

Antioxidants like vitamin E act like scavengers in the blood, neutralizing cancer-promoting chemicals known as oxidants.

The researchers speculate that sugary diets trigger lots of insulin production by the body. Insulin is needed to help body cells use the right amount of sugar.

But insulin also acts like a powerful fertilizer to tumor cells, greatly speeding up the growth of the harmful cells. The more insulin the body produces in response to a sugary diet, the more fertilizer is poured on cancer cells, the report suggests.

Backing up the suspicions about sugar, a statistical study in the same issue of *Clinical Nutrition* documents a strong link between sugar eating and breast cancer deaths.

Some of the same researchers checked records of average sugar consumption in 20 countries around the world. Then they cross-checked rates of breast cancer and deaths from breast cancer in those same countries for women between the ages of 55 and 74.

Sure enough, countries with the lowest sugar consumption per person — like Japan and Hong Kong — also have the lowest rates of death from breast cancer, the report says.

Those countries with the biggest hunger for sugar — like the United States and Great Britain — have the highest rates of breast cancer deaths. The average person in the United States takes in two pounds of sugar a week, the report says.

But the average Japanese citizen eats less than half that much sugar in a week — 14 ounces on average, the report says. The report notes that the death rate from breast cancer in Japan is about one-fifth that of the United States.

The statistical comparison took into account and adjusted for other factors, including average daily fat intake, the journal article says.

Underlying both reports is the suggestion that slower-growing tumors result in people living longer after diagnosis of breast cancer.

Based on their findings, the researchers suggest that women with diagnosed breast cancer should cut back on sweets and maintain a low-sugar diet.

Vitamin D treatment may slow spread of breast cancer cells

Investigators in England saw good results when they treated breast cancer cells in the laboratory with vitamin D three times a week. More than 80 percent of all breast cancer tumors contain chemical "sockets" that plug in with the vitamin D, said the report in *The Lancet* (1,8631:188).

Vitamin D in one form acts like a hormone in a woman's body and attaches to hormonally dependent tumors, they said. Once attached to a tumor, the vitamin D acts to halt spread of cancer cells and works to return cell activity to normal, the report said.

Long-term estrogen therapy linked to breast cancer

Many menopausal women take estrogen to prevent osteoporosis and heart and circulatory problems, but Swedish researchers have found a link between the hormone and breast cancer, leaving women and their physicians to decide whether estrogen's benefits outweigh the risks, suggest reports in *The New England Journal of Medicine* (321,5:293) and *Science* (245,4918:593).

Using prescription records, Swedish researchers identified 23,244 menopausal women taking estrogen and then compared the names with those of breast-cancer patients appearing in the national Cancer Registry. (In Sweden, physicians must report all newly diagnosed cases of cancer to the registry.)

After matching up the names, researchers compared estrogen brands, dosage and duration of use.

Long-term estrogen users had a 10 percent increase in breast-cancer risk, and the risk jumped to 70 percent after nine years of use, researchers said.

Estradiol, a potent form of estrogen, was the most commonly prescribed, and it was a higher risk factor for breast cancer than estriols, less potent forms of estrogen.

Many physicians — already aware of estrogen's link with uterine cancer — prescribe a combination of estrogen and progestin (another hormone) for menopausal patients.

Although progestin counteracts estrogen's negative effect on uterine cancer, women on combination therapy are more at risk of developing breast cancer, researchers said.

"Estrogen apparently has a [cancer-causing] effect because it stimulates the growth of cells of the breast and uterine lining. ... Progestin counteracts that effect on the uterine cells but acts with estrogen to stimulate breast cell growth. ... Progestin might therefore (increase) estrogen's effects on breast cancer."

Because American women generally take a different form of estrogen than do Swedish women, no one knows the impact of the study results in the United States.

For the moment, U.S. experts are siding with estrogen, arguing that "for every woman who might lose her life to breast cancer because of long-term estrogen use, another seven or eight might be spared from premature death by heart attack or stroke."

Upper-body fat may release extra hormones and trigger cancer growth

Ladies, if you can pinch much more than an inch on your waist, you may have a dangerous amount of upper-body fat.

And the more upper-body fat you have, the greater your risk for developing breast cancer, researchers report in the *Annals of Internal Medicine* (112,3:182).

Other scientists agree. Women past menopause who put on pounds around the middle were nearly twice as likely to develop breast cancer as those who gained weight elsewhere on their bodies, reports Dr. Rachel Ballard-Barbash in the *Journal of the National Cancer Institute* (82,4:286). Losing that fat may decrease your breast-cancer risk, they suggest.

Researchers at South Florida College of Medicine studied 216 overweight women aged 25 to 83 who had breast cancer but had not received hormonal or chemotherapy treatments.

They also kept records on another 600 women without breast cancer. They measured body fat at the neck, shoulders, arms, waist, hips and thighs. Women with breast cancer had more fat on the waist, arms, shoulders and nape of the neck than cancer-free women.

Researchers studying health records of 40,000 Iowa women also found the link between breast cancer and an "apple" shape.

"Pear-shaped" bodies, with fat distributed around the lower hips and thighs, had lower breast cancer rates. Luckily, women tend to gain weight below the waistline.

One of the first signs of breast cancer is a small growth in the breast. Scientists believe "out-of-control" estrogen — a hormone — might trigger breast tissue to begin growing too quickly, resulting in a lump.

Women with upper-body fat have more estrogen and lower levels of hormones that can fight excess estrogen, researchers say.

Upper-body fat may also contribute to gallbladder disease, high blood pressure and diabetes in women, they add. Similar links have been found among body shape, fat distribution and heart attack risks.

If you're concerned about your fat distribution and want to lose some weight, talk to your doctor about setting up a safe diet and exercise plan designed especially to meet your needs.

Fiber foils breast cancer

Eating more fiber might protect against breast cancer, suggests a study reported in *The American Journal of Clinical Nutrition* (51,5:798).

Scientists studied 24 Seventh-Day Adventist women between the ages of 64 and 83, half of them vegetarians for more than a quarter-century. Other than what they ate, both groups were very similar.

The vegetarians ate more fiber than the other group and had significantly lower levels of estradiol and estrone, two hormones that have been linked to cancerous tumor growth.

Lower levels of these hormones may translate into lower cancer risks, the researchers speculate.

They think that steroid hormones stick to bran fiber, oat hulls, cellulose and lignin and are tossed out of the body quickly.

A high-fiber diet also might protect against endometrial cancers, the report says.

Other studies have shown similar links: Eat more fiber and thus lower your risk of breast cancer, agrees a review in *Nutrition and Cancer* (13,1:1).

Broccoli and brussels sprouts might help prevent breast cancer

You might prevent breast cancer by eating more cabbage, broccoli and other cruciferous vegetables, suggests a new study published in the *Journal of the National Cancer Institute* (82,11:947).

Scientists are excited about the potential of a powerful cancer-fighting substance discovered in these vegetables. The substance — indole-3-carbinol — seems to convert one cancer-promoting form of the female sex hormone estrogen into a harmless form. That harmless form also may block absorption of the "bad" kind of estrogen by breast cells, suggests a report of the study in *Science News* (137,24:375).

The active forms of estrogen have been blamed by many scientists for triggering breast cancer growth. Anything that blocks active estrogen from breast cells could prevent the formation of cancerous growths, says the *SN* report.

Scientists fed volunteers 500 milligrams of indole-3-carbinol daily for a week. They used a manufactured form of the natural chemical. The daily dose was the equivalent of eating about half a head of cabbage a day.

The production of estrogen-blocker jumped by 50 percent after just one week, the study shows.

The results may explain why Asian women — who eat a lot of cruciferous vegetables — have much lower breast cancer rates than American women.

The problem is one of taste — many people just don't like to eat their veggies, especially broccoli and brussels sprouts. Dr. Jon J. Michnovicz, one of the researchers who found the cancer fighter, suggests that indole-3-carbinol could be sold in a pill form.

That would allow women who don't like cabbage to take a daily supplement to prevent breast cancer, suggests the report in *SN*. No such supplement currently exists.

Vegetables containing indole-3-carbinol include cabbage, broccoli, brussels sprouts, mustard greens, bok choy, kale, collards, turnip greens and cauliflower. All these are members of the cruciferous family of vegetables. The flowers of these vegetables resemble small crosses. Their Latin name means "cross-like."

Several studies have shown that eating a lot of vegetables protects against several other forms of cancer, notably colon and rectal cancers. But researchers until now had thought the protection came from the fiber contained in the vegetables.

This is the first study to show that a specific natural chemical may be responsible for at least part of the protective effect against breast cancer.

Prevents spread of cancer to lungs — Now, a new study in the journal *Nutrition and Cancer* (12,2:121) demonstrates that a diet including cabbage and collards protects against the spread of breast cancer to the lungs. This study, involving rats, is the first to show that a diet that includes a particular family of vegetables fights the spread of cancer cells from its original location to another site in the body.

"The metastasis, or spread of a tumor to a secondary site, is the cause of death of a majority of patients, despite removal or treatment of the primary tumor with chemotherapy or radiation," the report says.

All the animals got injections of live breast cancer cells. Then the researchers watched to see how many in each group would develop cancer of the lungs as a result of the spread of the cancer cells.

At the end of the two-month experiment, animals fed cabbages and collards had half as many lung tumors as the rats fed a control diet without the two vegetables.

The researchers said they felt collards and cabbage diets might be useful in treating active cancerous tumors in addition to fighting the spread of the disease. But they should be raw, not cooked, say researchers at the University of Manitoba in Winnipeg. That's because cooking, especially in water, drains the cancer-fighters out of the vegetables.

These leafy vegetables contain lots of anticancer compounds called indole glycosinolates, says a report in *Science News* (136,22:351).

Indole glycosinolates also trigger release of enzymes that take the sting out of cancer-causing chemicals in some foods we eat, according to the report.

Eating fish may lower breast cancer risk

Women who eat fish regularly may lower their risk of getting breast cancer.

Apparently, the omega-3 oils found in deep-water fatty fish help to cut levels of estradiol, a hormone that promotes cancer growth.

The fish oil itself seems to slow down tumor growth, reports a Rutgers University researcher in the *Journal of Internal Medicine* (225,731:197 Supplement).

A preliminary statistical study reported in the journal *Nutrition and Cancer* (12,1:61) also found a link between eating fish and lower rates of breast cancer.

Researchers at two Canadian cancer institutes analyzed how people eat in 32 countries around the world, including the United States.

They looked at each country's average daily intake of total fats, animal fat, meat, cereal, milk, sugar, animal oil, total oils of all kinds, fish, coffee, tea, cocoa and riboflavin (one of the B vitamins). Then they compared the diets with breast cancer rates for those countries.

They found what several other studies have shown — breast cancer rates go up where women eat more fats, especially animal fats. But the new study also indicated that in countries where fish consumption is high, breast cancer rates are lower.

"The observation that percent calories from fish is inversely related to [breast cancer] risk implies a protective role for this dietary component," says the report.

The scientists speculated that protection might come from the highly polyunsaturated omega-3 fatty acids contained in many kinds of fish from deep, cold waters.

Depression affects cancer survival rates

Women with breast cancer who got together in weekly group therapy sessions survived almost twice as long as women who received only regular cancer treatment, Dr. David Spiegel recently told the American Psychiatric Association. In addition to regular medical therapy, the women who lived the longest met weekly in "supportive group therapy," Spiegel says.

He studied 86 women with metastatic breast cancer over a 10-year period. (Metastatic means that the cancer has spread from the original site to another location.) All were receiving standard drug, chemical or radiation treatments.

About half the women participated in group therapy during the first year. Women in the weekly therapy group survived an average of 34.8 months.

But women who received conventional medical treatment alone, without the group meetings, survived just an average of 18.9 months, according to Spiegel's study.

"Furthermore, there was a trend linking group attendance with longevity among treatment patients," the doctor says.

These findings match those of other doctors who have found that "secondary depression can actually shorten survival," reports *Medical World News* (30,13:20). "When depression accompanies a medical problem, patients are sicker, need more medication, and spend more days in the hospital," the magazine report says.

Spiegel, an associate professor of psychiatry and behavioral sciences at Stanford University School of Medicine, says he hopes his research will encourage metastatic cancer patients to actively participate in group therapy.

Diagnosing and treating depression in cancer patients can affect the outcome of the disease, according to Dr. Charles Nemeroff in a speech to the American Psychiatric Association. Nemeroff, a professor at Duke University in North Carolina, warns that depression can impair the body's immune system.

"The last thing you want in cancer patients is an impaired immune response," Nemeroff said. "We need to aggressively diagnose and treat cancer patients with depression."

Breathing and Lung Health

Breathing fresh air may be harmful

Opening your windows for a breath of fresh air may be hazardous to your health. The fresher the air, the more it may harm you if you live in one of the 81 areas in the United States that flunk federal air-quality standards, according to reports in *Science News* (136,13:198) and *Medical World News* (30,18:39).

Bell Communications researchers in Red Bank, N.J., were baffled by laboratory equipment problems such as cracked power cords. Red Bank, incidentally, is just south of New York City, one of the nation's most polluted cities. To their surprise, the culprit was ozone, a type of oxygen.

To solve the mystery of the disintegrating equipment, Bell researchers measured indoor ozone levels continuously, noting how many times per hour outdoor air was flushed through the company's buildings. Surprisingly, the "fresher" the air, the higher the ozone levels.

If you open the windows in your home, fresh air will be flushed through five times an hour, says Charles J. Weschler, a Bell senior scientist. Inhaling ozone — whether indoors or out — for prolonged periods leads to lung inflammation and breathing problems. The effect of ozone and air pollution is like a sunburn, says Dr. Robert Phalen, who studies how dirty air affects health.

Air pollution destroys the protective lining of the respiratory tract, from the nose down to the lungs, allowing poisons to enter the body more easily. After a lot of ozone exposure, the lungs "become far more susceptible to infection and cancer," says Dr. Phalen.

Other health problems include coughing, headache, eye irritation, sore throat and chest discomfort.

The effects of pollution may be cumulative, meaning that illness may develop after years of exposure. Ironically, people with healthy lungs may be more sensitive to ozone pollution than asthmatics, whose lungs are protected by a mucous lining.

Also, people who exercise or do strenuous work outdoors or in well-ventilated buildings may be more at risk because strenuous exercise causes heavy breathing and inhalation of unfiltered air through the mouth. (The nasal passages serve to filter air taken in through the nose.)

Air pollution, once thought to be an urban problem, affects people living 100 miles downwind of a pollution source. The pollutants include ozone, sulfur dioxide and carbon monoxide. Weather patterns significantly affect air pollution across the United States. Generally, winds blow west to east, resulting in more pollution in the east, according to the *Medical World News* report.

Doctors report that the number of asthma cases in the United States increased during the 1980s because of air pollution.

Tips to protect yourself from ozone and air pollution

❒ Find out the daily pollution levels in your area from local newspapers, radio and TV stations. Call the National Weather Service Office or the nearest office of the Environmental Protection Agency to get more information on local pollution levels.

❒ If pollution levels are high, limit your time outdoors. Keep doors and windows closed during times of high levels of pollution.

❒ Consider installing air cleaning devices in your home, especially the devices that use activated charcoal to filter incoming air. Activated charcoal is a very good absorber of ozone. Don't confuse activated charcoal air cleaners with so-called "air purifiers." Most air purifiers don't trap ozone, radioactive radon gas or many of the other gases that cause health problems. Such devices do screen out larger airborne dust and pollen particles, but only while the particles are in the air, not after they've settled on furniture and carpets.

❒ Don't use ozone-producing devices inside your home. Some ozone-producing devices are marketed as "air fresheners." They just add to the ozone pollution problem. Avoid them.

❒ Check with your doctor or health care provider about other options to protect your lungs if you have asthma or other breathing difficulties.

Pollution slows body's defenses

Researchers at the University of Southern California caution that nitrogen dioxide, a common pollutant from auto exhaust, appears to damage lung cells and tissues. The damage makes the lungs more susceptible to cancer growth, says a report in *Science News* (137,14:221).

Nitrogen dioxide also damages the body's natural "killer" cells that help the immune system fight off other sicknesses.

Caution: Some humidified air pollutes home

If you have one of the newer "high-tech" types of home humidifiers, here's a caution. Fill your ultrasonic-wave humidifier with distilled or demineralized water, not water straight from your home faucet, according to a U.S. government scientist.

If you use tap water in an ultrasonic humidifier, you could be polluting your indoor air with tiny mineral particles, says a report in *Science News* (134:141).

In a test conducted by researchers at the Environmental Protection Agency, an ultrasonic device filled with ordinary tap water sprayed an average room with 40 times the recommended safe limit for breathable mineral particles, the report says. Those mineral particles may include lead, aluminum and asbestos, all harmful if inhaled in high concentrations, the report says.

Traditional kinds of humidifiers, which use impellers or fan blades to break up moisture into fine particles, produce about one-third that amount, the report says. Steam vaporizer units didn't generate any measurable particles.

Using the ultrasonic humidifiers with regular tap water to help people with asthma may backfire and actually do more harm than good, say the researchers. Most makers of humidifiers advise using distilled or demineralized water, but many homeowners seem to be ignoring those warnings, the report says.

Vitamin C, niacin beat bronchitis

If you're wheezing from repeated attacks of bronchitis, you may need more vitamin C and niacin, says a digest in *Modern Medicine* (57,10:17).

At the same time, a salty diet may be troubling your lungs. People who ate a tenth of an ounce of salt a day were 27 percent more likely to come down with bronchitis than those on a low-salt diet, the report says.

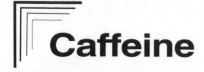

Caffeine

Coffee and caffeine: How much is too much?

If you're worried about your cholesterol levels or suffer from cardiovascular disease, put down your cup of coffee and take note.

Research indicates that drinking one to five cups of caffeinated coffee every day nearly doubles your risk of heart disease and stroke, compared with noncoffee drinkers, according to *U.S. Pharmacist* (14,6:28). Six cups a day of the regular brew increases your risk 2.5 times, the report says.

A "safe" daily intake of caffeine is about 200 milligrams (less than one-hundredth of one ounce), according to the report. But one regular cup of coffee contains at least 170 milligrams.

Excess caffeine can provoke arrhythmia, an irregular heartbeat. That can be dangerous for some people. Too much caffeine also seems to be linked to increased levels of blood cholesterol, which in turn can be very bad for your heart and arteries.

In one eight-week study, people with existing heart rhythm problems got worse after taking the equivalent of three to five cups of caffeinated coffee each day, says a report in *American Family Physician* (39,6:214).

Researchers haven't managed to tag coffee with directly causing cancer. One difficulty is that heavy users of caffeine also tend to be heavy smokers. Tobacco smoking has been established to be a proven, direct cause of lung cancer.

There have been some links discovered between caffeine and other cancers. "It appears that coffee drinkers are marginally more likely to develop bladder cancer than abstainers," says the *U.S. Pharmacist* report.

A 1981 study suggested a link between caffeine and cancer of the pancreas, but that has not been confirmed in other studies.

Coffee is the major source of caffeine for most Americans. Just two cups a day can put you over "the safe limit," defined in this report as 200 milligrams. But did you know that a cup of drip or percolated coffee has nearly 80 milligrams of caffeine more than the same cup filled with instant coffee?

If you don't like decaffeinated coffee (which contains five milligrams of caffeine), try instant coffee instead to cut your daily intake, the report suggests.

Some other caffeine counts to note are the following:

Brewed tea, 6 oz. cup — 50 milligrams of caffeine

Instant tea, 6 oz. cup — 30 milligrams

Cola drinks, 12 oz. — 30 to 50 milligrams

Hot cocoa, 6 oz. cup — 2 to 8 milligrams

Sweet dark chocolate, 1 oz. — 5 to 35 milligrams

Chocolate desserts — 10 milligrams

Note: Pain relief medication also can contain caffeine. One Excedrin tablet, for example, contains 65 milligrams of caffeine.

People who consume excess caffeine — 500 to 600 milligrams a day — may experience caffeinism, or "coffee nerves," and become addicted. You may be suffering from caffeinism if you have several symptoms like these: restlessness, insomnia, flushed face, stomach upset, nervousness and irregular heartbeat.

If you believe that you may be addicted, test yourself by not having your usual morning cup of coffee. If you have a severe headache later in the day, you probably have caffeinism.

Cutting back from large daily doses of caffeine all at once may cause you to experience severe withdrawal symptoms, like throbbing headache, fatigue, irritability and anxiety. Try to cut down your caffeine habit gradually, rather than quitting "cold turkey."

If you're drinking three cups of caffeinated coffee a day, try to cut back to two cups for a week or so. Then cut to one cup, and so forth.

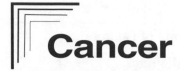

Cancer

Preventing cancer: Your diet can make the difference

Despite ever-increasing evidence that what we eat can play a major role in preventing many forms of cancer, only about one in five Americans regularly eats the right kinds of foods to get the highest protection.

Researchers at the National Cancer Institute in Bethesda, Md. surveyed 11,658 white and black adults about a typical day's diet. The study showed that only 16 percent of those surveyed ate high-fiber cereals or whole-grain breads.

Only 18 percent ate at least one green vegetable (high in cancer-fighting beta-carotene), and only 20 percent had any kind of fibrous vegetables. High vitamin C fruits and vegetables came out a little better (28 percent).

On the other hand, 55 percent of all adults ate red meat, rich in cholesterol, at least once a day. Processed lunch meats and traditional, fatty breakfasts, both high in many suspected cancer-causing preservatives, appeared on the menus of 49 percent of the males and 37 percent of the females surveyed.

The large study showed, in fact, that many of us tend to eat just those things that are worst for our health and avoid those foods that are best for us.

Income levels and where we live make a difference, the study showed.

Southerners balanced a plus with a minus, eating the least red meat but ignoring high-fiber cereals. Young white males seem to avoid foods that are good sources of vitamins A and C. The higher the income, the more red meat, produce and high-fiber cereals are consumed.

Numerous scientific studies advise us to eat fruits and vegetables, whole grains and foods rich in vitamins A and C and fiber, and to do it every day. The same studies say we should cut way down on red meats and fat and avoid any foods that have been salt-cured, nitrite-cured, smoked or pickled.

On the same lines, a report in *The American Journal of Clinical Nutrition* (49,5:993) outlines how your diet can mean the difference between healthy maturity and lingering illnesses.

About 35 percent of all cancers currently are linked to poor diet, according to the report. A high-fiber diet has been shown to reduce colon-cancer risk, and a high-fat diet increases breast-cancer risk.

The experts have devised dietary guidelines, which include a varied, well-balanced diet (fruits, vegetables, whole grains) with reduced fat, salt, alcohol and processed foods.

Fresh fruits and vegetables help prevent cancer

Eating a lot of fresh fruits and vegetables may help you prevent cancer, researchers report in *Food, Nutrition and Health* (13,9:2).

Almost all fruits and vegetables contain small amounts of acids called phenols, which stop cancer-causing agents from attacking healthy cells. Potatoes, grapes and nuts have especially high amounts.

Because phenols are surprisingly plentiful in the diet, scientists say that some people may take in more than one gram every day (although they haven't yet determined the ideal amount).

To get the anticancer benefits, you must eat fresh fruits and vegetables, because processing and storing plants destroy phenols.

Scientists are now looking for ways to "fortify" fruits and vegetables with phenols in the laboratory.

Onions and garlic may be natural cancer fighters

You may not like what onions and garlic do to your breath. But your stomach and colon may be dying for what these members of the allium family can contribute to your better health.

Scientists at the National Cancer Institute (NCI), working with colleagues in China, discovered that Chinese people who eat a lot of onions and garlic have only a fourth as many stomach cancers as other Chinese people. That's important, because the Chinese population has a high rate of stomach cancers, according to a report in *Healthline* (8,8:5).

Researchers are still trying to determine what it is about onions, garlic, chives, leeks and scallions that seems to slash the numbers of such deadly cancers.

One NCI official suspects that the protective agent is the smelly part of the vegetables, the allyl sulfides, according to a report in *Health* (21,5:16).

Scientists at the University of California, Berkeley, think the answer may lie with a turncoat chemical, quercetin. Quercetin switches sides in the cancer battle, sometimes acting like a powerful cancer causer, other times like a strong cancer fighter.

It's found in alliums and in deep green and yellow vegetables like broccoli and squash. It also turns up in red grapes and in common plants like ferns. Onions are extremely high in the substance.

In ferns and red wine (made from fermented grapes), quercetin seems to be a mutagen, a chemical that helps to trigger cancerous tumors. In fruits and vegetables, quercetin ties in with natural sugars and takes on a neutral stance, neither causing nor fighting cancer.

But once those sugar-linked quercetin molecules get into the digestive system, our natural enzymes break down the sugars and release quercetin into the stomach and intestines.

Some bacterial enzymes present in our digestive tract act differently or not at all with different foods. For example, some bacteria work only with milk products.

What quercetin does to our insides — whether it acts as friend or foe — may depend on what kinds of natural bacteria we have inside us and on what combinations of food we eat, the Berkeley scientists think. Apparently, the alliums and quercetin act as allies against cancer.

Anti-cancer agents are in the spice cabinet, not medicine cabinet

That delicious spicy stew that your grandmother taught you to make is not just a yummy meal and a family tradition. It might also be a valuable disease-fighter. Spices such as ginger, clove and cumin appear to have disease-fighting properties, reports *The Atlanta Journal/Constitution* (Oct. 25, 1990). Animal studies show that these spices might help fight cancerous tumors.

And the yellow stuff — known as curcumin — found in the spice turmeric, seems to halt tumor growth, to prevent new tumors from forming and to hunt down and neutralize cancer-causing chemicals in the blood, says a report in *The Journal of the American College of Nutrition* (8,5:450).

Turmeric is peppery and sometimes is substituted for saffron. It's used in curry recipes, on rice dishes, with yellow vegetables and, in Europe, even as coloring in some beverages like lemonade.

But, you don't have to go overboard with the spices. Small amounts are all that is necessary. For example, you don't even need a quarter of an ounce of ginger each day to get the health benefits it provides.

Drink low-fat milk instead of whole milk to help prevent cancer

Could the kind of milk you drink increase your risk of getting cancer? Researchers in Buffalo, N.Y., think that it could.

According to a report in *Nutrition and Cancer* (13,1&2:89), researchers at Roswell Park Memorial Institute compared the risks of drinking whole milk and the risks of drinking fat-reduced milk (2 percent or skim milk) and found some surprising results.

There were fewer cases of cancer among the patients who drank large amounts of fat-reduced milk than among the patients who did not drink fat-reduced milk.

These findings suggest that drinking whole milk may cause cancer, whereas drinking fat-reduced milk may actually help prevent cancer.

Whole milk and fat-reduced milk are both rich sources of calcium, riboflavin, vitamin A and vitamin C. However, whole milk is the fourth-largest source of calories and the second-largest source of saturated fats in the typical American diet. Whole milk is also a large source of cholesterol.

Researchers suggest you drink fat-reduced milk. It provides you with vital nutrients without extra fats and cholesterol and helps protect you from the cancer risks that seem to be linked to whole milk.

Natural cancer-fighting strategies

Many health-conscious readers already know there's a lot of evidence showing that carotenoids (relatives of vitamin A), vitamin A itself, vitamin E, the mineral selenium, omega-3 in fish oil, and dietary fiber seem to protect some people from various kinds of cancers.

But there's more good news about some natural cancer fighters you may not have heard much about.

❐ Getting more vitamin D may help people living in areas of high air pollution avoid cancers of the breast and colon, says a report in *Modern Medicine* (57,6:29).

Researcher Cedric Garland says excess sulfur dioxide in the air around industrial cities may block sunlight. Less sunshine means lower levels of vitamin D in the bloodstream.

Lower levels of serum vitamin D are linked with a five-fold increased risk of colon cancer and doubled risk of breast cancer, the report says.

After studying cancer rates in 35,000 men and women in Maryland and 18 Canadian cities, he recommends taking at least 400 IUs (International

Units) of vitamin D each day. That's the same as 10 micrograms (abbreviated either "mcg" or "μg") of cholecalciferol, the chemical name for vitamin D.

Instead of taking it in pill form, Garland's advice is to drink at least four glasses of vitamin D-enriched milk each day. That will give you the 400 IUs, he says.

Of course, as always, check with your doctor before taking any supplements or trying to medicate yourself.

❐　Eating strawberries, grapes and Brazil nuts may help your body ward off cell damage from cancer-causing chemicals known as carcinogens, according to researchers at the Medical College of Ohio in Toledo.

Many kinds of nuts and berries contain ellagic acid, says scientist Gary D. Stoner in *Science News* (133:216). Ellagic acid snoops out cancer-causing chemicals floating in the bloodstream and neutralizes them, the report says.

In tests on mouse and human lung tissue, the nutty substance also seems to help keep normal cells from becoming cancerous, Stoner reports. But it only works when added to the system just before or during the time the body is exposed to the carcinogens, the report says.

Supplements of pure ellagic acid don't work well, Stoner says, because the body has trouble absorbing the concentrated version. The natural stuff, in nuts and berries, is the most easily absorbed form, he says.

❐　Cheese, milk and even some kinds of cooked meats — including charbroiled hamburgers — contain a substance that burrows into your body tissue and sets up anticancer guardposts inside the cells themselves, according to researchers at the University of Wisconsin-Madison.

The anticancer substance is a form of linoleic acid, a kind of fatty acid present in large concentrations in cheese and grilled ground beef, says a report in *Science News* (135,6:87). Linoleic acid is one of three polyunsaturated fatty acids that seem to be very efficient killers of cancer cells, the report says.

But since this form of linoleic acid comes buried in a food's fat — including the saturated kind that can load up your blood with high levels of cholesterol — researchers advise against pigging out on cheese and hamburgers just to get the anticancer effect.

"But within a balanced diet ... [linoleic acid] may confer some protection against cancer — particularly when present in combination with other dietary anticancer agents ... found in many vegetables, including beans, rice and potatoes," the report concludes.

B vitamins may offer protection from cancer

The B family of vitamins may fight tumor formation and boost protection from cancer, according to a nutrition scientist. That's important "because 30 to 40 percent of cancers in men and up to 60 percent of cancers in women are related in some way to diet," *Food and Nutrition News* (61,3:15) reports.

"The B-complex vitamins appear to have supportive roles in maintaining immune system functions which can aid in preventing growth of initiated tumors, as well as having anticancer effects of their own," researcher Ronald Ross Watson writes in *Food and Nutrition News*.

"A balanced diet consisting of moderate amounts of a wide variety of wholesome foods, including those containing the B-complex vitamins ... will enhance health and offer protection against the devastating disease of cancer," Watson says.

❑ **Pyridoxine (vitamin B6)** — "Of all the B-complex vitamins, vitamin B6 appears to have the most important role in maintaining the normal functioning of the immune system," says Watson. Deficiencies of vitamin B6 possibly decrease resistance to cancer and other diseases. In addition, vitamin B6 is being tested as a treatment for melanoma skin cancer.

❑ **Folic acid** — Increased intake of folic acid might decrease the occurrence of cancer, some researchers believe. That's because people with folic acid deficiencies have higher rates of stomach cancer and cancer of the esophagus, the tube from the mouth to the stomach. Folic acid supplements have also been used to successfully treat cervical dysplasia, a precancerous condition of the opening to the womb, according to *Food and Nutrition News*.

❑ **Vitamin B12** — "A recent preliminary study in smokers who had potentially precancerous lung lesions implicated a role for folic acid and vitamin B12 in [lowering] the risk of lung cancer," Watson says. "Vitamin B12 is also thought to support immune system functions," he says, but its unique role is difficult to identify because vitamin B12 works and interacts so closely with folic acid.

❑ **Thiamine (Vitamin B1)** — "Animal experiments have shown that a deficiency of thiamine may cause immune system impairment," and could play a possible role in the development of human cancer, the study reveals.

❑ **Riboflavin (Vitamin B2)** — "Certain populations of people in China, Africa and Iran who have dietary deficiencies of vitamin B2 have shown a high incidence of esophageal cancer," says Watson. Riboflavin is important in the development and maintenance of certain cells in the esophagus. In some cases, riboflavin supplements helped shrink cancer sores, but more research is needed in this area, he says.

"Whole grains, nuts, beans, lean meats, milk, eggs and leafy green vegetables are good sources of B vitamins," according to the article.

"The risk of cancer may be expected to be increased if people avoid certain healthful foods, such as dairy products, lean meats and nuts," just because these foods are high in calories or fat, Watson warns.

In any diet you follow, make sure you get the recommended daily minimums of essential vitamins and minerals.

Too much iron may cause cancer

Iron supplements should be avoided unless people have a deficiency, new research suggests. A recent report says unusually high doses of iron have been linked to greater human cancer risks.

A report in *The New England Journal of Medicine* (319:1047) warns that excess amounts of iron stored in the body may cause an increased risk of cancer and death, particularly in men. In a study involving 14,000 people over 13 years, the researchers linked high body levels of iron with cancer of the colon, bladder, esophagus and lungs.

Unlike most other vitamins and minerals, iron is not automatically thrown off by the body, but is stored. Therefore, taking too much iron can cause unhealthy iron deposits in the body.

People with low levels of iron in their blood, known as anemia, often take several iron supplements daily. Supplements also are recommended after surgery, blood loss, for people with hemorrhoids, peptic ulcers or colitis, or for women with heavy menstrual periods.

The U.S. Government also recommends extra iron for women during pregnancy and breast feeding. Additional iron is very important for the health of these people.

However, other people take iron as part of their daily vitamin and mineral intake, or just because they feel that more iron will help keep them healthy. But iron supplements for people who are not anemic may be unwise, Dr. Richard G. Stevens stated in the journal article.

Many foods, like breakfast cereals, often have added iron. Because of the possible link with cancer, Stevens questions whether everyday foods should be "iron fortified."

Study links bone cancer to fluoride

Flying in the face of 50 years of government and scientific acceptance, a new federally sponsored study suggests that fluoride may have caused bone cancers in some laboratory test animals, reports *Medical Tribune* (30,31:1).

"Very preliminary data from recent health studies on fluoride indicate that fluoride may be a carcinogen," the *Tribune* quotes from a briefing paper prepared by staff scientists at the Environmental Protection Agency (EPA). A carcinogen is a chemical that harms body tissue and triggers cancer.

"If fluoride turns out to be a carcinogen, it will be the environmental story of the century," the story quotes an official of the American Water Works Association. The AWWA is a group that represents the nation's municipal and public water suppliers.

More than six out of every 10 public water suppliers routinely add fluoride to drinking water in a campaign to cut tooth decay. Many of them have been fluoridating water since the 1940s, the *Tribune* report says.

In addition, most toothpastes contain added fluorides, and dentists across the country routinely prescribe fluoride supplements for pregnant women and many children, the paper says.

The fluoridation campaign, despite outcries from various groups in the 1940s and 1950s, has gained wide medical and public acceptance.

In recent months, the EPA has come under criticism for seeming to ignore some studies that showed disturbing links between fluoridated water and increased cancer rates, the news report says.

For example, in the late 1970s, a scientific study showed that cities with fluoridated water supplies had a 5 percent increase in cancer rates. Other studies have been less clear.

Fluoride is a compound made from the gaseous element fluorine. It's a chemical cousin to chlorine, which is used in most public water supplies to kill bacteria in drinking water.

Fluoride gets into and chemically bonds with teeth and bones. It seems to strengthen teeth and make them less vulnerable to decay. Its reputation for fighting tooth decay has been the main justification for adding the chemical to more than half the nation's water supplies.

So far the strongest evidence linking fluoride to bone cancer comes strictly from animal tests. However, the government banned some artificial sweeteners during the past two decades based strictly on animal tests that showed links to cancer.

Vegetable variety a key to preventing lung cancer

To lower your risk of lung cancer, you should eat a variety of fruits and vegetables, such as tomatoes, broccoli and cabbage, researchers report in *Science News* (136,7:102) and the *Journal of the National Cancer Institute* (81,15:1158). Researchers say those foods contain substances that prevent tumor growth and can reduce your lung-cancer risk — even if you smoke.

In the lung-cancer study, females got big benefits from a wide variety of vegetables. Women registered a cancer risk decrease of seven-fold, while men were "only" three times less likely to get lung cancer by eating lots of different veggies, the *SN* report says.

Women seemed to benefit slightly more from a single substance, beta-carotene, than men. Women had a three-fold risk reduction, compared to two-fold for men.

Previous lung-cancer research centered on the anti-cancer properties of beta-carotene, a component of vitamin A found in carrots, papaya, mangoes, sweet potatoes and some other vegetables. But researchers have discovered that other substances related to beta-carotene — lutein, indoles and lycopene — seem to be just as beneficial.

Lutein is found in watercress, spinach, broccoli, green pepper and other dark-green vegetables. Broccoli also contains indoles. Researchers have known for some time that broccoli and cabbage, known as cruciferous vegetables, help prevent colon cancer.

Tomatoes (including tomato juice) contain lycopene and are the only fruit shown to have the same beneficial properties as vegetables, researchers say.

Researchers say eating a variety of vegetables is good for smokers as well. In their study of 230 men and 102 women with lung cancer and 597 men and 268 women without lung cancer, researchers found that eating vegetables reduced lung cancer risk the most in men who were heavy smokers or recent ex-smokers and women who were light smokers.

Milk sugar can be a cancer risk

Women who have trouble digesting a form of sugar found in dairy products may face higher risks of developing cancer of the ovaries, a study in *The Lancet* (2,8654:66) suggests. The study is the first to link dairy products to ovarian cancer, says *Science News* (136,4:52).

The researchers "found that women who ate yogurt at least once a month were nearly twice as likely to develop ovarian cancer as women who reported less frequent yogurt consumption," according to the *SN* report.

Eating cottage cheese at least once a month also raised the cancer risk, the report says. The culprit may be galactose, a type of dairy sugar, the researchers say.

Some women have trouble producing a digestive enzyme to break down the galactose, according to the study. Many don't even know they have the problem.

But if they eat dairy products, this disability may result in "potentially toxic galactose bathing their ovaries for longer than women who metabolize the sugar efficiently," says the *SN* report. "Women who consumed more dairy products than they could metabolize had the greatest risk of ovarian cancer," the report says.

People get the bulk of galactose during digestion of lactose, the main sugar found in milk products. A little galactose is found naturally in most dairy products.

Yogurt and cottage cheese contain very high amounts of galactose. That's because a natural bacteria process breaks down the lactose and releases galactose during the making of the two products.

If the surprising findings are backed up by other studies, "avoidance of lactose-rich foods by adults may be a way of primary prevention of ovarian cancer," says Harvard Medical School researcher Dr. Daniel W. Cramer, one of the authors of the study.

Vitamins that may fight cervical cancer

Women with abnormal cervical cells sometimes have low blood levels of vitamin A, vitamin C and folic acid, one of the B vitamins. These abnormal cells, known as cervical dysplasia, can develop into cancer of the cervix in women.

Research is now under way at the Albert Einstein College of Medicine in New York to see if adding these vitamins to the diet can help reverse the abnormal cell development and help prevent cervical cancer. Other studies have linked low levels of vitamin A to development of cervical cancer, according to reports in *Gynecology and Oncology* (30,2:187) and *American Journal of Obstetrics and Gynecology* (148,3:309).

But this new research will focus on the role of vitamin supplements in preventing cervical cancer.

Your job may increase your risk of bladder cancer

Painters, auto workers and drill press operators are just a few of the workers with an increased bladder-cancer risk, according to a new study in the *Journal of the National Cancer Institute* (81,19:1472).

Bladder cancer is the fifth deadliest cancer among men in the United States. It's four times more common in men than in women.

Researchers at the National Cancer Institute in Bethesda, Md., interviewed 2,100 white men and 126 nonwhite men with bladder cancer to determine the type of jobs they had held for six months or more since age 12.

They then compared that information with questionnaires completed by healthy men of the same age and race.

Among white men, high-risk occupations include driving trucks and taxicabs; grading and packing produce; performing railroad, lumberyard and insulation work; and broadcasting.

Among nonwhite men, auto workers, dry cleaners and clerical workers were at highest risk. The risk to petroleum workers was high in both groups.

Although researchers admit the relationship between job and bladder cancer may be coincidental in some cases, they estimate that "21–25 percent of bladder cancer diagnosed among white men in the United States is attributable to occupational exposures." For nonwhite men, that estimate jumps to 27 percent.

"Overall, our findings suggest that occupational bladder cancer among white and nonwhite men is similar," researchers say. Smoking among all high-risk workers increased the cancer risk even more, they add.

The high-risk occupations have one thing in common: They expose workers to cancer-causing agents, such as dyes, air pollutants and toxic fumes.

For example, painters are exposed to formaldehyde and asbestos, bootblacks to dyes in shoe polish, truck drivers to motor exhaust, machinery operators to coolants and lubricants used in cutting metal, and dry cleaners to petroleum-based cleaning solvents. Asbestos may contribute to insulation workers' increased risk.

Researchers failed to explain why the risk was high for workers such as clerks and broadcasters.

Among occupations studied, the length of time employed was significant in 16 categories. The odds of developing bladder cancer were greater for painters who began work before 1930 and who worked for more than 10 years. The same held true for petroleum processors.

Raw fruit lowers oral cancer risk

Cancer of the mouth is a devastating, disfiguring disease thought by many researchers to be linked to smoking, especially pipes, and to use of chewing tobacco and snuff.

It usually starts as a red or thickened white patch or a painless ulcer inside the mouth. The abnormal area, known as a lesion, is most common on the lips, tongue and floor of the mouth.

Cancer of the mouth and throat ranks number six on the most-common-cancer list among men and women combined. But men over 45 are twice as likely as women to develop it.

Some forms of oral cancer are increasing in the United States because of the popularity of chewing tobacco and snuff among younger men, says a report in *The Lancet* (2,8658:311).

Although lip cancer is detected easily (and treated more successfully than mouth cancer), most people wait too long before seeing a doctor.

Long delays before treatment usually mean that the single, local cancer has spread to other areas. The big delay results in a five-year survival rate of only 30 percent.

Oral cancer is preventable, if you observe the following guidelines:

- **Stop smoking.**

- **Decrease your alcohol intake.**

- **Improve diet and oral hygiene.**

See your dentist regularly because oral cancer screening is part of a routine dental examination.

Now there's also news from a recent report from the National Cancer Institute that indicates that if you eat more raw fruit you may lower your risk of getting cancers of the mouth and throat. The study says that people eating more than four raw fruit servings every day have about half the oral cancer risk of people who average eating one or fewer servings daily.

NCI researchers say that vitamin C, carotene and fiber present in generous amounts in raw fruits may be part of the reason for the protection, but not the only reason. They failed to find a similar preventive effect in vegetables, some of which contain those same nutritional ingredients.

Just eating some cooked vegetables without fruit failed to lower the risk of oral cancers. But chewing crispy vegetables did have a beneficial effect, but not as much good effect as the multiple servings of raw fruit each day.

The researchers think the extra anti-cancer action may be due to the mechanical cleansing action of the raw fruit during chewing and swallowing. Another reason might be the presence in fruit of ellagic acid, thought to be a cancer inhibitor. The same study says that drinking coffee and other hot beverages has no effect, either positive or negative, on mouth and throat cancer risks.

Vitamin A may prevent oral cancer

A recent study indicates that taking vitamin A or its "pre-vitamin" form, beta-carotene, may reduce the risk of getting oral cancer, even among heavy users of tobacco. Scientists from the British Columbia Cancer Research Center in Vancouver gave weekly doses of 200,000 international units (IU) of vitamin A to 21 people in a study in India. The people studied all chewed tobacco mixtures and showed signs of developing oral cancers.

The treatment shrunk precancerous white spots (called leukoplakias) on the tongue and mucous lining of the mouth in 12 of the people studied.

The vitamin therapy also prevented new sores from forming during the year-long study. That degree of prevention over such a long period impressed the researchers, the report said. The researchers worried about the possible toxic effects of megadoses of vitamin A over a year's time. Vitamin A is fat-soluble and is stored by the body. (On the other hand, vitamin C, which is water-soluble, passes quickly through the body and must be replenished daily.)

Because it's stored, vitamin A can build up to dangerous levels in the body and lead to serious health problems. To compare the vitamin doses involved, remember that the U.S. minimum dietary requirements of vitamin A for an adult add up to 35,000 IU in a week's time. The Indian patients received more than five times that amount every week.

The Vancouver scientists are looking for ways to avoid the overdose danger and still get the cancer prevention effects. One way, now being studied, may be to take smaller "maintenance" doses of vitamin A, the report said. Another may be to eat red palm oil, which is rich in beta-carotene, the study said.

Using beta-carotene to prevent oral cancer shows promising results in other research as well. A report on a study of beta-carotene benefits was recently presented to the American Society of Clinical Oncology at a meeting in San Francisco, says *Medical World News* (30,16:19).

In the study, each of 23 people with precancerous patches in their mouths received a 30-milligram daily dose of beta-carotene. Within six months, the beta-carotene treatment apparently caused the sore-like areas to shrink by half in 17 of the 23 people.

Beta-carotene is a yellowish substance that the body converts into true vitamin A.

You can reap beta-carotene's anti-cancer benefits by eating more leafy, dark-green vegetables and deep-yellow fruits such as kale, spinach, carrots, peaches, papayas and cantaloupe, according to *Medical World News*.

Normal servings of these sources can provide five to six milligrams of beta-carotene daily. That allows your body to produce about one milligram of vitamin A, which is within the range recommended for good health, according to *The Merck Manual* (15th edition).

Previous studies have found that vitamin A-type compounds seem to fight formation of several kinds of cancers, including those of the larynx, esophagus, stomach and bladder. Ongoing studies are measuring beta-carotene's potential for preventing lung and skin cancers.

Cancer treatment Catch-22

It seems that treatment for one form of cancer may eventually cause another kind of cancer. Women who undergo chemotherapy for ovarian cancer have a higher risk than usual of developing leukemia later on, says a report in *The New England Journal of Medicine* (322,1:1).

Studies in Europe, England and Canada have identified several factors that work together to increase a woman's leukemia risk:

❏ **Age** — The older a woman is when she's diagnosed for ovarian cancer, the higher her leukemia risk. During the studies, at least half the women were 58 or older at the time of diagnosis.

❏ **Stage of cancer** — Women in an advanced stage of ovarian cancer are more likely to get leukemia after chemotherapy because they need more chemicals to fight advanced cancer. An early cancer diagnosis cuts the leukemia risk, the report says.

❏ **Type of treatment** — Women with ovarian cancer who are treated with surgery alone have the least chance of developing leukemia later on. Those who are treated with radiotherapy have a slightly higher risk. Chemotherapy alone presents the highest risk, researchers say. The risk of radiotherapy and chemotherapy combined is a bit lower, possibly because smaller doses of chemotherapy drugs are used.

❏ **Type of chemotherapy drug used** — During the study, researchers identified some chemotherapy drugs that increase the leukemia risk including chlorambucil, cyclophosphamide, melphalan and thiotepa. The risk depends on dosage and whether the drugs are used in combination — the current trend in ovarian cancer treatment, researchers say.

❏ **Time elapsed after chemotherapy** — Women are most likely to get leukemia four to six years after beginning chemotherapy (or one to four years after finishing it), although the risk is still significant even 10 years later.

Researchers point out that chemotherapy is becoming a popular treatment for women with ovarian cancer. At this point, they aren't sure whether the benefits outweigh the leukemia risks, the report says.

There are no set rules or guidelines about cancer-therapy risks. Each woman is treated individually. If you have ovarian cancer, ask your doctor to fully explain the risks and side effects of each form of treatment.

Be persistent. You need all of the facts before you and your family can choose the therapy that will give you the greatest benefit with the lowest risk.

Nasal sprays and cancer

People using nose sprays were nearly four times more likely to develop cancers of the nasal passages and sinus areas than nonusers, according to a study reported in the *Journal of Epidemiology and Community Health* (42:243).

The study showed that cancer risk rose as nose spray usage increased. The longer people used the preparations and the more weeks out of the year that they sprayed themselves, the greater the risk of developing cancer, the report said.

People who had been using sprays or drops for 10 years faced a cancer risk six times greater than those who had used sprays or drops less than one year. Those who used sprays or drops up to 26 weeks each year had a risk factor 3.8 times greater than those who used the preparations less than one week a year. Many of those studied used the nose drops and sprays to fight nasal congestion and runny noses brought on by hay fever and colds.

The preparations included decongestants and corticosteroids and contained a mixture of over-the-counter medicines and prescription drugs.

The researchers said most of the cancer tumors were squamous cell type, the kind that develop in the surface layer of tissues lining the nasal and sinus passages.

The study compared a group of 53 people with sinonasal cancers with a larger group of 552 people without cancer who had no history of nasal medication use. The study was done in western Washington state.

Even if nose spray wasn't a cancer risk, it's not a good idea to use it often. Over-the-counter nose spray can be addictive, reports *Healthline* (7,4:14).

A doctor at Stanford University Medical Center Allergy Clinic says that prolonged use of decongestants causes nose tissues to swell up even after both the spray and the condition that caused the nose irritation are removed. This "rebound" effect makes a person's nose feel stuffed up even when the cold or flu has long gone, the study said. The clinic's advice: Don't use nose sprays for more than three days at a time.

Where you live can cause cancer

Does your home state increase your risk of developing cancer? In fact, if you live in the northeastern United States, you are at higher risk of developing breast and colon cancer than Southerners or Westerners, according to research from the American Cancer Society.

Benzopyrene, a pollutant generated by automotive exhaust, tobacco smoke, and power and industrial plants, seems to promote cancer development, says a study by biochemist Jack Bartley in Berkeley, Calif. It is found in higher concentrations in the Northeast.

Even if you don't live in an area with air pollution, where you live can still be dangerous. Radon gas in homes may be the second leading cause of lung cancer, according to the Environmental Protection Agency (EPA).

Radon gas is a radioactive by-product of uranium and radium that has been found in over 30 states. It is a colorless, odorless gas that can seep undetected into a house through concrete floors, floor drains, cracks, or even through your water if you have a private well. You absorb radon into your lungs when you breathe contaminated smoke and dust particles.

To check your home's radon gas level, call your local health department or the Radon Information Service sponsored by the EPA at 1-800-334-8571. Some "do-it-yourself" radon testing kits are now available on the market so you can test your own home for contamination.

Also check your neighborhood for large chemical plants, polluted water or waste disposal areas. Living close to these places increases your risk of getting cancer.

Common U.S. fern linked to high cancer rates

The bracken fern, one of the world's most common plants, has been linked to cancer in animals who eat it and to high rates of cancer in people who live or work in bracken-covered areas, the *Medical Tribune* (30,6:2) reports.

Two field guides to edible wild plants in America recommend eating this plant, either cooked or raw. A recent report from Europe, however, accuses the same plant of being a potent cancer-causer. "Deer, cattle and sheep that graze on bracken develop mouth and stomach cancers," the article says.

Studies from Costa Rica and Venezuela showed that people who drink milk from cows that have grazed on bracken, in turn, develop more cancers of the stomach and esophagus, the *Tribune* article says.

The fern under fire is known scientifically as Pteridium aquilinum and is commonly known in this country as pasture brake, eagle fern, brakes, hog brake and brake fern. It is the single most common wild fern in the United States. It grows easily in "full sunlight, in woods, old pastures, new roadsides, burned-over regions, sandy and partially shaded areas and in thickets," according to *Field Guide to Edible Wild Plants* (Stackpole Books), a manual still being sold in many bookstores.

Still another manual, *Field Guide to North American Edible Wild Plants* (Outdoor Life Books) lists bracken as a "related edible species" to ostrich fern. In that guide, bracken was considered a nonpoisonous plant.

Even getting close to bracken may be hazardous, the *Tribune* report suggests. One expert recommends that anyone who goes often into areas in which bracken covers the ground should wear a face mask to limit exposure to bracken spores. The spores are thought to contain several powerful cancer-causing substances such as shikimik milk, quercetin and ptaquiloside.

People who should wear face masks include "shepherds, forestry workers, and even hikers and backpackers," says Dr. Jim Taylor of University College in Wales (Great Britain) and chairperson of the International Bracken Group.

"People may also be affected by drinking water from bracken-covered slopes" and by drinking milk from cows who have eaten bracken, he warns.

Bracken is one of the first ferns to appear in the spring. It grows to a height of from one to four feet, adding new leaves throughout the warm months. The darkly green fronds look heavy and leathery. The fern spreads by oozing a toxic chemical into the ground that poisons all surrounding plants competing for the same space. These same poisons can affect both animals and people, according to the *Tribune* report.

The potentially dangerous spores are released from the maturing plant from June through October, Taylor says.

A further note: Much research has been done on cancer-causing chemicals in recent years. Anyone who relies on field guides for safely stalking wild asparagus and other such wild delicacies should be sure the material has been printed very recently and contains the most up-to-date scientific information.

Check with your doctor or an expert in plant-produced chemicals about questionable plants. Safest bet of all: If it's wild, don't eat it. And, in the case of bracken fern, don't even get near it.

Amazing fish oil fights deadly cancer of the pancreas

New research suggests that a diet high in fish oil may do double duty in fighting cancer of the pancreas. First, the omega-3 fatty acid in the fish oil seems to prevent the formation of precancerous tumors, based on animal studies reported in *Science News* (135,25:390). Second, the oil also may hinder the spread of a tumor that's already turned into cancer. The fish oil that the scientists used in the animal study was from a common deep-sea fish called menhaden.

Cancer of the pancreas is the fifth leading cancer killer in the United States. Scientists suspect that high-fat diets are a major risk factor for getting this disease. The pancreas is a banana-sized gland behind the stomach that produces digestive juices and hormones.

Researchers are finding out that what kinds of fats you eat could make a lot of difference in your cancer risk. In this animal study, rats were injected with a powerful chemical that is known to trigger pancreatic cancer. The rats then were fed a high-fat diet containing either 20 percent corn oil or 20 percent fish oil, according to a report on the study published in the *Journal of the National Cancer Institute* (81,11:858).

The rats fed fish oil developed only about one-third as many precancerous tumors as the corn-oil-fed rats, the report says. After tumors turned into cancer, the researchers were able to slow their growth and spread by lowering the total amount of fat in the diets.

Other studies suggest that the omega-3 itself, not just a reduction in fat, slows down the spread of cancer cells from their original site to other parts of the body.

"There's no doubt about it. Something about fish oil puts it in a separate category from the average oil," agrees Leonard Cohen of the American

Health Foundation in Valhalla, N.Y. But, he notes, you have to eat a "hefty" amount before seeing the anti-cancer effects.

How much omega-3 should be eaten daily is still up in the air. One recent nutrition study suggests that the government should develop a recommended minimum daily dietary amount for average Americans. No such MDA (minimum daily allowance) for omega-3 currently exists.

Many doctors recommend that you get the benefits of omega-3 oil by eating cold water fish rather than by taking capsule supplements containing fish oil. People with diabetes and those who take aspirin or blood thinners or have recently had surgery should be especially careful about taking fish oil supplements. The omega-3 acts like a blood thinner itself. Such combinations of blood thinners and fish oil could cause excessive bleeding.

Cancer prevention tips

- Avoid drinking or cooking with chlorinated water.
- Avoid using talcum powder in the genital areas.
- Avoid drinking coffee, either regular or decaffeinated.
- Avoid contact with asbestos.
- Avoid excessive exposure to the sun.
- Avoid fried foods.
- Avoid processed foods containing carcinogenic additives.
- Avoid barrier forms of contraception.
- Eat foods rich in vitamin D, calcium, molybdenum and selenium, such as fish, whole grain foods, wheat germ and beans.
- Include lysine, an amino acid, in your diet.
- Eat crunchy, yellow and dark-green leafy vegetables.
- Reduce sodium and increase potassium in your diet.
- Eat foods rich in dietary fiber.
- Avoid cigarettes.
- Avoid excessive amounts of alcohol.

Source: *Natural Health and Wellness Encyclopedia,* FC&A Publishing

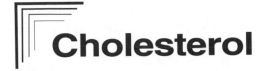

Cholesterol

The cholesterol controversy

Millions of Americans are confused by the controversy regarding cholesterol. Can cutting cholesterol really help you live longer? Or is it an overblown myth that has no scientific basis? *Nutrition Action,* a newsletter that is published by the Center for Science in the Public Interest, has asked experts on heart disease to respond to these questions.

The experts say that many factors contribute to heart and artery disease: heredity, smoking, high blood pressure, diabetes, lack of exercise and being overweight.

But the fact also remains that heart disease is a problem only in those countries where the typical diet is high in cholesterol.

There is no getting around the fact that for every one percent reduction in serum cholesterol in the blood there is a two percent to four percent reduction in the risk of heart attack. And it's difficult to ignore the famous Framingham Heart Study, based on 5,200 residents of Framingham, Massachusetts.

That study shows that high levels of LDL (low-density lipoprotein, the "bad" cholesterol) and low levels of HDL (high-density lipoprotein, the "good" cholesterol) place the elderly at greater risk of heart attack. It has also shown that after menopause, blood cholesterol levels are clear indicators of coronary risk for women.

Dr. August Watanabe, chairman of the International Scientific meeting of the American Heart Association, stated in an article in the *Saturday Evening Post*, "The recent data regarding cholesterol pretty convincingly show that it is an important risk factor, and that if you lower the cholesterol you'll reduce the risk for cardiovascular disease. ... I think it's important for the public to be aware that we are making substantial progress in decreasing mortality from cardiovascular disease. This is very different from any other major category of disease.

One reason is better awareness by the public of risk factors such as smoking, dietary factors, cholesterol, etc. I think there is generally a better awareness and people are changing their lifestyles."

True, there is a minority of respected researchers and physicians who question the value of cholesterol reduction in preserving health and preserving life.

But, since progress is being made against heart disease, the nation's number one killer, and since reducing cholesterol is a big factor in that progress, it seems unwise to abandon these facts.

The facts about cholesterol

The first step in reducing the risk of heart and artery disease is to have your cholesterol level checked.

A recent survey by the Centers for Disease Control in Atlanta reports that "only 47 percent of persons surveyed have ever had their blood cholesterol level measured, only 19 percent have ever been told their cholesterol level, and only 6 percent actually know their blood cholesterol level."

The National Cholesterol Education Program recommends that every adult should have a total blood cholesterol level measurement at least once every five years.

Until recently it was thought that if your total cholesterol level was below 200 milligrams per deciliter (mg/dl), you were within the accepted standard and considered "safe."

However, a large number of patients whose total cholesterol levels were within the "safe" range have been found to have diseased heart arteries, researchers at the Johns Hopkins Medical Institutions in Baltimore report.

This discovery has prompted the scientists to question whether current guidelines need revision.

We "were curious to find out if, in fact, there were lipid abnormalities that were prevalent in a patient group that otherwise would not be detected by the present guidelines," said Dr. Michael Miller, one of the researchers.

The Johns Hopkins scientists evaluated the blood lipid (fat) content of 1,000 patients who had undergone diagnostic coronary angiography, an X-ray of their heart arteries, to search for obstacles that might interfere with blood flow to the heart.

Of the 1,000 patients, there were 185 men and four women who had coronary artery disease even though their total cholesterol levels were less than 200, well within the so-called "desirable" range.

Patients with a recent heart attack were excluded from the study because the heart attack would have altered their lipid levels. This left 138 men and three women with coronary artery disease and total cholesterol levels less than 200 in the investigation.

Sixty-eight percent of the men and 32 percent of the women had HDL-cholesterol levels of less than 35 milligrams per deciliter. (HDL is the "good" cholesterol.)

Earlier studies have shown that the risk of heart disease increases as the HDL levels fall. An HDL level of 35 translates into a 50 percent higher risk than an HDL level of 45, according to the Framingham Heart Study.

Medical statistics show, and the Johns Hopkins study confirms, that a low HDL level is a strong predictor of coronary heart disease — even better, some scientists believe, than the presence of high levels of LDL. Scientists believe that HDL helps lower the risk of heart disease by transporting cholesterol to the liver to be processed for excretion.

LDL is the category of cholesterol that many doctors call the "bad" cholesterol. It circulates in the blood, depositing fat and cholesterol in the tissues, contributing to the buildup of plaque in the artery wall.

This can lead to "hardening" or narrowing of the arteries and increases the risk for high blood pressure and heart problems.

Regardless of the total cholesterol level, doctors should measure and analyze the fasting blood levels of total cholesterol, HDL cholesterol and triglycerides of everyone with heart disease, the researchers recommend. Cholesterol levels of 245 mg/dl were associated with "a twofold greater risk of dying of coronary artery disease in six years," in the Multiple Risk Factor Intervention Trial. Total cholesterol levels of 300 mg/dl quadrupled the risk.

The following chart shows the accepted standard for total cholesterol levels and the new standards for LDL and HDL cholesterol levels:

Total cholesterol levels	Guidelines
less than 200 mg/dl	desirable
200 to 239 mg/dl	borderline high
240 mg/dl and over	high

LDL-cholesterol levels	Guidelines
less than 130 mg/dl	desirable
130 to 159	borderline high
160 mg/dl and over	high

HDL-cholesterol levels	Guidelines
less than 35 mg/dl	too low

Source: *The Western Journal of Medicine* (150,3:562)

According to Miller, one way to increase HDL levels is to lose weight, particularly for obese patients. If you lose weight, not only will your HDL levels go up, but your triglyceride levels may go down. (Some researchers think that high triglyceride levels in the blood may also be a risk factor for heart disease.)

Weight loss also reduces the risk of diabetes, which is itself a contributing factor to heart disease. Regular exercise and quitting smoking will also help to raise HDL levels.

Dietary changes commonly reduce blood cholesterol levels. Polyunsaturated fats, such as those in corn or safflower oil, decrease total cholesterol levels, but they also lower HDL levels. However, Miller says, recent studies have shown that monounsaturated fats, such as olive oil, will reduce the total cholesterol without adversely affecting the HDL level.

A recent study by the Centers for Disease Control in Atlanta found that between the ages of 20 and 60, men's cholesterol levels increase an average of 50 points. In that same period, women's increase about 70 points.

The researchers hope this discovery will help alert younger adults to their future risk of heart disease, so they can choose a healthy diet and lifestyle at an early age.

Low cholesterol can be just as dangerous as high cholesterol

Is it possible to have cholesterol levels that are too low? The answer, especially if you are over 70, is yes, says a report in *The Lancet* (1,8643:868).

Research indicates that, for some people, extremely low levels of cholesterol in the blood may be just as dangerous — and as deadly — as extremely high levels of cholesterol.

If you're over 70 years of age and have blood cholesterol levels of 156 milligrams per deciliter (mg/dl) or lower, you're at high risk for a stroke, a French research team suggests.

A long-term Japanese and U.S. study indicates that extremely low blood cholesterol can actually increase the risk of a fatal stroke known as a cerebral hemorrhage, according to a report in *Science News* (135,16:250). A cerebral hemorrhage happens when an artery in the brain bursts open.

Cholesterol is an important ingredient in cell walls, and ideal levels of cholesterol help keep cell walls strong and healthy. Abnormally low blood cholesterol levels weaken cell walls and damage arteries.

High blood pressure puts extra stress on the damaged arteries and may cause a "blowout" — a hemorrhagic stroke.

Another possible factor adding to the high death rate among those with low cholesterol levels and high blood pressure may be polyunsaturated fatty acids, the studies suggest. Older men and women who are on diets to avoid saturated fats may eat large amounts of polyunsaturated fatty acids.

Normally good for you, these polyunsaturated fatty acids thin the blood and lower the blood's ability to clot. When you've already got weak cell walls, the polyunsaturated fatty acids greatly increase the risk of a stroke by hemorrhage, according to the reports.

If you're concerned about your cholesterol levels, high or low, ask your doctor before you change your eating habits or medicines.

Change your eating habits to lower cholesterol

You can make a big change for the better in your blood cholesterol levels just by changing your eating habits. Eating a well-balanced diet is the easiest and least expensive method to reduce cholesterol.

Your goals should be to lower saturated fat intake, which accounts for 40 percent of our daily calorie count; lower your dietary cholesterol, found in meats, dairy products and animal fats; and count calories.

Overweight people are more likely to have higher cholesterol levels than normal-weight people. While you diet, be careful to keep on getting proper nutrients.

Below are some guidelines to help you choose the healthiest foods to eat.

- ❐ **Dairy products:** Choose skim milk instead of whole milk; low-fat plain yogurt instead of fruit yogurts made with whole milk; low-fat cheeses (farmer's, mozzarella), and ice milk or sherbet instead of ice cream. Limit egg yolks to less than three per week; use egg whites in place of whole eggs in recipes.

- ❐ **Meats and seafood:** Think lean. Choose chicken, turkey and well-trimmed cuts of lean beef. Eat at least two servings of fish per week. Fish from deep, cold waters are best because they're high in essential omega-3 oils. Fresh or frozen fish are better than canned. If you do eat canned fish, choose fish packed in water, not oil.

- ❐ **Fruits and vegetables:** Eat three servings of fresh fruits daily (except coconuts). Avoid fruit canned in heavy syrup. Read the labels on jams and jellies and choose a low-sugar product. Most vegetables and preparation methods are fine, but avoid avocados, olives and cheese, cream and butter sauces. Restrict starchy vegetables, such as potatoes.

❐ **Cereals, nuts, breads:** Most hot and cold packaged cereals are fine, but watch the sugar and salt content. Also check the labels and buy those that are highest in dietary fiber, vitamins and minerals (remember that dietary fiber is not the same thing as crude fiber). Although pecans, walnuts and peanuts are good for you, remember that they're loaded with calories. Avoid hydrogenated peanut butter. Choose whole-grain breads, and avoid commercially baked goods, such as cakes and pastries, which are loaded with fat. Instead of egg noodles, choose pastas and rice.

The above guidelines are from *Postgraduate Medicine* (85,6:243) and are based on recommendations from the American Heart Association and the National Cholesterol Education Program Expert Panel.

How you prepare food also will affect your cholesterol levels. You may freely use vinegar, soy sauce (but watch the sodium) and most spices and herbs.

Cooking oils are another matter. Choose polyunsaturated vegetable oils, such as safflower, corn and sesame oils. Avoid lard altogether. Instead of butter, try polyunsaturated margarine instead.

How to eat less fat

Saturated fats, found in red meats and dairy products, should be reduced to less than 10 percent of total calories. Unsaturated fats, such as fish and vegetable oils, may constitute as much as 10 percent of total calories. Your entire fat intake should be less than one-third of your total daily calories.

❐ Eliminate or drastically reduce consumption of egg yolks, organ meats and most cheeses.

❐ Reduce your consumption of butter, bacon, beef, whole milk, cream, chocolate, almost any food of animal origin, hydrogenated vegetable shortenings, coconut oil and palm oil.

❐ Use monounsaturated oils like olive oil or peanut oil, or polyunsaturated oil like corn, safflower, sesame seed, cottonseed, soybean or sunflower oils. Use soft margarine instead of butter.

❐ Never eat beef, lamb or pork more than three times per week. Choose lean cuts of meat and cut off all visible fat before cooking.

❐ When preparing chicken or turkey, be sure to cut off the skin before cooking because much of the fat is contained in the skin. Eat the light meat because it contains less fat than the dark meat.

❏ Eat smaller portions of meat by using dishes that combine meat with vegetables (especially legumes like beans), pasta or grains.

❏ Avoid duck, goose, gravies, sauces, casseroles, pot pies, bacon bits, croissants, fried fast foods, prepackaged cake mixes, biscuit mixes, pancake mixes, ice cream, whole milk, evaporated milk, artificial or non-dairy creamers and sweetened, condensed milk.

A lifestyle change that can reverse heart damage

Diet and lifestyle changes can actually reverse damage to your heart and arteries, a new study by Dr. Dean Ornish at the University of California, San Francisco, confirms.

"Changing your lifestyle can actually begin to reverse coronary blockages," Dr. Ornish told the American Heart Association.

However, Ornish believes that the lifestyle changes have to be strict and major for drastic improvements in the arteries.

In a year-long study, people with artery problems who practiced meditation, exercised, quit smoking, participated in group counseling and ate a vegetarian diet with less than 10 percent fat had dramatic improvements in their arteries and cholesterol levels.

However, Ornish warned that the people in a comparison group, who consumed a regular, low-fat diet with just 30 percent fat, exercised and quit smoking, did not experience improvement in their arteries — their blockages actually got worse.

Ornish admits that "there is no way to know for sure" how faithfully the patients followed the strenuous regimen. They fill out questionnaires, but "the most objective evidence we have that people are following the changes are the striking reductions in total cholesterol and LDL-cholesterol levels, despite the fact that we are not using cholesterol-lowering medications," the scientist explained.

The major-lifestyle-change group not only experienced a significant decrease in cholesterol levels but also a measurable widening of the coronary arteries that had been narrowed before, Ornish reported.

Total cholesterol declined from a median 227 mg/dl to 136 mg/dl, and the average extent of coronary artery narrowing decreased from 38.8 percent to 34.9 percent.

However, in the comparison group, there was no significant change in cholesterol levels and the narrowing of the patients' heart arteries continued to get worse, from an average of 44.8 percent to 50.6 percent.

Remember, Ornish was trying to help people *reverse* heart disease. To do this, you have to make major lifestyle changes. You can *slow down* the progression of heart disease with even minor changes in lifestyle.

A little lean meat may not hurt your heart

A diet including lean meat may be "almost as effective" as a vegetarian diet in reducing your risk of heart disease, Australian researchers report in *The American Journal of Clinical Nutrition* (50,2:280). More of us would stick to a diet that includes lean meat, the scientists believe.

In the study, 26 men from a fitness center ate one of three different diets — a high-fat "typical Australian" diet, a lean-meat diet, and a milk-egg-vegetable diet — for six weeks so researchers could compare the risk-reduction benefits.

The diets varied from 2,100 to 3,000 calories per day, based on individual needs as determined by metabolic tests. Only among the milk-egg-vegetable group was there a small loss of weight.

The researchers found that the milk-egg-veggie eaters cut their cholesterol levels by ten percent. The lean-meat eaters cut their total cholesterol by five percent. Both "healthy" diets had a slight effect on blood pressure, lowering diastolic pressure an average of two to five points.

Participants on the lean-meat diet ate about nine ounces — slightly over a half-pound — of lean meat every day. The lean meat included processed ham, corned beef, chicken sausage, fresh beef and chicken. This lean-meat diet replaced 60 percent of the plant protein in the milk-egg-vegetable diet with meat protein.

Incidentally, the high-fat Australian diet was also high in cholesterol and low in fiber — similar to the typical American diet. Not surprisingly, men on this diet did not do as well as their counterparts on the other two diets.

During the study, researchers checked the participants' heart rate, blood pressure and serum cholesterol levels every two weeks. They also checked HDL cholesterol and LDL cholesterol levels.

Although men on the milk-egg-vegetable diet had the greatest reduction in blood pressure and cholesterol levels, the lean-meat diet "did not negate" the lowering of those two risk factors. Men on the high-fat diet had the least reduction, and, thus, the least benefit.

However, as the researchers expected, the lean-meat diet also reduced "good" cholesterol levels. The researchers believed the decline in HDL cholesterol would level off and stabilize over longer periods.

Although the lean-meat diet was less effective than the milk-egg-vegetable diet, researchers believe a diet including some lean meat is more acceptable to most people and would stand the best chance of long-term compliance.

High-fiber cereals for breakfast can help control cholesterol levels

Your cholesterol levels throughout the day seem to be directly affected by the food you choose for breakfast, researchers suggest in *The Journal of the American College of Nutrition* (8,6:567).

Adults who "break the fast" with ready-to-eat cereal "have significantly lower fat and cholesterol intakes than those who [eat] other foods at breakfast" or even those who skip breakfast altogether, says the report.

The five-year study, called the National Health and Nutrition Examination, analyzed the food intakes of 11,864 Americans. To determine whether breakfast really is the most important meal of the day, researchers divided respondents into one of these three categories:

- **cereal eaters**

- **breakfast eaters (but without ready-to-eat cereal)**

- **breakfast skippers**

The noncereal breakfast eaters had the highest fat intakes, followed by breakfast skippers.

Among men and women aged 50 to 74, the study indicates that serum cholesterol levels were lowest for those people eating breakfasts that include cereal and highest for those who skip breakfast altogether.

Having cereal for breakfast seems to help keep cholesterol levels under control — an important factor in controlling your heart-disease risk. The breakfast skippers apparently ate higher cholesterol meals later in the day, the study indicates. In addition, they don't get the cholesterol-lowering benefits of the high-fiber breakfast cereal.

Eating a high-fiber cereal for breakfast can result in weight loss, too, according to a study reported in *The American Journal of Clinical Nutrition* (50,6:1303). Men and women who eat high-fiber cereal for breakfast tend to feel less hungry throughout the day compared to those who eat other breakfast foods or cereals with low amounts of fiber. Therefore, high-fiber-cereal eaters tend to eat less food during breakfast and lunch, the report says.

Researchers asked men and women between the ages of 24 and 59 to eat a 7:30 a.m. breakfast of orange juice and cold cereal with milk.

They ate either Post Toasties (lowest in fiber), Shredded Wheat, Bran Chex, All Bran or Fiber One (highest in fiber of the five). Three and a half hours later, they ate a buffet lunch. The high-fiber eaters consumed about 100 fewer calories at breakfast and about 50 fewer calories at the lunch buffet than those who had eaten lower-fiber cereals, according to the report.

Saving 50 calories at lunch doesn't seem significant, but "theoretically could result in substantial weight loss if continued long-term," the researchers conclude.

By the way, a high-fiber hot cereal like oatmeal probably would give many of the same benefits.

The good news about apples

A French study has found that eating two apples a day can lower your cholesterol level by at least 10 percent and by as much as 30 percent, reports the *Medical Tribune* (30,6:14).

Apples long have been recognized as healthful food, but their beneficial effect on cholesterol levels has only recently been discovered.

Researcher David Kritchevsky contends that pectin, the fiber naturally found in apples, is the important cholesterol-lowering ingredient.

Kritchevsky, a professor at the University of Pennsylvania School of Medicine, has conducted several studies on fiber and feels that pectin's benefits have often been overlooked, the *Medical Tribune* reports.

Because apples are naturally low in calories, high in pectin and have been shown to help lower cholesterol, Dr. Kritchevsky believes they are an excellent snack and an important part of a good diet.

Fish oil and rice bran

Recent research shows that rice bran plus fish oil appears to reduce fat in the blood better than wheat bran plus fish oil.

According to a report in *The Journal of Nutrition* (120,4:325), rice bran plus fish oil does a better job of cutting blood cholesterol. So, if you're watching your diet to lower your cholesterol, try some tuna and rice.

A well-known natural laxative that cuts cholesterol

Millions of people have used a common over-the-counter natural laxative to get relief from occasional constipation. By taking a dietary fiber called psyllium, they probably were helping their hearts at the same time. Psyllium is the main ingredient in laxative products like Metamucil and Fiberall.

A recent study on the cholesterol-lowering effects of psyllium shows that psyllium lowers both total cholesterol levels and LDL cholesterol levels, says the *Southern Medical Journal* (83,10:1131).

The people who volunteered for the study took psyllium twice daily. They mixed three packets of instant Metamucil into a 12-ounce glass of water. The volunteers each drank one glass of Metamucil before breakfast and one after dinner. They also drank a 12-ounce glass of water after each glass of Metamucil.

The volunteers participated in the American Heart Association diet while they tested the psyllium. The AHA diet promotes good health by lowering weight and cholesterol levels.

The combination of the AHA diet and the psyllium drinks resulted in a 17.3 percent decrease in total cholesterol in men and a 7.7 percent decrease in total cholesterol in women. The study also showed a 20 percent decrease in LDL cholesterol in men and an 11.6 decrease in LDL cholesterol in women.

Researchers suggest that psyllium is probably most effective in lowering cholesterol when it is combined with the American Heart Association diet. (You can contact the American Heart Association for a copy of this diet.)

Other researchers found that daily doses of just three teaspoons of psyllium can lower cholesterol levels in the blood by 5 percent and can slash levels of "bad" cholesterol by 10 percent or more. The results are reported in *The Journal of the American Medical Association* (261,23:3419).

For every percentage point you lower your total cholesterol level, your risk of heart attack drops by two percentage points, the report says. In addition, the fiber supplements can raise the proportion of "good" HDL cholesterol while it lowers the "bad" LDL cholesterol. That also fights your risk of heart disease.

The researchers gave the psyllium to people who had mild to moderate cases of hypercholesterolemia, the medical name for too much cholesterol in the blood.

The 75 people had already been put on low-fat diets to treat their condition. Most received some benefit from just that step alone. In addition to the low-fat diet, half of them took the extra psyllium daily for up to 16 weeks during the experiments. The ones who took the fiber laxative were the ones who had the dramatic additional cuts in cholesterol levels.

They took each teaspoonful of psyllium with eight ounces of water. Besides the beneficial effects of lowering cholesterol, the psyllium supplements had no serious side effects.

About one out of six people reported minor discomforts such as temporary feelings of fullness with some abdominal cramping. One in 12 had bloating and increased amounts of intestinal gas being passed.

Only one experienced a significant laxative effect. "All of these events were transient and minor in nature, and none required discontinuation of treatment," the *JAMA* article says.

The psyllium fiber worked even better than oat bran, according to the report. Overall, eight out of 10 people who took the psyllium (in the form of Metamucil) had lower "bad" cholesterol and total cholesterol levels after eight weeks. That compared to almost no changes in the control group, which had been given a fake supplement.

Psyllium is the fiber part of seed husks from the common plant, English plantain. The fiber dissolves in water and forms a kind of gel in the digestive system. Doctors still aren't sure how the fiber fights cholesterol, only that it does.

Nearly 25 percent of the American adult population — one out of every four of us — has unhealthy cholesterol levels, the study says. Many doctors prefer to use natural means — particularly changes in diet — as the first stage of treatment in lowering blood cholesterol levels.

Swelling and itching blamed on allergic reaction to psyllium

Psyllium is great for lowering cholesterol — if you're not allergic to it, that is.

Recently, a 43-year-old woman had to see a doctor because of an allergic reaction she had to the psyllium contained in the cereal Heartwise, reports *The New England Journal of Medicine* (323,15:1072). The woman developed swelling and itching around the mouth and eyes, and she began vomiting and coughing. Her doctor treated the allergic reaction, and the woman had a satisfactory recovery.

Allergic reactions to psyllium are rare, but they can occur. If you develop a strange allergic reaction after eating or handling psyllium, be sure to check with your doctor right away.

A vitamin that fights cholesterol

A daily doctor-prescribed supplement of niacin can help lower dangerously high cholesterol levels, according to *Mayo Clinic Nutrition Letter* (2,10:1). "Daily doses of 0.5 to 6 grams of niacin decrease levels of total cholesterol and LDL cholesterol," according to the report. That's 31 to 375 times the officially recommended daily allowance (RDA).

Niacin, a member of the vitamin B complex, is prescribed in some cases because it stops the production of LDL cholesterol and helps the body absorb carbohydrates. Experts have known of the vitamin's cholesterol-lowering abilities for more than 30 years and often prescribe it in conjunction with other medications. If you're tempted to self-medicate yourself, don't. The report offers a few reasons:

❑ When taken in such large doses, niacin acts like a powerful drug and can cause side effects, such as flushing and upset stomach. The higher the dosage, the more severe the side effects. Even 500 milligrams can be very harmful.

❑ Niacin is not a cure-all. You must change your diet and exercise more to lower cholesterol successfully.

❑ Your doctor may think that another treatment would work better for you.

In a recent article of the *Saturday Evening Post*, Dr. Kenneth Cooper also warns about the care that must be taken when using niacin to control cholesterol. He says, "It works in some cases, but you've got to follow patients at least at six-week intervals, because a certain number will develop severe liver problems in conjunction with it. I've hospitalized at least six patients as a result of niacin problems."

Chromium shines as guard against cholesterol

Chromium does more than just put a bright shine on your car bumper. One form of this mineral is a vital nutrient that helps your body turn sugars and fats from food into energy for cells all the way from your brain to your big toe. New research shows it also might help lower cholesterol levels, especially LDL cholesterol, the "bad" type that clogs heart arteries and raises the risk of heart attacks, says a study reported in *The Western Journal of Medicine* (152,1:41).

Researchers at San Diego's Mercy Hospital and Medical Center studied 28 people who ranged in age from 25 to 80. They tested a supplement called chromium picolinate, a form of chromium that is believed to be easily absorbed by the body. The daily supplements provided 200 micrograms of biologically active chromium. Among those taking chromium supplements for six weeks, total cholesterol levels dropped 7 percent, and LDL cholesterol plunged more than 10 percent. The chromium supplements also raised by 7 percent the levels of a protein that forms HDL cholesterol.

The Recommended Dietary Allowance for chromium is not precise. Instead, the RDA is a range of 50 micrograms to 200 micrograms daily. Some studies show that the typical American diet provides less than 50 micrograms of chromium per day.

The researchers point out that many people might not be getting enough "bioavailable" chromium in normal diets or even in other forms of chromium supplements.

Adding to their worry is the finding that infection, pregnancy, stress, high glucose intake and just plain aging deplete blood levels of chromium. Natural sources of chromium include brewer's yeast, calf's liver, American cheese, corn, mushrooms and wheat germ.

Unlike some other mineral nutrients, chromium in its biologically available form appears to be safe even in amounts several times the RDA, and few problems have been reported with chromium overdoses, says the official "bible" of nutrition, *Recommended Dietary Allowances, 10th Edition*, published by the National Research Council.As always, check with your doctor before taking any kind of nutritional supplement.

A natural sugar that could harm your heart

If you're concerned about lowering your cholesterol levels and decreasing your heart attack risk, you should watch your fructose intake, researchers report in *The American Journal of Clinical Nutrition* (49,5:832). Fructose is a natural, simple sugar found in fruits and honey.

You get fructose another way, also. Your digestive system breaks down regular table sugar — sucrose — into about equal parts fructose and glucose. Of every 1,000 calories we eat and drink, about 100 calories — 10 percent — end up in the form of fructose, says a report in *Science News* (133:196).

Many doctors recommend fructose as a partial replacement for regular sugar in their diets, *SN* says. Researchers were curious about the effects of fructose because it's becoming a popular sweetener in many soft drinks and processed foods. The researchers did a 10-week study to find out what would happen if the fructose intake were increased to 20 percent of a person's daily calories. For the first five weeks, the research team fed 21 men a typically American high-fat diet with the added fructose.

Each man consumed more than 3,200 calories a day on the non-weight-loss diet. The foods they ate exceeded limits of fat and cholesterol recommended by the American Heart Association. During the last five weeks, they replaced fructose with high-amylose cornstarch. The fructose increased one heart-disease risk factor — uric acid levels — by 13 percent among all participants. Although the increases in triglycerides and cholesterol "were small to moderate," researchers believe they signal a disturbing trend.

Perhaps the most ominous finding of the study was that "most cholesterol and triglyceride increases occurred in the very-low-density lipoproteins and low-density lipoproteins — the so-called 'bad' lipoproteins that increase the risk of heart disease," says the *Science News* report. People who already have high triglyceride levels are at highest risk. Ten of the 21 men in the study met this criterion.

Good fat, bad fat

Watch out for "bad" cholesterol if you have a fat belly or a chubby chest, warns a report in *The New England Journal of Medicine* (322,4:229).

Upper body fat, high levels of insulin in the blood and a weakened ability to turn blood sugar into energy seem to work together to lower your level of "good" HDL cholesterol. Less HDL means a worse risk for heart disease, the report says.

It's smelly, but it works

Although many physicians turn up their noses at the very idea, garlic for medicinal purposes is making a comeback, according to *The Lancet* (335,114:1990).

In recent studies, garlic helped prevent heart disease by lowering "bad" cholesterol, raising "good" cholesterol and keeping blood flowing freely.

The problem is, you'd have to eat much more garlic than you (or anyone living with you) could stand. The good news is that health food stores sell deodorized garlic in pill form.

Cholesterol and cancer

High levels of cholesterol in the bloodstream represent more than an increased risk of heart attack and stroke, according to a report in the *British Medical Journal* (298,6690:26).

A massive statistical study of 17,718 British men indicates that a high cholesterol level is a risk factor for developing cancerous brain tumors. A rise of just one millimole per liter in plasma cholesterol levels represents a larger risk for brain tumors than age, weight and social/financial status, according to the study authors. The exact relationship between raised cholesterol levels and brain cancer has yet to be figured out, the report says.

Researchers also believe that cholesterol-lowering drugs may help block colon and pancreatic cancer, according to *Science News* (136,5:70).

The body goes through several chemical steps when it makes cholesterol. Cholesterol-lowering drugs such as lovastatin work by blocking one of those chemical steps. Scientists knew that cholesterol seemed to influence cancer, so they injected unfertilized frog eggs with cholesterol-lowering drugs to see what would happen. It turns out that when the drugs block one of the chemical steps the body goes through when making cholesterol, they also keep a protein involved in cancerous cell division from working. This protein is involved in colon and pancreatic cancers.

These studies have established a link between cholesterol and cancer.

How effective is high-cholesterol treatment?

People with high cholesterol do not respond equally well to cholesterol-lowering treatment (whether diet or drugs), say New Hampshire researchers, who advocate individual treatment for every patient.

According to a report in *Archives of Internal Medicine* (149,9:1981), the researchers evaluated data from several high-cholesterol studies and noted these trends:

- **Elderly men benefited less from high-cholesterol treatment than younger men. Age might influence the response to drug therapy and dietary change, researchers said.**

- **Smokers do not respond as well as nonsmokers.**

- **The data for men and women are conflicting. Some studies show men at greater risk, while others show women at greater risk.**

- **Lowering cholesterol benefits people who have high blood pressure more than people with normal blood pressure.**

Researchers also point out that cholesterol treatment has a price. "For most Americans, dietary intervention requires substantial and possibly life-long changes in eating habits. Drug therapy requires long-term compliance, is costly, and may produce unpleasant side effects."

Chronic Fatigue Syndrome

Chronic fatigue syndrome: exercise to get rid of fatigue?

It's hard to pinpoint, and even harder to treat. But fatigue is almost as rampant as the common cold.

Millions of people pay for yearly visits to their doctors, complaining of vague forms of fatigue — everything from loss of concentration to low energy levels that persist in spite of adequate rest.

Chronic fatigue syndrome (CFS) has been linked most often to the mononucleosis and Epstein-Barr viruses. But recent studies seem to suggest that CFS has been around for many years, often changing names, but presenting its sufferers with the same problems.

The routine advice given to CFS patients has been to rest. But now doctors are trying a new approach, and it shows great promise, reports *Drug Therapy* (20,8:29).

Carefully planned, regular exercise — instead of an inactive life-style — is now recommended. The idea is to break the vicious cycle of fatigue and its inevitable results of poor fitness and poor cardiovascular health.

CFS sufferers are warned not to expect immediate results, but to gradually increase their activity until a level of fitness is achieved that cancels out most of the symptoms of fatigue.

As with most problems, a healthy diet plays an important role in recovery. The American Heart Association recommends a low-fat diet as a wise choice.

It provides your heart with the proper fuel to do its job, while supplying much-needed energy to tired muscles.

As frustrating as CFS might be, people experiencing it can bring about healthy results if they maintain a positive attitude and follow their doctor's suggestions completely.

Colds and Flu

A better remedy for cold symptoms?

British doctors think they may have come up with a better remedy for the common cold. Their approach calls for inhaling moist, hot air for 20 minutes, according to the research report in *British Medical Journal* (298,6683:1265).

The report says that inhaling humidified air at just under 110 degrees Fahrenheit shortens the course of the cold and brings many patients next-day relief.

In a controlled study, those who breathed in moist, hot air improved faster than those who inhaled "steamy" air. The warm, steamy air was at about 86 degrees Fahrenheit. Such warm, steamy air can be produced by a common vaporizer. Vaporizers are widely used by cold sufferers to ease their symptoms.

Researchers studied two groups of patients. They found that the "hot-air" patients did better than the "warm-air" patients. On the fourth day of medical checkups, 21 of the hot-air patients said their colds were gone.

But only one of the warm-air patients reported no more cold symptoms. However, people in both groups reported their symptoms had been cut nearly in half by the treatments.

In another, follow-up study, volunteers received one 20-minute hot-air treatment on the first day and 10-minute treatments each morning after that until their cold symptoms disappeared. The first treatment seemed to benefit them, but the additional treatments didn't seem to do any good, the *BMJ* report says. Treatments of 10 minutes aren't long enough to do any good, researchers concluded. They must be 20 minutes or more to have a beneficial effect.

The hotter-air treatment also helped hay fever sufferers, leading researchers to suggest the hot, moist air treatments may have some kind of anti-inflammatory effect. No bad side effects were reported by any of the patients, the report says. If you try a homemade version of the "warm-air" treatment, be careful not to get burned.

Air when it immediately comes out of a vaporizer is very hot, but inhaling unregulated hot air or placing your face near a vaporizer could scald your face, mouth or nasal passages. Trying to "do-it-yourself" could result in painful, possibly dangerous burns. The people who took part in the experiments did so under careful medical supervision and used specially designed breathing apparatus.

So far, we know of no commercially available machine that will deliver moist air at exactly 110 F safely to your mouth and nose. But, remember that the experiment showed that even warm, moist air — like that found in a hot shower or a few feet away from a home vaporizer unit — also can produce good results.

How to halt your hacking

From a dry tickle at the back of your throat to a never-ending hacking to a gut-wrenching, sputum-producing heave — coughing is one miserable symptom that seems to accompany a variety of health problems. Colds, flu, heartburn, even some drugs such as ACE inhibitors cause coughing.

Coughing can lead to serious health problems like urinary incontinence and rectal and vaginal muscle strain. But even without the additional problems, coughing is irritating enough in itself to warrant some cures.

Here are some ways to relieve your discomfort when coughing strikes:

❏ **Get that chicken soup comfort.** — If you are coughing up phlegm, you need to let nature take it's course and even help it along. Warm soup will help speed up the process of coughing up the phlegm and mucus caught in your lungs, reports *Health Letter* (6,2:1). When your body coughs "productively," it can clean out unwanted substances in your lungs.

❏ **Drink warm liquids and plain water.** — Warm liquids and water are the best way to loosen the mucus in your lungs so that it's easier to cough up. If your cough accompanies other cold and flu symptoms, try to drink at least eight to 10 glasses of liquids a day. Liquids will help keep a fever down, soothe a sore throat and help your body flush out germs.

❏ **Take the right kind of cough medicine.** — If you are coughing up phlegm, you need to take an expectorant that will help you cough. If you have a "dry" cough that doesn't bring up any mucus, you can use a cough suppressant. Suppressants are also called antitussives, and they come in both liquid form and lozenge form.

❏ **Take a hot shower or a steamy bath.** — Use a humidifier or sit in a steamy room to help loosen the mucus in your lungs, suggests the *British Medical Journal* (298,6683:1280).

❑ **Eat a banana.** — Heartburn is the culprit for about one in every 10 chronic coughers, reports *The Lancet* (336,8710:282), and researchers have found that bananas are a great natural solution for heartburn. Banana powder, a dried, ground-up form of the fruit, also works well. Other heartburn remedies are raising the head of your bed, avoiding food and drink before bedtime, losing weight and eating more slowly.

❑ **Put down that cigarette.** — Have you ever met a smoker who doesn't have a chronic cough? Even if you don't smoke, if you work or live with people who do, passive smoke could be the culprit for your cough. Put your foot down about your smoky environment, or you could be coughing and wheezing forever.

If your cough goes on and on and gets worse instead of better, make sure you see a doctor. Coughing up blood, shortness of breath when you cough or sharp pains in your chest when you cough are all sure signs that a doctor's visit is in order.

Fend off infections with moderate exercise

Walking may help your body fight off flu and other serious infectious diseases, according to new studies from Australia.

Moderate exercises like walking seem to boost the body's natural defenses against infections, reports *Medical Tribune* (31,9:9).

The boost to the immune system especially benefits the sensitive mucous membranes in the mouth, throat and breathing passages, the report says. Those are areas vulnerable to colds and influenza attacks.

Moderate exercise may trigger production of more "killer cells" in the bloodstream, the equivalent of sending more fresh "soldiers" into battle against invading disease germs, suggests Laurel Mackinnon, a professor of exercise physiology and wellness at the University of Queensland in Australia.

But the key is moderation, the report says. Too much heavy exercise seems to have the opposite effect, cutting back numbers of immune system "soldiers," immunoglobulin A (IgA), for up to two days, says Professor Mackinnon. That may be why very fit athletes seem to come down with an unusually large number of upper respiratory infections following intense training, the report suggests.

Before you start or change your exercise program, be sure to check with your doctor about what exercises will be appropriate for you.

Colon Cancer

'Stress' causes cancer?

Stress is usually caused by hectic schedules, rush hour traffic and other situations that seem to be out of your control.

But you may be creating the most dangerous kind of stress at your supper table!

Recent studies show that you may be putting dangerous stress on your body by eating certain foods, by not eating the right proportion of foods, and by eating the wrong kinds of foods.

According to a report in the *Journal of the National Cancer Institute* (82,6: 491), the hidden stress caused by this "stress diet" may actually encourage cancer to begin growing in your intestines.

What is a "stress diet"? Unfortunately, it is typical of the diet of most people in the United States. The "stress diet" has four problem areas that you should watch for:

❑ **Not enough calcium.** Some sources recommend up to 1,500 milligrams per day, but the average American only gets 500 to 600 milligrams per day.

To increase your daily calcium intake, eat more foods that contain calcium, such as milk, cheese, yogurt and molasses. You may consider taking calcium supplements.

❑ **Not enough vitamin D.** Vitamin D helps your body absorb and use calcium. So a vitamin D deficiency also can cause a calcium deficiency.

Studies show that if you get enough vitamin D, you are less likely to get colon cancer. Vitamin D is found in egg yolks, organ meats and bone meal.

You also can get vitamin D by spending a few minutes each day in the sunlight. Sunlight produces vitamin D naturally in the body.

❑ **Too much phosphorus in relation to calcium.** You need equal amounts of phosphorus and calcium in your diet. The Recommended Daily Allowance (RDA) for phosphorus and calcium is 800 milligrams for each.

Many Americans get 1500 milligrams of phosphorus or more per day and only 500 to 600 milligrams of calcium per day. Although phosphorus is good for you, too much phosphorus can keep your body from using the calcium it needs. Foods that contain phosphorus are meats, poultry, fish, eggs, grains, nuts, dry beans and peas.

❐ **Too much fat.** Most people in the United States get about 40 percent of their calories from fat. Animal fats and some polyunsaturated vegetable oils (such as corn oil) contain fats which promote the development of cancer.

Scientists recommend that you decrease your intake of red meats and polyunsaturated vegetable oils. Then increase your intake of "good" fat such as safflower, sunflower, soy and canola oils.

If your diet contains one or more of these four "stress" factors, you may be creating extra hidden stress in your body that could eventually lead to colon cancer. Eliminating the "stress" from your diet could decrease your risk of cancer. But remember, you should discuss any drastic changes in your diet with your doctor to guarantee your best health.

Antacid stops 75% of colon cancers?

Taking twice the current Recommended Dietary Allowance (RDA) of calcium every day might prevent nearly 75 percent of all colon cancers, says a cancer researcher in *Medical World News* (31,4:22). That's equal to about eight regular nonprescription calcium carbonate antacid tablets.

Evidence of calcium's prevention power is snowballing, with 60 studies worldwide now reporting the mineral's natural benefits. In light of these encouraging study results, some researchers are suggesting a change in the RDA of calcium for adults.

It takes 1,200 milligrams of calcium a day to prevent colon cancer in people under the age of 49, some pro-calcium researchers say. People over age 49 need 1,500 milligrams daily to get the prevention effect, they suggest.

Check with your doctor before taking supplements of any kind, and especially before taking more than the RDA.

Colon cancer is the second deadliest cancer in the United States, and each year, 145,000 new cases are diagnosed. Most of its victims are middle-aged or beyond. The disease can be controlled and even cured if caught in its early stages.

Researchers really don't know how calcium works, but some believe it fights the effects of a high-fat diet on the colon wall, according to a report in *Preventive Medicine* (18,5:672). Studies have shown that fatty foods speed up cell growth in the colon, and such spurts are the first step to tumor development.

Calcium travels throughout the digestive tract, working to keep cell growth under control. It gets there by way of vitamin D — a rapid transit system of sorts — which transports energized calcium to the intestines, primed for preventing bad cell growth.

Taking eight carbonate tablets (such as Tums) a day would provide about 1,600 milligrams of calcium. (One regular Tums contains about 200 milligrams of calcium.)

If you take calcium supplements, you should drink at least two liters of fluid every day, recommends Dr. Cedric Garland, a professor at the University of California at San Diego. Too much calcium and not enough fluids could add up to a case of painful kidney stones.

Check with your doctor before taking antacids or any supplements. There's a limit to how much calcium you can take safely, and calcium antacids have their own set of side effects.

You may do better taking regular calcium supplements than calcium antacids. Calcium antacids taken for more than a few days may cause acid rebound. Your stomach is stimulated to produce even more acids and excess gas. If you have heartburn, it could get worse.

Milk provides essential cancer-fighting elements

Mother was right when she told you to drink your milk. It could help save your life.

Just two eight-ounce glasses of fortified milk a day provide enough calcium and vitamin D to help lower your colon-cancer risk, according to *Medical World News* (31,1:41).

In a recent study, seven men at high risk for colon cancer took 1,250 milligrams of calcium every day for one week. In four men, extra calcium cut the amount of a cancer-causing enzyme in the colon by 50 percent.

This finding confirms several previous studies.

Researchers also found that people with high levels of vitamin D — at least 20 nanograms per milliliter of blood serum — had a 70 percent smaller colon-cancer risk compared with people with low vitamin D levels (lower than 20 ng/ml). (A nanogram is one-billionth of a gram.)

Does colon cancer thrive where the sun doesn't shine?

To protect yourself from colon cancer, get more winter sunshine, a new study suggests.

For several years now, scientists have noticed that colon cancer rates are higher in parts of the world that receive less sunshine.

In fact, a recent government study shows that the highest death rates from colon cancer in the United States occur along a line from Maine to Iowa. Six researchers in Maryland and California wondered if the unexplained differences might be related to the "sunshine" vitamin — vitamin D.

In 1974, 25,620 volunteers in a Maryland county were tested for their blood levels of vitamin D. After nine years, the researchers checked back to see who had come down with colon cancer out of that group.

They found that people with blood concentrations of 20 nanograms of vitamin D per milliliter or higher were three times less likely to develop colon cancer. People with lower levels of activated vitamin D were at greater risk for colon cancer, indicates the report in *The Lancet* (2, 8673:1178).

Vitamin D levels in the blood vary from season to season, especially in colder climates that receive fewer hours of sunlight. Sun rays activate a forerunner of vitamin D in the skin and turn it into a form that's usable by body tissues.

In Britain, vitamin D levels in blood vary from an average of about 13 nanograms per milliliter in March to over 20 nanograms per milliliter in August, according to the *Lancet* report. In elderly British people, winter vitamin D blood levels were even lower — in some cases one-sixth the summer levels, the report says.

It's important to note that you can drink a lot of vitamin-D-fortified milk, eat a lot of vitamin-D-rich foods like fish and eggs, and even take vitamin D supplements and still have a shortage of activated vitamin D in your system because of a lack of sunlight.

"Anything that blocks sunshine from penetrating the skin will reduce the amount of vitamin D that the body makes," according to *Vitamin and Mineral Encyclopedia* (FC&A Publishing). It's the ultraviolet rays that trigger the vitamin D into action in the body.

You should certainly avoid sunburns and too much ultraviolet exposure for fear of higher skin cancer rates. The body needs some ultraviolet rays to activate needed vitamin D, but not so much sunshine exposure that it would harm the skin. Generally speaking, you should try to get more sunshine during autumn and winter months to keep blood levels of vitamin D closer to summer levels.

Only ultraviolet rays of a certain wavelength will produce the necessary vitamin D. Very little ultraviolet light of the correct wavelength reaches the earth's surface in northern latitudes in the winter months even when the sun is at its highest point at midday. But just a few minutes of midday sun exposure during the summer produces all the vitamin D the body can use.

A caution — don't overdo the sun seeking. Only a little activated vitamin D over the recommended dietary allowance (RDA) can produce side effects ranging from mild (headache, ringing in the ears, nausea) to severe (damage to heart and kidneys, even death).

"Of all the nutrients analyzed ... [including fat, total calorie intake and dietary fiber], only vitamin D and calcium affected the incidence of colon cancer," the *Lancet* study reports.

Sitting down to a steak dinner may be dangerous for your health

If you sit down to a meal of cheese steak very often, your colon may be paying a high, even deadly, price. Those two actions — sitting a lot and consuming a lot of fatty meats and dairy products — are the very highest risk factors for developing colon and rectal cancers, says a major new study in the *Journal of the National Cancer Institute* (82,11:915).

The study of hundreds of Chinese people in America and in China pointed at two main villains: saturated fat and a sedentary life-style. In fact, the study found, your cancer risk increases as you spend more time sitting.

Eating more than 10 grams a day of saturated fat, along with physical inactivity, "could account for 60 percent of colon and rectal cancer incidence among Chinese-American men and 40 percent among Chinese-American women," the report says. Ten grams is slightly more than one-third of one ounce.

Researchers compared the two groups because they wanted to find out why colon and rectal cancer rates are four to seven times higher among Chinese people who move to America than rates among the general population in mainland China. They took into account the difference in diets in the two countries. For example, a typical mainland Chinese person will eat more calories per day than his Chinese-American cousin. But more of those native-country calories will come from carbohydrates and starches.

In China, the average person will get about 54 percent of his protein requirements from grains like rice, and only 20 percent from meat (mainly pork) and fish, the report says. Over here, however, the Chinese-American will reverse that — 60 percent of his protein will come from meat and fish, and only 17 percent from rice and other grains.

Both groups got about four to five grams a day of crude fiber. Chinese-Americans took in more daily calcium and beta-carotene, a forerunner of vitamin A. The two nutrients plus fiber seemed to give some protection against the two bowel cancers.

After accounting for diet differences, the two culprits of saturated fat and sedentary lifestyle stood out in the lineup as the major risk factors for developing colon and rectal cancer.

Interestingly enough, people living in two mainland Chinese cities also had higher cancer rates, suggesting that city diets might not be as healthy as country diets.

Saturated fat is the stuff that makes butter and animal fat solid at room temperature. Vegetable fats, on the other hand, usually contain monounsaturated and polyunsaturated fats and are generally liquid at room temperature. Vegetable fats like corn oil and soybean oil make up most of the liquid cooking oils these days.

Nutritionists recommend that you eat foods low in saturated fats. They suggest that you try to get less than a third of your daily calories from fats of all kinds, and less than one-tenth of your total calories from saturated fats.

Dietary fibers differ in fighting colorectal cancer

"High intakes of fruits and vegetables had a beneficial effect on the colon," says a group of researchers from the University of Utah School of Medicine. In fact, of all the food groups the researchers examined, "fruit appeared to have the greatest protective effect."

Other studies in the *Journal of the National Cancer Institute* (55:15) and the *Journal of Epidemiology* (109:132) have shown a direct link between high fiber and a lower incidence of colon cancer. Despite those findings, doctors were not sure what type of fiber was most effective.

For this study, the Utah team evaluated "various types and sources of fiber in the diet" of more than 500 men and women for five years. Crude fiber was the most important fiber-type in the study, as it consistently decreased the risk of colon cancer in both men and women.

The average person consumes "only 15 to 20 grams of fiber a day, when they need 25 to 40 grams," according to Dr. Denis Burkitt, one of the most respected researchers in the field of dietary fiber.

By increasing daily intake of soluble fiber and insoluble fiber to at least 25 grams, adults and children can help prevent colon cancer as well as "digestive disorders such as constipation, irritable bowel syndrome (IBS), hemorrhoids, and diverticular disease," Dr. Burkitt said.

Soluble fiber, like pectin in apples, is easily dissolved in water. Soluble fiber bonds chemically with certain substances like cholesterol and moves them quickly through the digestive tract.

Insoluble fiber, like cellulose (in whole grains) and hemicellulose (in vegetables) doesn't dissolve in water. Instead such fiber absorbs water like a sponge, softening waste products in the intestines and speeding it out of the body.

Both kinds of fiber are needed for healthy digestion.

Another report in *Nutrition and Cancer* (13,4:271) says, "vegetable fibers may generally be more protective against colorectal carcinogenesis [cancer] than cereals."

Vegetables are more "fermentable" than cereal fibers. Fermentation refers to the process in which the body (particularly the stomach and intestines) breaks down foods into usable compounds necessary for proper nutrition. A fiber source that is highly fermentable appears to be a strong warrior against cancer.

Fermentation takes place when the "good" bacteria in the intestines break down vegetable or animal matter. During that process, nutrients are released into the intestines. This process supplies the body with important nutrients. And, equally important, fermentation helps resupply the intestinal bacteria with vital nutrients. The bacteria help keep the bowel healthy and functioning properly and help protect the colon from cancer.

Put the starch back into the diet

Years ago, starch was something other than what you spray on shirts to be ironed. Starches were considered a distinct food group, and youngsters were encouraged to eat something from that group two or three times a day to ensure a healthy diet.

Come the 90s, and starches are now "complex carbohydrates."

Despite the trendy name, starchy foods are still the same ones we knew as children: potatoes, rice, breads and foods made from grains.

One British researcher believes that starchy foods may be what's missing in our search for foods that protect against cancers of the colon and rectum. No, it's not the fiber in those foods, either. Instead, believes K.W. Heaton of the Bristol Royal Infirmary in England, it's the starchy foods that "escape" digestion in the stomach and small intestine that may do us the most good.

Those "escaped" starches are quickly fermented in the large intestine (colon) and pass rapidly on through the bowel. The fermentation and quick passage protect the colon from being exposed for too long to harmful substances in foods.

One finding supporting this theory is that people who develop a lot of precancerous growths in their colons also seem to be unusually efficient at digesting starch before it gets to the colon, says Heaton.

Even those people could help themselves by eating starchy foods in less digestible forms, the researcher suggests. For example, instead of using baked flour products, eat a lot of whole grains like rice.

Dietary fiber may actively fight cancer

Scientists have discovered an active ingredient in dietary fiber that may help to prevent cancer and treat established cancer. According to the journal *Carcinogenesis* (10,3:625), fiber contains inositol hexaphosphate (InsP6), which was effective in significantly reducing the size and number of colon and rectal cancers in rats and mice.

Inositol hexaphosphate, also known as phytic acid, is found in wheat, corn, oats and rice. It is "an abundant plant seed component present in many, but not all, fiber-rich diets," researchers report in the journal *Cancer* (56,4:717).

Doctors have known that dietary fiber helps reduce the risk of cancer, but they believed it was only because fiber helps move waste through the body and reduces the amount of time that cancer-causing substances can build up in the colon.

Dr. Abulkalam Shamsuddin of the University of Maryland in Baltimore decided to study the effects of InsP6 when he noticed that different groups who ate high-fiber diets often had different rates of cancer. The only difference in the diets seemed to be the amount of InsP6 the diet contained, so Dr. Shamsuddin decided to test InsP6's effectiveness without the fiber content. He removed InsP6 from fiber and gave it to test animals in their drinking water.

Besides this fiber ingredient, the test animals had no other fiber in their diet. Even without the roughage, "the treated animals developed significantly fewer cancers, and their cancers were two-thirds smaller than those of untreated controls," Dr. Shamsuddin said.

Tablets or capsules of InsP6 could one day be used in the treatment of human cancer because InsP6 can be extracted easily, Dr. Shamsuddin says.

Other studies by Graf and Eaton reported in *Cancer* (56,4:717) have backed up Shamsuddin's findings. The studies have shown that InsP6 suppresses colon cancer and other inflammatory bowel diseases.

Research by Dr. Lillian Thompson at the University of Toronto has also shown that InsP6 has an anti-cancer effect in mice. Other studies showed that InsP6 given after five months of cancer helped to slow the cancer growth.

Dr. Shamsuddin found in an earlier study that inositol hexaphosphate reduced the effects of cancer in the large intestine as well as in the colon and rectum, he reported in *Carcinogenesis* (9,4:577).

"Large intestinal cancer is the second most common cancer in the United States with an expected 147,000 new cases" per year, *Carcinogenesis* reports.

High-fiber diet slashes rectal cancer rates

A high-fiber diet can slash your risk of rectal cancer, a four-year scientific study indicates. It can do this by reducing the number of noncancerous tumors of the rectum, according to encouraging results reported in the *Journal of the National Cancer Institute* (81,17:1290).

People got the best results with dietary fiber levels of nearly one ounce every day. That's about twice what most Americans eat regularly.

The high-fiber diet seems to fight formation of benign rectal polyps. These are little tumors on stalks. Sometimes polyps look like tiny mushrooms growing out of the walls of the rectum and lower intestine.

These benign polyps, if not discovered or if left untreated, almost always turn into cancer, the report says.

Previous studies have shown that high-fiber diets decrease risks of getting colon cancer, so researchers studied 58 people to determine whether they would reap the same benefits farther down the digestive tract.

Before the study began, patients were given a baseline examination to calculate the size and number of polyps. There were three groups: Sixteen took vitamin C and vitamin E with a low-fiber supplement (vitamin group); twenty were given the vitamins with a high-fiber supplement (high-fiber group); and 22 received only a low-fiber breakfast cereal supplement (control group).

On the average, the vitamin group took in 11.3 grams of wheat fiber per day; the high-fiber group, 22.4 grams; and the control group, 12.2 grams. One ounce equals just over 28 grams.

Researchers chose wheat fiber and vitamins C and E because they have shown the best results in anti-cancer studies. The wheat fiber — a non-water-soluble kind of dietary fiber — came from a common brand of breakfast cereal.

Every three months, researchers examined all the groups to see if the number of tumors rose or fell. In addition, nurses counseled people having trouble following the diet.

After six months, polyp size and numbers had been cut in half in the high-fiber group, researchers said. Those who took vitamins with a low-fiber cereal generally broke even — no increase and no decrease in tumors.

"A high prescribed fiber intake and, to a lesser extent, a high vitamin intake, were associated with lower polyp number ratios," according to the report. This is good news, especially for people with a family history of rectal tumors.

Compliance in the study was low, meaning that the people being studied failed to stick strictly to their diets.

That surprised the researchers, since the patients were aware of their cancer risk. Compliance was highest overall for the high-fiber group, which also showed the best results, followed by the vitamin group and the control group.

In addition to diet therapy, treating polyps in the colon with nonsteroidal anti-inflammatory drugs (NSAIDs) shows promising results, according to *Medical World News* (30,18:23).

NSAIDs are effective because they limit the production of prostaglandins, a type of fatty acid found in large amounts in tumors.

Taken daily, an NSAID called indomethacin stopped polyp formation in 11 patients who had already undergone surgery to remove colon tumors. More studies are planned.

Common bean and pea help reduce the risk of cancer

It's no longer a secret — the food on your dinner plate can greatly influence your health. In fact, if you choose your menu wisely, you can actually build a line of defense against cancer.

The common bean and pea are two kinds of those cancer-fighting foods, reports *Nutrition and Cancer* (14,2:85). In a recent study, people who frequently ate legumes (beans, peas, lentils, soybeans, etc.) cut their risk of colon and rectal cancer in half.

The secret behind the anti-cancer effects of legumes is a substance known as protease inhibitor (PI). Protease inhibitor is a strong anti-cancer ingredient, and legumes contain high concentrations of this cancer-fighting substance.

Another plus: Adding more foods with a high PI content to your diet helps protect you from colon and rectal cancer without causing any adverse side effects.

'Skin tags' provide clues for detecting colon cancer

Just about every second person over the age of 50 has skin tags. These are little tumor stalks or flaps that protrude from the skin surface in the armpits, neck and groin area.

Usually skin tags cause no problems. But, researchers are beginning to wonder whether the little stalks and flaps might be an early clue to tumors of the colon and rectum.

Colorectal tumors, of course, often turn into colon cancer. Cancer of the colon or rectum is a slow-growing disease that will kill 60,000 people in the United States this year, reports Dr. J.R. Varma in *The Journal of the American Board of Family Practice* (3,3:175).

Colon cancer, caught in its early stages, is curable 90 percent of the time, the report says.

Those with skin tags were twice as likely as the general population to have tumorous growths, called polyps, in the colon, according to the article. People under age 50 with skin tags were six times more likely to have colon polyps.

"Skin tags need to be considered a significant risk factor for polyps of the colon," says Dr. Varma. "I believe that [people] with large skin tags should be evaluated more closely."

That would include tests of bowel movements to look for hidden blood, X-rays using barium enemas and colonoscopy (viewing the inside of the colon through a tube).

Depression

A vitamin deficiency may lead to depression

Low levels of the B vitamin, folic acid, have been linked to depression by A. Missagh Ghadirian of McGill University in Montreal, says a report in *Psychosomatics*. Dr. Ghadirian found that folic acid supplements relieved depression in people who had a folic acid deficiency.

Depression, loss of appetite, dizziness, fatigue and shortness of breath are the first signs of a folic acid deficiency. Folic acid is a water-soluble vitamin, so extra amounts are usually passed out through the kidneys into the urine within 24 hours. Without regular folic acid, deficiency symptoms may occur after just 100 days of low folic acid intake.

Adults require 200 micrograms of folic acid daily. In addition, pregnant women need 400 micrograms to help prevent birth defects. Nursing mothers should have 280 micrograms each day.

Folic acid is found naturally in yeast, liver, lima beans, whole-grain products, leafy green vegetables, oranges, asparagus, turnips, peanuts, oats, potatoes and beans. Folic acid dissolves in cooking water when foods are heated, so raw foods are a better source of this vitamin. Many things can interfere with the body's proper absorption of folic acid. Even if you are getting the daily requirement, your body may not be able to use it.

Oral contraceptives, aspirin, acetaminophen (like Tylenol and Panadol), Dilantin, primidone, phenobarbital, methotrexate, pyrimethamine, triamterene and high doses of vitamin C reduce the amount of folic acid available for the body to use.

The percentage of depressed people who are actually suffering from a folic acid deficiency is not known, the report said.

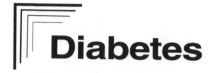

Diabetes

You may be diabetic and not know it

The American Diabetes Association (ADA) estimates that five million Americans have diabetes and don't know it. Here are the warning signs the ADA lists:

- Overweight and over the age of 40
- Excessive thirst
- Easily tired
- Diabetes history in the family
- Change or blurring in vision
- Frequent urination
- Sores heal slowly

If you or anyone you know shows these symptoms, the ADA advises you to get a doctor's help immediately.

Check your feet for blood sugar disorder

The ulcer that has developed on your foot recently may be a blessing in disguise. It could be the telltale sign that your doctor needs to diagnose a blood sugar disorder that has gone undetected for years.

According to a report in the *British Medical Journal* (300,6731:1046), about 15 percent of all diabetic people develop foot ulcers, and most foot ulcers are directly associated with diabetes. So, if you develop a foot ulcer, you have a strong chance of having diabetes.

Some studies have indicated that foot ulcers may be associated with smoking, although many scientists doubt this theory. Foot ulcers have also been linked with other disorders such as vascular disease (blood vessel disease).

Because a foot ulcer could have various causes or even several causes, it is important for you to have it evaluated right away to avoid further complications.

Researchers recommend that if you develop a foot ulcer, you should check with your doctor immediately for a diabetes test and possibly go to a special diabetic service for a full evaluation.

A little table sugar may be safe for some diabetics

There may be sweet news on the horizon for some diabetics. Adding sucrose to their restricted diets had no bad effects on a small group of Type-II (non-insulin-dependent) diabetics, according to an Australian study. Sucrose is a natural sweetener that most of us know in its refined form as table sugar.

"Our study suggests that the controlled use of sucrose can be considered in certain [diabetic] individuals," researchers report in *The American Journal of Clinical Nutrition* (50,3:474). The results of this and other studies may redefine the traditional dietary guidelines for diabetics.

Diabetics cannot process natural sugars efficiently. So, until now, they have been told to avoid table sugar completely. Diabetics regularly use artificial sweeteners such as aspartame.

The researchers studied nine people whose diabetes was well under control. None were taking insulin, and all were in good health. Three were treated with diet only, and six were treated with diet and a drug used to control diabetes.

Researchers randomly assigned participants to one of two groups for six weeks. One group received one and one-half ounces of sucrose daily, and the second received about five and one-half ounces of aspartame, the amount equivalent in sweetness to sucrose.

The participants did not suffer any harmful effects from the supplements and were able to process sugar effectively, even without the drug.

Total cholesterol, high-density lipoprotein (HDL or "good") cholesterol and triglycerides (a type of fat in the bloodstream) "were not significantly different" at the end of each study period, compared with the levels measured before the study began. The same held true for blood-sugar and insulin levels.

Researchers "caution against overinterpreting the results," emphasizing the following:

❏ The form of sucrose used is important. Participants used sucrose as an additive, only in coffee or tea or on breakfast cereal. High-fat, high-sugar baked goods were not evaluated.

❏ Participants must be followed up for long-term side effects.

❏ Regular "diabetic-type" diet is important. Studies in which sucrose supplemented a high-carbohydrate diet had poor results.

❏ The study size was small, only nine people. Much larger studies are necessary for more precision in determining accurate results that might apply to most Type-II diabetics.

If you are a diabetic, don't try this experiment on your own. Check with your doctor before making any change in your diet or treatment program.

New sweetener safe and ideal for diabetics

Diabetics and dieters! Have you ever wanted a sweetener that is safe, sweet and tasty? Well, thanks to some Danish scientists, you may soon have one, claims *The American Journal of Clinical Nutrition* (52,4:675).

The Jerusalem artichoke can provide a kind of natural sugar called fructan that might fulfill all of your requirements for a sweetener.

This new sweetener has two main benefits:

❏ Low in calories. Fructan has long molecules instead of the short molecules found in most common sugars. Your body cannot absorb the long fructan molecules very well. This means that you may take in a lot of calories by using the sweetener, but you won't have to suffer the consequences because your body can't "use" the sugar.

❏ Stabilizes blood sugar levels. Fructan does not appear to cause a drastic change in blood sugar levels.

Eating carbohydrates usually raises blood glucose levels. But, when fructan is used, the blood sugar levels appear to be lowered instead of raised. And fructan seems to reduce the body's need for insulin, which is great news for diabetics!

Scientists are still researching and studying fructan, but some forms of fructan are already on the market. If you are on a special diet or are taking insulin or other medicines, check with your doctor before using fructan products.

Diabetics die from excess of fat

Diabetics are dying "from an excess of fat," according to *The Journal of the American Medical Association* (262,3:398). Heart and artery disease are the leading causes of death among diabetics.

Research shows that high cholesterol levels as well as weight problems are a danger to diabetics. Despite these facts, most diabetics are not aware of their own cholesterol levels. Even some diabetics who know they have high cholesterol levels are not being treated correctly, a University of Texas study reveals.

More than 40 percent of the people with diabetes had high levels of blood lipids (a cholesterol measurement), says a study in *The Journal of the American Medical Association* (262,3:360). Less than one-fourth of the nondiabetic population has blood-lipid levels that high.

Twenty-three percent of the diabetics also had additional risk factors — high triglyceride levels or low levels of HDL (high-density lipoproteins). The problem is compounded because less than a fourth of the diabetics with cholesterol problems knew that they had problems.

What's worse, only 10 percent of the diabetics studied were receiving treatment for their cholesterol problems, notes Dr. Michael Stern, who led the study. "We suspect that the low level of awareness and treatment … is probably a general phenomenon," says Stern.

"An excess of fat, an excess of fat in the body [obesity], an excess of fat in the diet, and an excess of fat in the blood" were considered a cause of heart and artery disease in diabetics as early as 1927, an editorial in *JAMA* notes.

"Despite the seven decades that have passed and the considerable knowledge that has been gained since that time, physicians continue to pay little attention to the control of plasma lipid disorders in their diabetic patients," *JAMA* says.

The study by Dr. Stern and an editorial by Dr. George Steiner warn that doctors and diabetic patients must become more aware of the dangers of high cholesterol.

Both patient and doctor must learn to treat the dangerous condition through proper diet, through weight reduction, or, if necessary, with prescription drugs. "Important though it may be, glycemic [blood sugar] control is not sufficient to provide the best treatment for a diabetic patient," Steiner says.

The American Diabetic Association now recommends that all diabetics have their cholesterol levels checked regularly. The test should produce a fasting lipid profile, including total cholesterol levels, high-density lipoproteins (HDL), low-density lipoproteins (LDL) and triglycerides.

Each person should keep a personal record of each cholesterol test result to help increase awareness and to provide information in case of an emergency. If your levels are not within the National Cholesterol Education Guidelines, work with your physician to reach safe levels.

High-carbohydrate diet
may be risky for diabetics

To lower heart-disease risk, the American Heart Association (AHA) recommends a low-fat, high-carbohydrate diet for all Americans. Some researchers contend a high-carbohydrate diet may be harmful for people who are insulin-resistant — namely, diabetics — and cannot process large amounts of carbohydrates, says a report in *Science News* (136,12:185).

Both the AHA and the American Diabetes Association (ADA) recommend that carbohydrates make up 50 to 60 percent of daily caloric intake. Some researchers believe that percentage is too high.

"When patients who have non-insulin-dependent diabetes are given this so-called 'good' diet, they have marked increases in triglycerides and a significant decrease in HDL cholesterol," says diet researcher Ann M. Coulston of Stanford University. "And in patients with diabetes, a rise in triglycerides is associated with an increased risk of cardiovascular disease."

Coulston advocates a diet of 40 to 45 percent total carbohydrates. She and her colleagues conducted a six-week study, giving 12 diabetics two diets for six weeks at a time. Carbohydrates made up 40 percent of total calories in the first diet, and 60 percent in the second (the recommended amount).

"Diabetics on the 60 percent diet had a 30 percent rise in serum triglycerides and a 9 percent decrease in HDL," according to Coulston's report at an ADA meeting.

Pea fiber: good news for diabetics

Danish researchers say the kind of dietary fiber found naturally in peas helps smooth out the usual sharp rise in blood sugar levels right after a meal. That's good news for diabetics because they sometimes have trouble controlling their levels of "postprandial glycemia" (sugar in the blood after a meal).

An added bonus: Used in regular baked products, the pea fiber tastes OK too, says the report in *The American Journal of Clinical Nutrition* (50,2:324). "Because the palatability is good, it may prove a valuable food additive for diabetics," the report states.

The researchers compared the beneficial effects of a commercial brand of pea fiber available in Denmark to comparable amounts of wheat bran and beet fiber. "The postprandial blood glucose response was markedly reduced by the pea fiber," the report says.

The wheat bran and beet fiber had almost no effect on either blood glucose or serum insulin levels, the researchers say.

The pea fiber used is a white, almost tasteless granulated powder that is easily baked into bread. About two-thirds of pea fiber is the water-soluble type. The added pea fiber had no effect on normal bowel movement schedules, the study says.

Only one patient reported any side effects: a feeling of fullness after eating the test meal. The meal contained 30 grams (just over one ounce) of pea fiber in a mixture of ground beef and two kinds of sugar.

Pass the pasta to conserve chromium and avoid diabetes

The spaghetti you eat today may help keep you healthy tomorrow! Researchers now believe that eating a diet that conserves the mineral chromium may prevent the development of a form of diabetes called Type-II diabetes.

This form of diabetes usually affects adults over forty who are overweight. The people who risk developing this non-insulin-dependent form of diabetes are not able to absorb the blood sugar (glucose) from their bloodstreams properly and are said to be "glucose intolerant."

Your doctor can give you a simple test that will reveal whether you have mild glucose intolerance, the condition that precedes Type-II diabetes. If you are mildly glucose-intolerant, don't worry! You may still be able to avoid diabetes with certain changes in your diet.

The key is to increase the amount of chromium in your body. According to *Science News* (137,14:214), chromium can improve your ability to use blood sugar and help prevent the development of Type-II diabetes.

Unfortunately, it's not that easy to increase your chromium. You can eat high-chromium foods like meat, cheese, whole-grain breads and cereals, broccoli, potatoes, and some fruits, wines and beers. But your body can't easily absorb the chromium from all these natural sources.

Researchers suggest another approach to try in combination with a chromium-rich diet: Stay away from foods rich in simple sugars such as fructose and glucose. These foods cause your body to excrete large amounts of chromium.

On the other hand, eating foods that are high in complex carbohydrates, such as pasta, will help you conserve the chromium in your body.

Ask your doctor's advice. If you have mild glucose intolerance, or even if you have already developed Type-II diabetes, you may be able to improve your glucose tolerance just by changing your diet.

Magnesium helps lower blood pressure in Type-II diabetes

It seems that eating a fresh green salad with lunch every day may help lower your blood pressure if you suffer from high blood pressure and Type-II diabetes.

What's so great about a green salad? you ask.

Green, leafy vegetables found in fresh salads are good sources of the mineral magnesium. Magnesium is an important mineral in the human body, and studies show that a magnesium deficiency may contribute to high blood pressure, reports *Science News* (138,12:189).

Eating green vegetables every day helps increase the amount of magnesium in the body. And a magnesium-enriched diet may help lower high blood pressure by relaxing constricted (tightened) blood vessels.

Recent studies suggest that people with high blood pressure and Type-II diabetes have low levels of magnesium in their red blood cells. So, researchers think that many Type-II diabetics could help control their high blood pressure by taking magnesium supplements or by eating foods rich in magnesium.

However, they warn that magnesium supplements could be dangerous for some diabetics. Apparently, some people with diabetes experience kidney problems that could result in dangerously high levels of magnesium in the blood. Therefore, researchers recommend that all diabetic people consult their doctors before taking any magnesium supplements.

Blood pressure drugs may trigger some diabetes cases

Diabetes in middle-aged men may be brought on by prescription drugs used to lower high blood pressure, according to a new report in the *British Medical Journal* (298,6681:1147).

Men treated for high blood pressure were more likely to develop diabetes than men with normal blood pressure who were not taking medication, says Dr. Einar T. Skarfors, leader of the nine-year study in Sweden.

Treatment with blood pressure drugs seemed to be most harmful in men who were "predisposed" to diabetes, Skarfors explained. Men with high risk factors for diabetes, like an immediate relative with diabetes, a low insulin index or an extremely high blood pressure (before the drug therapy), were most likely to develop diabetes while on blood-pressure-reducing drugs.

The study focused on the second number in a blood pressure reading, known as the diastolic pressure. It measures the pressure of blood in the arteries while the heart rests between beats.

According to the *BMJ*, "the incidence of diabetes was seven times higher among men whose diastolic blood pressure had been greater than 105 mm Hg [prior to drug therapy] than among those in whom it had been less than 85 mm Hg." A diastolic level of less than 85 mm Hg is considered normal. But a reading of more than 105 is considered high and a potential health risk.

Today's most commonly prescribed blood pressure drugs "may cause a decrease in insulin sensitivity which does not disappear with time," according to the report. Continued use of these blood-pressure-reducing drugs may actually trigger diabetes, the report says.

The study "does not prove" that this drug therapy causes some cases of diabetes. But it does support the theory that long-term treatment with blood-pressure-reducing drugs may increase the chance of developing diabetes, Skarfors writes.

The prescription drugs taken by the men in the study were propranolol, hydralazine, atenolol, metoprolol and thiazide diuretics (also known as water pills).

A way to slow the onset of diabetic blindness

Some degree of vision loss is inevitable for nearly every diabetic, according to Dr. Ronald Klein, ophthalmologist at the University of Wisconsin Medical School. The vision problems facing 11 million American diabetics result from a condition known as diabetic retinopathy. It's the leading cause of new blindness in the United States for people between 20 and 75.

But there's new hope for lessening the damage caused by the disease, says a report in *Medical Tribune* (30,20:1). Aspirin and a tight control of blood sugar levels seem to put the brakes on the progress of retinopathy, says Dr. Harold Rifkin, clinical professor of medicine at New York's Albert Einstein College of Medicine. That's especially true in the early stages of the disease.

Researchers in British and French studies found that giving a diabetic an aspirin tablet (330 milligrams) three times daily slowed the deterioration of tiny arteries feeding the eyes. Also, diabetics who stick close to doctor-recommended dietary guidelines and keep blood sugar levels under tight control have less vision loss.

Severe cases of retinopathy now are treated by laser flashes that promote clotting of tiny eye hemorrhages. Untreated retinopathy can lead to blindness.

One symptom of the problem is cotton-wool spots — white spots with fuzzy borders — in the field of view. Others include blurred vision and small black spots ("floaters") that move in the field of vision as the eye moves.

Every diabetic patient should get regular eye checkups from an ophthalmologist who has a special interest in diabetes, recommends Dr. Jeanne L. Rosenthal, attending surgeon at the New York City Eye and Ear Infirmary.

Check with your doctor about the benefits of aspirin for diabetics.

This 'hot' cream gives pain relief

For people who haven't been able to find relief from the pain and discomfort of diabetic neuropathy and pain after surgery, scientists have a "new" remedy.

The "new" is actually a reproduction of the old, only a little stronger and more effective. The new remedy is a stronger formula of nonprescription capsaicin cream. Capsaicin is made from one of the natural ingredients that makes peppers hot.

According to a news digest in *Geriatrics* (45,8:19), most people who use the new, stronger cream report improvements in sleeping, walking, working and recreation. The only drawback — capsaicin may cause stinging and redness of the skin for the first few days of use. However, those minor problems disappear within three or four days.

An extra benefit is that capsaicin gets into the skin but not into your system, so it is safe to use even if you are taking several other medications, says the report.

Digestive Disorders

Blood with bowel movements

One of the more unsettling personal experiences is discovering the presence of blood after a bowel movement. The important question is: When is blood mixed with bowel movements only a minor irritation, and when is it potentially very serious?

"Rectal bleeding of any degree is always alarming," says *The Lancet* (1,8631:195), "with the fear of cancer being uppermost in the patient's mind."

However, the report went on to note that traces of blood on toilet paper are relatively common and should not be cause for great worry. "A little blood on the paper after defecation is noticed by about one in seven of the adult population," the report states. But, "blood in the lavatory pan [toilet bowl] or mixed with the stool [bowel movement], a far more important observation, is seen in only 2 to 3 percent and generally leads to hospital referral," the researchers said.

The general rule of thumb is that if the blood is actually mixed with the bowel movement or is in amounts great enough to stain the water in the toilet bowl, in all cases a doctor should be consulted. But, *The Lancet* said, even most of those cases turn out to be more worrisome than dangerous, and most will not require further treatment. In other words, using the report's statistics, out of 1,000 people, about 142 people occasionally will notice a little blood on the toilet paper after a bowel movement.

Of that 142, only about 20 or 30 people will have blood mixed with the fecal material itself, an indication of bleeding higher up the anus or intestinal tract and a sign that a doctor's examination is needed.

Of those 30, doctors' examinations and hospital tests will show about nine will have "sizable," noncancerous polyps (benign tumors) in the bowel or colon. Of those same 30 persons, three will be found to have cancerous growths in the bowel tract, according to the figures given in *The Lancet* report.

Dealing with diarrhea

The most important thing you can do if you're suffering from diarrhea is to replace the fluids your body is losing, says a report in *Medical Abstracts*

(10,2:2). Even if you're nauseated and sick at your stomach, you need to try to force some liquids down.

Try to take frequent small sips of liquids such as Gatorade, fruit drinks, chicken broth without fat, and nondiet, noncaffeinated soft drinks. Try to drink at least two quarts of liquids a day. And drink three quarts if you have a fever, the report suggests.

Do you abuse laxatives?

Do you have diarrhea, cramping, nausea and vomiting, but your doctor can't find anything wrong with you? If you use laxatives, you may be overdoing it, says a report in *Medical World News* (31,1:19).

Regularity doesn't necessarily mean daily bowel movements, the article points out. Many people don't realize the dangers associated with laxatives and thus use them much too often.

Laxative abuse is commonly defined as using a laxative at least once a week over a period of several months, according to the report.

"Patients risk nutritional deficiencies, metabolic disorders, and potentially severe damage to the gastrointestinal tract with regular, long-term use of laxatives," according to experts at an American College of Gastroenterology meeting. Over-the-counter laxative abuse is very hard to diagnose because the symptoms are similar to those of other common intestinal disorders. And doctors often fail to ask about laxatives when questioning patients about medication use.

If you think you are overusing laxatives, experts suggest that you eat more foods high in dietary fiber, drink more fluids and begin a progressive exercise program. That combination will give you the same results as the laxatives without the harmful side effects of laxative overuse.

How to put brakes on breaking wind

Benjamin Franklin called it, "Breaking wind." Some say, "Passing gas." The technical term is flatulence, and it has been the source of everything from off-color fraternity jokes for college students to serious attacks of pain — and social embarrassment — for some sufferers.

Almost everybody experiences up to a dozen episodes daily of passing gas. It's the normal by-product of healthy digestion. Unfortunately, in some cases, that gas also can become trapped in folds of the colon and cause mild to severe pain. "It may feel like a knife stabbing the chest or abdomen," says Dr. John H. Renner. Because the pain can be severe and occurs in areas close to the heart and stomach, many sufferers fear the pain may signal more serious problems like heart disease and ulcers, even cancer.

The gas itself is caused by fermentation, the same process that makes wine. Bacteria are normally present in the digestive tract, according to a report from the American Digestive Disease Society. When the bacteria work on the undigested parts of a big meal, one by-product is a mixture of gases, including hydrogen sulfide (the familiar rotten egg odor) and smelly residues of fatty acids.

Several things contribute to excess flatulence and gas pain, Renner says. Here are the main ones:

❑ **The kinds of food we eat.** Almost everybody gets gas from eating beans. That's because beans contain two kinds of starches that bacteria love to ferment and that the body can't break down and absorb first. Other problem foods include onions, brussels sprouts, raisins, prune juice, apricots, celery, carrots, bananas, bagels, wheat germ and pretzels, not necessarily in that order.

Sometimes a combination of otherwise innocent foods will trigger excess gas. Keep track of what you eat, compare that with when you experience gas discomfort, and tailor your diet accordingly.

❑ **Sudden switch to more high-fiber foods.** Most of us need more fiber in our daily diet. But one of the prices we have to pay may be increased flatulence. "Start with a small dose of fiber so the bowel gets used to it," advises Dr. Michael Mogadam of Georgetown University. "That lessens the increase in flatus." After about two weeks on an increased fiber diet, most people's gas production returns to normal levels.

❑ **Lactase deficiency.** Some people lose the ability to digest milk and milk products efficiently because of a shortage of a digestive enzyme, lactase. Undigested milk sugar gets to the colon and becomes a ripe target for gas-producing bacteria. Try a milk-free diet for two weeks to see if episodes of excess gas decrease. Your doctor can help you zero in on the cause.

❑ **Swallowing air.** Some people actually gulp down large volumes of air while smoking, chewing gum, eating or drinking. Taking smaller bites, chewing them longer, and swallowing smaller amounts of liquid smoothly, without gulping, will help solve that problem. If chewing gum or smoking are the culprits, abandon the guilty habits. And if you feel like belching, don't help the process, Renner says. Trying to belch just draws in more air, adding to the problem.

❑ **Anxiety.** Being over-anxious or "stressed out" can bring on flatulence. Doctors think stress gives rise to overeating, poor eating habits and impaired digestion processes, all combining to produce excess gas.

When avoiding certain foods or beverages doesn't solve the problem, Renner suggests an over-the-counter product containing simethicone. Simethicone breaks down large gas bubbles trapped in colon folds and may ease painful flare-ups.

The doctor suggests that activated charcoal tablets, available without prescription at most druggists, may also help by absorbing excess gas.

The problem with charcoal is that it also absorbs needed minerals and interferes with many medications. Check with your doctor before using either product.

Bananas for indigestion pain?

Bothered by indigestion pain? Eat a banana!

That's the essence of a study by researchers in India, reports *The Lancet* (335,8689:612).

They took 40 people — each of whom had experienced many months of stomach pain and nausea but who had no ulcers — and tried a natural remedy on half of them.

The researchers gave 20 of them capsules containing banana powder — eight capsules a day for eight weeks. The second group of 20 took nothing for the discomfort. All of them stayed away from antacids or ulcer medicines. By study's end, half of those who took banana pills reported complete relief, and another one-fourth received at least some relief from their constant indigestion problems. In the other group, 16 out of 20 (80 percent) still had indigestion problems.

Bananas are a common food in India, and many Indians also use banana powder, a dried and ground-up form of the fruit, the report says.

Banana powder also protects the stomach lining from irritation by aspirin and some other drugs, say the report authors, and has been used with some success in treating ulcer symptoms. No side effects were reported.

Spice for life

Ginger is believed by some to be one of the better natural stomach "medicines" around.

Ginger seems to help prevent stomach ulcers, says a digest in *HerbalGram* (20:23).

It also is used commonly to prevent or calm motion sickness, morning sickness, or just general nausea.

A real-life home health story — the wonders of psyllium

Here is a personal story about the healing power of soluble dietary fiber in the digestive tract.

A friend of mine, Susan, had a serious problem with bleeding from the rectum. She had much pain, and it seemed that the problem was more than simply hemorrhoids. She went to her doctor, and his diagnosis was anal fissure, a serious tear or slit in the rectum. He recommended that she have an operation to correct the problem, but he couldn't guarantee that it would be completely successful.

Susan asked her doctor if there was an alternative to surgery, and he suggested that she try a natural soluble fiber dietary supplement containing psyllium, sold in every drug store.

Susan chose the natural treatment. She mixed a spoonful of orange-flavored psyllium powder in water to make a tasty beverage which she drank once a day. With the soothing effect of the supplement, her body healed, and she has experienced no more pain, bleeding or discomfort.

Drinking Water

What you can do about fluoride in your water

Because having fluoride in drinking water is thought by many people to be beneficial, most water filter manufacturers don't buck prevailing wisdom by advertising products that remove fluoride.

Removing fluoride from your water probably isn't a good idea unless you know that your water contains unusually high or possibly toxic levels of fluoride. Some areas of the country have more fluoride in the water than others because of the presence of mineral deposits near rivers, streams and lakes. While municipal water supplies are required by the state and federal government to be monitored regularly, no one is required to keep a check on private well water.

What can you do if you find out you are consuming harmful amounts of fluoride? There are no products available in the United States specifically designed to remove fluorine compounds from home tap water, according to Tom Snee, an official of Intec Corp. of Eagan, Minn.

The company makes whole-house units that combine electronic and absorption methods to filter various materials from drinking water. "There's nothing on the market right now just for fluorine," Snee says. But, even though manufacturers don't advertise it, activated charcoal units remove some of the fluorides in drinking water, Snee says. If you want to cut down the level of fluoride in your tap water, a simple activated charcoal filter is about as good as anything currently available, Snee indicates.

The truth about 'bottled water'

If you are trying to drink more water every day, you may be among millions of Americans who want something other than what comes out of your home faucet. But, much bottled water may not be any better than water straight from your own tap. In fact, some bottled water comes straight from somebody else's tap.

Bottled water is defined by the U.S. government as "water that is sealed in bottles or other containers and intended for human consumption," according to the *Journal of Nutrition for the Elderly* (8,1:73).

Twenty-five percent of bottled water doesn't come from protected springs and wells at all, but from municipal water systems, reports the June 1993 *FDA Consumer* (27,5:10). That water may not even be as good for you as your own tap water.

In January 1993, the FDA announced proposed regulations that would set strict standards for bottled water products, reports the June 1993 *FDA Consumer*. You should read the label and the list of ingredients on the bottled water carefully to determine which of the following FDA-defined categories the water falls into.

Many brands use as part of their brand name the word "spring," but that may have nothing to do with the origin of the water in the bottle.

- ❐ **Spring water** — If the list of ingredients says spring water, the U.S. Food and Drug Administration requires that the bottled water come from a deep underground source that flows naturally to the surface, or would flow naturally to the surface if it weren't collected underground through a bore hole first. Again, forget the brand name. Look at the list of ingredients on the label.

- ❐ **Artesian water** — This is water from a rock formation in which the water level stands above the natural water table.

- ❐ **Distilled water** — This is water that is "distilled" (vaporized then condensed) to remove its dissolved mineral content.

- ❐ **Purified water** — This is distilled water that meets the standards of the U.S. Pharmacopeia. It is commonly used in laboratories and for medical purposes.

- ❐ **Mineral water** — Under the newly proposed FDA regulations, mineral water will, for the first time, have to meet bottled water standards. Mineral water must come from a geologically and physically protected underground water source.

The FDA's regulations don't include "carbonated" water, "seltzer" water, "soda" water and "tonic" water. These water types are considered soft drinks.

- ❐ **Club soda** — This is just tap water that has artificial carbonation added to it, as well as mineral salts added for flavoring. It also probably has been filtered.

- ❐ **Seltzer** — Like club soda, this is artificially carbonated, filtered tap water, except it has no mineral salts added. Usually, it's also salt-free.

- ❐ **Sparkling water** — May be either naturally or artificially carbonated.

Some naturally carbonated water has carbonation added to it during bottling to keep the carbonation level consistent.

❑ **Flavored water** — May be any of the above types with either natural or artificial flavoring added to it, including sugar or sweetening. Under the new FDA regulations, certain types of flavored bottled water will have to comply with regulations limiting the amount of contaminants in the water.

Drink more water to fight confusion

Everyone dreads senility and the destruction of the mind that comes with Alzheimer's disease and some kinds of strokes. But not all mental confusion is so hopeless and incurable.

The signs and symptoms of dementia can, in some cases, be cured just by drinking water, according to reports in *Gerontological Nursing* (16,5:4) and *Senior Health Digest*.

Simple dehydration — loss of too much of the body's water supply — can bring on mental confusion, disorientation, seizures and other problems. As many as four out of 10 elderly people admitted to hospitals for dehydration die from complications brought on by fluid loss. The treatment is fairly simple: Drink at least two-and-a-half pints of fluids, especially water, every day, says the report.

Some seniors stay in a constant state of dehydration, simply because their mouths don't tell them that they need water. They don't feel thirsty even though their bodies may be suffering from lack of fluids. The thirst response gets rusty with increased age, lagging by two or three days. In other words, your body might need water on Monday, but you might not get the thirst message until Wednesday.

That's bad any time of year, but hot weather raises the danger level. During hot weather, you need to drink more fluids to keep your body properly cooled and to make up for fluid lost in sweating. In addition, blood flow to the skin can be 50 percent lower in people over 65, says the *Digest*. That further lowers the body's cooling ability.

To be on the safe side, suggests *New Health Tips Encyclopedia* (FC&A Publishing), drink enough fluids to keep the urine a pale yellow in color, not dark. Dark or cloudy urine might indicate you're not getting enough water.

During hot weather, weigh yourself daily, and drink a pint of water for every pound that you lose, whether you feel thirsty or not, researchers suggest.

Check with your doctor about your fluid needs and how best to meet them.

Exercise and Fitness

Why aerobic exercise is so good for your heart

Exercise reduces your risk of heart disease because it speeds up the removal of triglycerides, a common form of fat, from the bloodstream, says new research from Rockefeller University.

In one study, carefully controlled workouts reduced fasting blood levels of triglycerides by 16 percent. Exercise reduced levels of triglycerides in the blood by 32 percent after a fat-containing meal.

Triglycerides flood the bloodstream after a meal and deposit part of their unneeded fatty load onto the walls of arteries. That dumping of fat onto the artery walls sets the stage for a heart attack, the scientists say in a report in *Circulation* (79,5:1007).

The men in the study completed 29 half-hour sessions of jogging on a treadmill over a period of seven weeks. The men jogged an average of 15 miles per week. "Based on our results, we think the primary effect of exercise training on lipoprotein metabolism is to increase clearance of triglyceride-rich particles from the blood," says Dr. Jan L. Breslow, head of the university's biochemical genetics and metabolism laboratory. "This may be one mechanism whereby exercise might reduce the risk of coronary heart disease."

The investigators noticed that exercise caused a significant increase in activity of an enzyme, lipoprotein lipase. This enzyme breaks down the triglyceride in the dietary fat particles.

In addition, a test to evaluate the men's physical fitness showed their maximum oxygen consumption increased 43 percent as a result of the exercise program. The test results showed that the men developed better fitness at the same time they decreased their blood-fat levels, the scientists say. This is the first study that separates the effects of exercise from those of diet change and weight loss, which can also reduce blood levels of triglycerides, says Breslow. "During the exercise phase of the study, we increased the calories in their diet slightly so they wouldn't lose weight."

Weight loss is well-known as a means of lowering lipoprotein levels, the researchers note, so "from a clinical view, the great benefit [to patients] would be to combine exercise and weight loss."

Doctors have known for years that exercise helps prevent heart disease. But until this study, scientists didn't know exactly how exercise helps to do that.

Just a little exercise goes a long way

People who completely avoid any physical activity run a 30 percent higher risk of developing coronary heart disease than more active people, according to Martha L. Slattery, a researcher at the University of Utah Medical School.

Slattery found that even the lightest physical activity has a protective, beneficial effect on health in general and the heart in particular. "Small amounts of activity offered protection, and ... little increase in protection is noted for larger amount of physical activity," says the study in the journal *Circulation* (79: 304). The benefits of exercise were not limited to heart disease protection — light physical activity reduced death from all causes. "Increasing physical activity, particularly of light-to-moderate intensity, is appropriate to prevent disease and promote health," the authors say.

Since the late 1950s, Slattery and her research team have been studying the health history and leisure-time physical activity of 3,043 white, male railroad workers whose jobs ranged from strenuous physical activity to desk work. Their leisure-time physical activities were classified as light, moderate or intense.

Light activity ranged from walking for pleasure to bowling or raking the lawn. Ballroom dancing and gardening were considered part of the moderate activities, while backpacking, jogging and snow shoveling, among others, were classified as intense activities.

In a follow-up period that lasted 17 to 20 years, the researchers looked at the leisure-time physical activity habits of the men and compared them to causes of death among those who died. They found that people who reported higher levels of physical activity had lower rates of heart disease.

And their findings confirm what other researchers have also seen. "You do not require a lot of activity to get a protective effect," Slattery says.

Statistics show that death rates from diseases of the heart and blood vessels were lower for men who used 1,000 or more calories a week in leisure-time physical activity. That is the equivalent of spending 30 minutes a day in some moderately intense activity, such as playing softball or weeding the garden.

But after taking into account such primary heart disease risk factors as smoking, high blood pressure and elevated cholesterol, the researchers concluded that "the greatest increase in protection was between those men who were sedentary and those who had some activity," Slattery says.

In other words, desk jockeys and couch potatoes get a great deal of added protection against heart attacks and other diseases just by hoeing weeds in the yard or taking a brisk walk several times a week.

Another study reported in *The Journal of the American Medical Association* (262,17:2395) and *Medical World News* (31,5:20) confirms that moderate, regular exercise decreases heart-attack risk.

Regular exercisers also are less likely to suffer from stroke, high blood pressure and some forms of cancer, the study says.

A person "does not need an athletic level of fitness to get a lot of benefit in terms of preventing early death," stated Dr. Steven Blair, director of epidemiology at the Institute for Aerobics Research in Dallas, at a seminar sponsored by the American Heart Association.

Dr. Blair believes the medical profession needs to recognize that poor physical fitness is a leading cause of early death. To prove his theory, he conducted a study of 10,224 men and 3,120 women and the effects of their exercise habits. None of the participants had ever had a stroke, diabetes, heart attack or high blood pressure — conditions that would have influenced the results.

Before the study began the men and women were given treadmill tests to determine their beginning level of fitness, then divided into three categories — low, moderate or high fitness groups. The three groups were studied for about eight years.

Over the eight year period, there were 240 deaths among the men and 43 deaths among the women. Without exception, the men and women in the low fitness categories experienced a higher death rate.

Among men, the primary causes of death were heart disease and cancer. Among women, cancer was the biggest killer, followed by "other illnesses." Heart disease ranked third for women.

The findings even showed that exercise provided extra protection for smokers and those with higher levels of cholesterol.

An editorial accompanying the *JAMA* report points out that time saving technology has decreased our activity levels, especially at home.

Do you use the remote control to change TV channels rather than get off the sofa to change them yourself? Use a riding lawn mower? An electric snow blower? Electric garage door opener? Conveniences such as these are turning Americans into couch potatoes.

Dr. Blair concludes that most men and women could reduce their risk of heart disease with the addition of very modest exercise. He recommends walking as the exercise that is easiest to mold into your lifestyle.

Of course, you should talk to your doctor before starting an exercise program, especially if you have health problems.

Personalize your walking time

As with any exercise, walking must be done regularly to get the greatest effects. Here are a few suggestions for developing a lifelong habit.

❑ First and foremost: Check with a doctor before establishing your walking routine!

❑ If you enjoy walking with others, choose a partner who shares your interest and will help you resist the temptation to occasionally "cut your walk short."

❑ If quiet moments are hard to find at your house, use your walk as special time apart from the crowd.

❑ Choose a route that offers either the comfort of familiarity, or the challenge of a different view, depending on your motivation.

❑ Use a miniature tape-player to listen to music, learn a new language, or "read-a-book" from the many available selections on cassettes.

❑ Make a personal commitment to "stick-to-it." It just might mean a longer life.

Choosing just the right 'equipment'

Like every sport, walking requires the right equipment. But since there are no balls, bats, rackets or clubs, we often overlook the one thing that is needed — proper shoes.

Here are a few suggestions from orthopedists, podiatrists and serious walkers on how to buy shoes that will help you put your best foot forward.

❑ Because it is recommended that you wear two pairs of socks (thin socks as a liner against the skin, and then a pair of thicker outer socks) to reduce friction and unwanted blisters, you should be wearing your socks when you test the new shoes for the proper fit.

❑ Never shop at a store that won't let you "get the feel" of your new shoes. Take your time. Walk around the store. Make sure you have the support and flexibility you'll need to keep you walking in comfort.

❑ Resist the urge to try on only one shoe. Since our right and left feet rarely match (they're usually slightly different sizes), it's best to put on both shoes. Remember, you need enough room to wiggle your toes — all ten of them!

❐ Don't shop for your shoes in the morning, since swelling feet can cause you to wear a half size larger by evening.

Finding your target heart rate and taking your pulse

To maximize your aerobic benefits from walking, it is best to find your target heart range and maintain it for at least 20 minutes.

1. Start with the number 220:	220
2. Subtract your age (50, for example):	-50
3. The answer is your maximum heart rate	170
4. Multiply your max. heart rate by 0.6:	170
(Low end of the target range; 60 percent)	x 0.6
	102
5. Multiply your max. heart rate by 0.8:	170
(High end of target range; 80 percent)	x 0.8
	136

If you are a beginner, always work at the lower end of your range. Only those already physically fit should attempt to achieve the 80 percent range.

Checking your pulse is easy if you have a watch with a second hand. Place your index and middle finger along the side of your neck, just below the jaw. Count the number of beats you feel for 15 seconds, then multiply by four to arrive at your heart rate.

If you have already determined what your target heart rate should be, you can then compare your walking heart rate with the rate you hope to achieve.

In this way you can keep your heart rate within safe limits without sacrificing your aerobic benefits.

No age limit on exercise benefits

Even elderly people who are frail can improve their overall health and mobility with appropriate exercises, say researchers at the University of Michigan School of Medicine. Such exercises may even keep some aged people out of nursing homes, says Tom Hickey, one of the researchers.

Seventy-five patients ranging in age from 65 to 98 tried a simple exercise program for six weeks. They tried "gentle neck and shoulder rolls, spinal twists, side stretches, feet and arm extensions, flexes and circles, and slow, deep breathing," according to the report in *Geriatrics* (44,6:13).

"Most of the patients were overweight and never exercised regularly," says the report. In addition, many of them suffered from arthritis, high blood pressure, diabetes, heart disease or a combination of the diseases.

They exercised twice a week in the program called SMILE, which stands for So Much Improvement with Little Exercise.

After six weeks, most of them reported less stiffness in the joints and said they had more energy. The researchers noted some drops in high blood pressure readings and in the times required to walk a certain distance.

"Regular exercise may prolong independent living and help keep frail older persons out of nursing homes," the researchers say.

Keep your brain young — walk!

Moderate exercise will increase your ability to reason and remember. And those abilities increase as activity levels increase, according to a report in *Psychology and Aging* (4,2:183).

"If people want to maintain mental abilities as they get older, they should exercise on a regular basis," says Dr. Louise Clarkson-Smith, an author of the report.

Scientists from the University of Southern California agree. Routine, easy aerobic exercise like walking may help the brain perform better as we get older, according to a new study. In animal tests, Dr. Mohamed A. Fahim found low levels of neurotransmitters in inactive animals and higher levels in animals that had exercised regularly.

Neurotransmitters help the brain communicate with muscles. With adequate levels of neurotransmitters, your brain can communicate with and control your muscles properly. But uncoordination and other signs of advanced aging will occur with low levels of neurotransmitters, Fahim discovered.

However, all is not lost if you have been leading an inactive life. Regular aerobic exercise can help restore the levels of neurotransmitters in about five months, Fahim concluded.

Aerobic exercise doesn't necessarily mean exhaustive workouts in a gym. Walking is one of the best overall aerobic exercises and is recommended for people of all ages. Just walking for 20 minutes, three times a week, will provide excellent aerobic activity.

Be sure to check with your doctor before starting a new exercise program.

Start jogging to boost levels of HDL cholesterol

If you have been trying to lose weight to control your cholesterol levels, you should consider taking up jogging. Men who have lost weight and started jogging show a marked boost in their HDL cholesterol levels, according to *Science News* (138,12:177).

HDL cholesterol is known as the "good" cholesterol, and high HDL levels help prevent coronary heart disease.

Interestingly, joggers who used to be overweight enjoyed higher HDL levels than joggers who had started out lean.

This does not mean that lean men should gain weight, then start jogging and lose weight just to get higher levels of HDL. It's simply an additional bonus for overweight men who become joggers.

Exercise raises risk of sudden death from irregular heartbeats?

Exercisers, you may face increased danger of sudden death from irregular heartbeats. It's not the physical activity itself that's the problem. It's the air you breathe while exercising.

You may be breathing in a variety of pollutants, including carbon monoxide and ozone. And that could trigger skipped heartbeats or irregular heart rhythms, says a report in the *Annals of Internal Medicine* (113,5:343). This increase in cardiac arrhythmias is dangerous because it increases a person's risk of sudden cardiac death.

These irregular heartbeats kill an estimated 350,000 people each year in the United States and represent the leading cause of sudden deaths from heart attack, says a digest in *Science News* (138,10:149).

The main sources of carbon monoxide in the environment are automobile exhaust and cigarette smoke, says an article in *The Physician and Sportsmedicine* (18,9:153).

Cigarette smoke is dangerous even if you don't smoke. Apparently, the secondary smoke from a cigarette contains more carbon monoxide than the directly inhaled smoke.

When carbon monoxide and ozone enter the blood, they decrease the body's ability to transport oxygen effectively. So, the heart has to work harder and beat faster to overcome the disability. This process is magnified during exercise, when the heart has to work harder anyway.

You also absorb a lot more pollutants as you gulp in lungfuls of air during vigorous exercise. However, the solution is not to stop exercising.

In fact, deep breathing of clean air during vigorous exercising can help clear the bloodstream of carbon monoxide.

To help avoid the dangers of air pollutants, observe the following safety precautions:

- Avoid exercising during peak traffic hours.

- Avoid exercising in bright sunlight. Ozone levels increase on sunny days.

- Exercise in open areas where the wind can disperse pollutants.

- Avoid resting under trees for long periods of time. Pollutants can get trapped under trees, making shady air "dirtier."

- Consider exercising indoors or in the country where pollutant levels are lower.

- Avoid smoking immediately before or after exercising. If you smoke after exercising, wait until you are breathing normally.

Help reduce dizziness with easy exercises

Dizziness is an irritating and ongoing problem that usually is caused by damage to one or both of your ears. The doctors tell you to get used to it because there's nothing you can do about it. They say the only thing you can do is avoid the motions or activities that bring on the dizziness.

That's all changed now, reports the *Medical Tribune* (31,20:2). Doctors recently have discovered that simple home exercises can help most people control or even eliminate their dizziness.

The best time to start exercises for dizziness is right after your ears are injured. Your ear doctor can test you for dizziness and choose special exercises for you to do at home. The exercises may be as simple as tilting your head from side to side as you sit in a chair, alternating standing on one foot at a time and then the other, or passing a ball back and forth above your head.

These exercises help reduce dizziness and increase physical strength. Although the exercises are not considered a cure, they may be the very best way for you to manage your dizziness and get back into a normal routine.

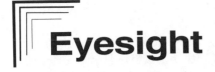

Eyesight

Set a date to save your sight

If you're over fifty, there's more reason to look at your calendar than just to remember an important date! Looking at the grid pattern on your calendar can reveal important changes in your vision that may actually help you save your sight.

After you reach 50, an important part of your eye called the macula may begin to break down a little bit. The macula is located at the back of your eye in the center of the retina, and it is the area of your eye that is most sensitive to light.

If the macula deteriorates, the middle of your field of vision becomes blurred or dark. This condition is called age-related macular degeneration (AMD). According to *Health After 50* (2,2:2), it affects about 25 percent of people over age 65 and 33 percent of those over 80.

If you have AMD, you may notice blurring or haziness in the center of your vision. Straight lines may look wavy, and you may not see colors as well as you used to. Fortunately, most people do not have serious vision loss from AMD.

However, people with AMD have about a 10 percent chance of developing a more serious condition called "wet" AMD. In wet AMD, tiny blood vessels at the back of the eye begin to leak, causing scarring and loss of central vision.

Health After 50 reports that wet AMD may develop suddenly at any time and cause rapid and severe vision loss within days or weeks.

This is where your calendar comes in. By monitoring your vision regularly, you can detect changes in it early enough to see your ophthalmologist right away and stop the damage caused by wet AMD.

Your doctor can give you an Amsler grid that looks much like a calendar to use when checking your vision.

Cover one eye and look at the Amsler grid or a calendar to see if the area on which you are focusing is clear or distorted. Then cover the other eye and check it.

If the center of the grid pattern looks broken, distorted or wavy to either eye, visit your doctor right away. An ophthalmologist can use laser treatment to stop the blood vessels from leaking and slow down the progress of wet AMD.

People suffering from AMD often are declared "legally blind" (less than 20/200 vision), says *The Merck Manual* (15th edition). However, these people usually have good peripheral vision and useful color vision, and they should be reassured that they won't lose all their vision.

There's no cure for AMD yet. But you can do two things to protect yourself from this cause of blindness.

See your eye doctor every year, and check your eyes with a calendar or an Amsler grid regularly. It could save you from serious vision loss.

(For information on devices for people with poor vision, write to American Foundation for the Blind Consumer Products Division, 15 West 16th Street, New York, N.Y. 10011.)

Prevent cataracts naturally

People who take regular daily doses of either vitamin C or vitamin E may slash by more than half their risk of developing blinding cataracts, a new scientific study suggests.

Those results come from a Canadian study of 175 cataract patients and 175 people without cataracts, according to a report in *Science News* (135,20:308). All those studied were over age 55.

"The scientists found that the only significant difference between the two groups, other than the presence of cataracts, was that the cataract-free individuals had taken at least 400 international units (one regular capsule) of vitamin E and/or a minimum of 300 milligrams of vitamin C per day over the last five years," the report says.

Most of the cataract-free people took only one of the two vitamins in the form of supplements.

Those who took extra vitamin C showed a risk reduction of 70 percent, the report says. Those who took vitamin E supplements had a 50 percent reduction in cataract risk.

This study backs up other recent research that shows dramatic blindness prevention benefits for people using these two vitamins.

One doctor, Charles Kelman, recommends taking 1,000 to 2,000 milligrams (one to two grams) of vitamin C (ascorbic acid) daily to help prevent cataracts. Scientists don't know for sure why the vitamins prevent the cloudy formations in aging eyes that are called cataracts.

Those clouds across the field of vision are caused by proteins being oxidized in the lens of the eye and then clumping together. (Proteins are "oxidized" when they combine with oxygen.) Some researchers believe that vitamins C and E, both of which are antioxidants, neutralize the lens proteins before they can clump together.

Two out of every 10 people between the ages of 60 and 75 in the United States have cataracts. The condition, which can lead to blindness, accounts for a half million surgical operations every year.

"If you could delay cataract formation by just ten years, you would eliminate the need for half of the cataract extractions," according to Allen Taylor, who works for the USDA Human Nutrition Research Center on Aging in Medford, Mass.

Cataracts may be caused or triggered by several things, including sunlight (ultraviolet rays), diabetes, steroids and X-rays.

However, vitamins C and E aren't the only powerful natural cataract fighters available. Beta-carotene, also an antioxidant, and riboflavin (vitamin B2) also may help prevent the eye-clouding growths.

People with higher than average intakes of vitamin C, vitamin E and beta-carotene "are at a reduced risk of cataract development," according to H. Gerster in a German study reported in *Z Ernahrungswiss* (28,1:56).

Studies by P. Jacques add that people with "high levels of at least two of the three vitamins [C, E and B2]" are at reduced risk of developing cataracts compared to people with low levels of these vitamins, reports *Archives of Ophthalmology* (106,3:337).

Harold Skalka has found that a deficiency of riboflavin (vitamin B2) can lead to cataract development, especially in older adults. "Older cataract patients had more riboflavin deficiency. An absence of riboflavin deficiency was found in our older patients with clear lenses," Skalka reports in *The American Journal of Clinical Nutrition* (34,5:861).

In earlier studies reported in *The Lancet* (8054:12-3), Skalka suggested that cataracts "may be corrected by dietary restrictions or supplements" of riboflavin.

Milk causes cataracts?

That second bowl of ice cream after supper could be increasing your risk of cataracts, warn researchers in *Science News* (137,12:189). The danger lies in the milk sugar galactose, which is found in most dairy products. This kind of milk sugar may hurt the lens of the eye if the sugar is not properly digested.

People who lack the ability to break down galactose run a four times greater risk of developing cataracts than those who digest it normally.

Even people who consume small amounts of dairy products risk cataract development if they cannot metabolize milk sugars. Ask your doctor about your chances of developing cataracts from dairy products.

Sun lovers more prone to cataracts

The more time you spend in the sun, the greater your risk of developing cataracts, researchers report in *Good Health Bulletin* (2,3:3).

Golfers, sailors and gardeners, for example, are exposed to more ultraviolet (UV) radiation than usual and should always wear sunglasses when outdoors — even on cloudy days. Look for sunglasses that block 100 percent of UV radiation.

Fatigued? It may be your eyes

With the fast-paced life of most Americans, many people seem to be suffering from fatigue. But the reason for your tiredness may be directly related to your eyesight.

People should make sure they are getting adequate sleep, daily exercise and a well-balanced diet before considering other causes of fatigue. However, many doctors warn that the eyes may be the key to unusual tiredness.

Old prescription glasses, improper contact lenses, or deteriorating eyesight can cause extreme fatigue, doctors warn. If you are tired, get an eye exam.

Using glasses or contacts that are not strong enough for your needs can put great strain on your eyes and zap your energy. An eye exam may uncover a visual problem that has been causing your tiredness.

People with high blood pressure, diabetes or a history of vision problems should have an eye exam by an ophthalmologist once a year. Everyone should see an eye doctor at least once every two years, according to the National Society to Prevent Blindness.

For elderly people on modest budgets or fixed incomes, a helping hand for eye treatment is available. The Eye Care Project Helpline is a toll-free number sponsored by the Foundation of the American Academy of Opthalmology. Call 1-800-222-EYES if you are over age 65 and have limited financial means.

An advisor will refer you to a participating local eye doctor who will charge no more than Medicare or insurance limits for an eye examination and treatment.

Keep your eyes young with shades

Sunglasses are stylish with the youngsters, but they will keep your eyes "looking" young in more ways than one. Wearing the "correct" sunglasses can cut certain aging processes in your eyes by up to six times, according to a report from Research to Prevent Blindness (RPB), a leading voluntary organization in support of eye research.

"Correct" means lenses that block out a high percentage (at least 90 percent) of the harmful ultraviolet (UV) light present in natural sunlight, and frames that position the lenses so that little sunlight seepage occurs around the edges and over the top. UV light is light at the shortwave end of the color spectrum and is responsible for suntanning, vitamin D production in the body, and other effects.

UV light "appears to accelerate aging of receptors of human vision, and cumulative exposure speeds up aging of the lens of the eye, contributes to cataract formation and possible changes in the retina [the screen of the eye], leading to macular degeneration," said Dr. John S. Werner, professor of psychology and neurosciences at the University of Colorado.

Macular degeneration, the impairment of the central area of the retina, is the major cause of blindness in those over age 60.

Normally, the eye's natural lens filters out much of the UV light we get in sunlight, even on cloudy days. If the natural lens is removed — for cataract surgery, for example — the UV rays speed through to hit and damage the retina, the main vision area of the eye.

Dr. Werner and associates studied eight patients who had cataractous lenses removed from both eyes and then had plastic lenses implanted.

On each patient, one eye was implanted with a plastic that absorbed 90 percent of the UV light hitting it, while the other eye got a plastic lens that filtered out only 14 percent.

Five years later, while both eyes appeared superficially healthy, on the eye that received more UV light, "our psychophysical tests showed loss in the shortwave cone sensitivity from chronic exposure to UV [radiation]," Dr. Werner reported to a RPB seminar on new findings about UV hazards. "Five years of chronic exposure to UVR [ultraviolet radiation] produced an average loss in shortwave cone sensitivity equal to about 30 years of normal aging."

While UV damage to the eyes is long-term and cumulative, experts are now warning all who spend any time outdoors to wear properly fitting sunglasses to avoid further bad effects. "You can't ignore the hazard in any season or location," Dr. Werner said.

Good UV-shielding sunglasses don't have to be expensive, according to *American Journal of Public Health* (78,1:72). Researchers tested 32 pairs of sunglasses, each costing less than $7, and found that most of them filtered out 98 percent or more of the harmful UV rays in sunlight. Glass and plastic lenses were equally effective in blocking UV, the study showed.

The problem was in the fit of the glasses on the head, particularly in whether the glasses allowed some sunlight (and UV light) to "seep" around the edges of the lenses into the eyes.

Using a mannequin and light detectors in place of eyes, researchers discovered that UV light leaked around the tops and sides of the frames. They also found that wearing the sunglasses even a third of an inch down the nose increased UV penetration by as much as 45 percent.

The lesson: Check the labels to make sure the sunglasses will block out almost all UV light (check with the merchant to be sure), and buy large-framed glasses contoured to your face to block out UV seepage from the sides and top. Wear them as close to your eyes as possible.

At the same time, be aware of the "sunglasses syndrome," as reported by three Harvard Medical School doctors in the publication *Your Good Health*.

Sunglasses syndrome includes numbness and unpleasant sensations beneath the eyes, inside the nose, over the cheeks, and eventually around the upper front teeth and gumline.

Such symptoms may indicate that your sunglasses, if large and heavy, are compressing a sensory nerve. That nerve emerges from the bone about a half inch away from the nose and a little under each eye.

Heavy sunglasses, worn for long periods, may pinch that nerve, producing numb gums and other uncomfortable sensations in the facial area. Get relief by removing the glasses. Padding also may help.

Migraines may cause vision loss

One of every three migraine-headache sufferers loses her peripheral vision, according to a new study in *Ophthalmology*.

Peripheral vision is "corner of your eye" sight. In other words, if you focus on an object straight ahead, you can still see things in a wide arc off to the sides. Elderly people are at the highest risk for losing this ability, the report says.

Ten to 12 million Americans suffer from migraines, and they are three times more common among women than men. Researchers are studying why migraines cause the loss of peripheral vision.

Unseen bathroom visitors may endanger your eyesight

Your bathroom may be the vacation home of vision-threatening pseudomonas germs. If you wear contact lenses, you may be doubly at risk.

"Pseudomonas love warm, moist environments," says Dr. Louis Wilson, professor of ophthalmology at Emory University in Atlanta, Ga. "Aside from their natural habitat in soil, grass and foliage, the bathroom is probably this bacteria's idea of heaven."

The germs are brought in from the outside in a variety of ways, usually on shoes or clothing. They thrive in and around the bathroom sink, the shower and the toilet.

A good germ breeding area is in the gooey underside of soap bars in the soap holders of the shower and sink. Unfortunately, the bathroom is also where most people put in and take out their contact lenses.

"People get pseudomonas on their hands, then contaminate their [contact lens] solutions," Dr. Wilson says. The germs grow quickly in homemade saline solutions, the liquid soaking mixtures made by dissolving salt tablets in distilled water, the doctor says. That's because the sterile distilled water may become contaminated with germs once it's opened and other things are added to it.

The germs get in large containers of saline solution when the contact lens wearer frequently opens and pours the solution, offering many chances for contamination. You are really risking germs when you pour the soaking solution from a large bottle into a travel-sized bottle that may have been used for other purposes earlier and may contain germs.

Even with all the chances for bacteria to get into your eyes, you probably are pretty safe unless you scratch the surface of your eye. That scratch provides an opening for the germs to get in and cause an infection. And, unfortunately, contact lens wearers are more likely to get eye scratches than people who don't use contacts, Dr. Wilson warns.

The danger arises when a germ-contaminated lens is put into an eye that has a scratch. Pseudomonas grow quickly, and within 12 hours, the eye will be painful. By the 24-hour mark, the infected eye will have reached the "big trouble" stage, according to Dr. Wilson. Left untreated, loss of vision and even loss of the eye itself is possible after 36 to 48 hours, Dr. Wilson said.

Symptoms of serious infections requiring immediate medical care include redness, sensitivity to light and a pain that becomes an ache. "If you think you have an eye infection, see an ophthalmologist immediately," Dr. Wilson says.

Preventive measures include careful handling of contact lens solutions and use of only medically sterilized containers. Buying solutions in bulk may not be wise, especially if you open and close the bulk container a lot. Better to use smaller, sterile containers, and steer clear of homemade solutions. An expensive alternative is the new, disposable contact lenses. Wear them a week, then throw them away.

Even if you don't wear contact lenses, be careful about rubbing your eyes with unwashed hands, especially if you may have scratches on the eye surface. And since germs multiply in the gooey part underneath the soap bar, use a platform on the soap dish to keep the bar dry, and wash off the bar first in hot water before washing your hands.

The danger of soft contact lenses

Nearly 13 million Americans enjoy the convenience of soft contact lenses, but physicians warn that long-term wear and poor hygiene may lead to a number of eye diseases and illnesses. The warning is especially important for the five million people who use extended-wear lenses.

A special report on ocular diseases in *Postgraduate Medicine* (86,4:90) recently outlined contact-lens injuries and ways you can prevent eye injuries.

❑ **Conjunctivitis.** Conjunctivitis, the most common eye disease, is inflammation of the mucous membrane lining the eyelid and part of the eyeball. It results from poor hygiene and affects ten percent of soft contact lens wearers each year.

There are many types of conjunctivitis, but generally, symptoms include irritation, itching, puffiness, burning and mucous discharge. You may have the sensation of a foreign body in the eye and may awake with swollen eyelids and matted eyelashes. The infection may start in one eye and quickly move to the other.

Proper hygiene will prevent conjunctivitis. Your eye doctor will probably remind you of the importance of soaking lenses in enzymatic solution every week to kill bacteria.

❑ **Corneal abrasions.** Abrasions or scratches usually occur when inserting or removing lenses. Symptoms include irritation, redness, pain and tearing.

Physicians prescribe antibiotic drops or ointment to use for four or five days until symptoms disappear.

❑ **Corneal ulcers.** "Trauma, underlying [eye] disease, and contact lens use are the three principal causes of bacterial corneal ulcers," which may cause permanent scarring and blindness if an ulcer erupts. Seven thousand people suffer corneal ulcers each year, and the number will increase as more people try extended-wear lenses.

The disease comes on quickly. Symptoms include pain, discharge, diminished vision, eyelid swelling and sensitivity to light. Physicians treat corneal ulcers with topical antibiotics (a cream or ointment) until the infection clears up. Some patients need hospitalization for further antibiotic treatment, and corneal transplants may be necessary if scarring is permanent.

❐ **Keratitis.** Keratitis is another form of corneal ulcer, caused by resistant bacteria that contaminate homemade saline solutions and contact lens cases. People who wear soft contact lenses overnight are ten to fifteen times more likely to get keratitis than daily wearers. Long-term wear cuts off the eye's oxygen supply, causing cells on the surface to die and form an ulcer, which may become infected, says a report in *Science News* (136,13:197).

Keratitis is becoming more common because the use of extended-wear lenses is increasing. Symptoms include pain, sensitivity to light and some loss of vision. Often, patients do not respond to early treatment. Keratitis is difficult to treat because the bacteria can transform itself into antibiotic-resistant forms. Corneal transplants are often necessary, and even after transplantation, the infection may recur.

If you have any of the symptoms described above, remove your lenses and see your eye doctor.

Tips on preventing contact-lens injury

- **Practice good hygiene. Wash your hands before inserting your lenses, and use sterile, commercially prepared saline solution. Follow disinfection guidelines, and never use homemade preparations. If you have extended-wear lenses, remove them at least every seven days for cleaning. (Some physicians recommend cleaning extended-wear lenses every day.)**

- **It may be best not to wear your lenses overnight.**

- **If your eyes are irritated, don't wear your lenses.**

- **If you have pain, eyelid swelling or a discharge, see your eye doctor.**

Avoid dangerous look-alikes that may cause serious eye injuries

Before you apply your eye drops, double-check that bottle — you could be making a sticky mistake!

The glue containers in "do-it-yourself" artificial nail kits are often identical to bottles used for prescription eye drops. As a result, *The Journal of the American Medical Association* (263,17:2301) reports that a large number of people have applied the fingernail glue to their eyes instead of medicine, causing painful injuries. When you have an eye infection or when you're not wearing your contacts or eye glasses, you tend to go by how things feel instead of reading labels.

You can avoid a mix-up by taking the following precautions: Try putting colorful labels on glue containers, eye drops and other medicine bottles to help you tell them apart. You may also find it helpful to store the artificial nail kits separately from your medicine.

Watch the clock for best eye therapy results

If you're using prescription eye drops to help treat your glaucoma, watching the clock makes a big difference in how effective your treatment is.

Researchers are finding that eye-drop drug therapy may be most effective at certain times of the day and less effective at other times.

Using the glaucoma eye drops at special times in the day may increase the effectiveness of the drug and cut down on the adverse side effects at the same time, according to a report in *Medical Tribune* (31,18:4).

Researchers used lab animals to test the effectiveness of timolol (a common glaucoma drug) at 6 a.m., noon, 6 p.m. and midnight. They found the drug to be most effective, with the fewest bad side effects, at noon.

Human testing is on the way. Researchers are excited about improving glaucoma treatment just by keeping an eye on the clock.

For safety's sake, don't change your eyedrop schedule without checking with your doctor first.

Common household products can cause severe eye injury

If liquid automatic dishwashing detergent splashes in your eyes, get to a doctor quickly, according to a report in *Emergency Medicine* (21,15:53).

Granular dishwashing detergents scratch and irritate the cornea, a transparent coating over the iris and pupil, and may cause serious injury.

Dr. Edward P. Krenzelok, director of the Pittsburgh Poison Center at Children's Hospital in Pittsburgh, "analyzed all cases of exposure to liquid automatic dishwashing detergent reported to the Pittsburgh Poison Center over a 15-month period."

Twenty-three cases involved the eyes, and the injuries were more serious than skin exposures or ingestions.

"More than 90 percent of the ocular exposures resulted in symptoms," according to the report. "The irritations were minor corneal abrasions in 74 percent of the cases, but four adults had more extensive corneal abrasions."

Shampoo is another household product to look out for. Getting shampoo in your eyes may mean more than just momentary stinging. A particular detergent contained in many shampoos could also cause damage to the cornea.

The detergent, sodium lauryl sulfate (SLS), is a common ingredient in soaps and shampoos, and even a drop of SLS is absorbed quickly by the cornea, according to Dr. Keith Green, professor of opthalmology at the Medical College of Georgia.

The chemical accumulates in the clear tissue and stays there for up to five or six days, Dr. Green said in a report to Research to Prevent Blindness, a leading voluntary organization devoted to eye research and vision protection.

The absorbed SLS causes changes in the amounts of some proteins in the eye, and creates a new kind of protein, not yet identified, in the eyes of rabbits treated in experiments. This raises questions about long-term effects on the normally clear cornea.

A further danger is that SLS in the eye delayed healing of the corneal epithelium — the surface layer of the cornea — when it was damaged. Tissue that would have healed in two days instead took ten.

While there are no signs of damage to the eye from SLS immediately after shampoo use, far more subtle effects may show up over a long period.

"Our findings lead us to call for more judicious use of detergents such as SLS by both manufacturers and users of soaps and shampoos," Dr. Green reported.

"This is particularly true when possible accidental exposure to SLS could occur in infants, where growth is occurring, and in any instance where a healing process is taking place."

The eyes of very young people and eyes in a healing stage are most susceptible to SLS damage. For adults, especially in middle and later years, SLS is suspected to be a factor in causing cataracts.

Not all shampoos or soaps contain SLS, so read the labels on such products and use those without the suspect ingredient, Dr. Green advises.

Contaminated mascara blinds Georgia woman

A 47-year-old Georgia woman was blinded when she accidentally scratched her cornea as she was applying mascara, her doctors report in *The Journal of the American Medical Association* (263,12:1616).

She complained of "pain, light sensitivity, redness and swelling of the eye," according to their report. She was given an eye ointment, and the eye was patched.

Three days later, the woman's conditioned worsened. She developed an infection in her eye and her vision was severely impaired. Doctors admitted her to the hospital. After treatment, the infection cleared up, but the woman failed to regain her sight.

The woman lost her sight because her mascara was contaminated with the bacteria, *Pseudomonas aeruginosa*. The report points out that "new mascara is rarely contaminated with bacteria but can become contaminated ... after use."

The lesson: Don't use a tube of mascara for more than a few months, and always apply makeup carefully. If you suffer any type of eye injury, see your doctor right away.

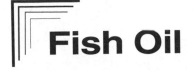

Fish Oil

Fish oil as a natural healer

An increasing number of researchers and physicians are discovering the many healing benefits of a natural ingredient called omega-3 fatty acids by scientists and simply "fish oil" by the rest of us.

Population studies show that people who eat substantial amounts of cold-water fish have lower rates of coronary artery disease than other people, even though the fish-eaters have about the same amount of fat in their diets as other people.

Recent studies suggest that the addition of fish to the diet, especially replacing red meat and dairy products with fish, will have a positive health benefit. Norwegian researchers, led by Kristian Bjerve, discovered that your body needs omega-3 fatty acids to process normally another kind of dietary oil, omega-6 fatty acids. Omega-6 oils are close relatives of omega-3 oils and are found in things like safflower oil and other cooking oils.

The Norwegians found a direct relationship between daily doses of omega-3 oils and healthy levels of certain substances in the blood such as plasma and lipids. "Omega-3 fatty acids possibly also have some specific function in the retina [in the eye] and in the central nervous system," Bjerve says.

"Dietary fish oils are rich in eicosapentaenoic acid (EPA), a polyunsaturated fatty acid of the omega-3 series," according to *Postgraduate Medicine* (85,4:406). Essential fatty acids such as EPA have been discovered to play important roles in preventing and controlling heart and artery disease, lowering high blood pressure and preventing unnecessary blood clotting.

Current research is also investigating fish oil's potential to help in angina (heart pain), rheumatoid arthritis and other inflammatory disorders, kidney disease and breast cancer, *Postgraduate Medicine* reports.

It's hard to say exactly how much fish oil you need. A study at the Pennington Biomedical Research Center in Baton Rouge, La., found that fish oil's anti-clotting action in animals "depends on the dosage of fish oil in relation to other kinds of polyunsaturated fats — not the absolute amount of fish oil consumed," *Science News* (135,12:183) reports.

The Norwegian researchers say that most people need 350 to 400 milligrams of omega-3 acids in the form of purified fish oil every day to maintain normal plasma and lipid levels.

But since a daily requirement has not been set, and safe levels of fish oil supplements have not been established, "the consumption of fresh fish two to three times weekly is likely a reasonable recommendation," says the *Postgraduate Medicine* report.

Here are some ways that fish oil helps to prevent artery disease:

❑ **Provides healing inside blood vessels.** The insides of arteries suffer injuries, sometimes from turbulent blood flow. Sticky platelets in the blood collect around the injured area and send chemical signals for more sticky helpers, including germ-fighting white cells. The result, sometimes, is too much help.

Cholesterol, a natural part of blood, collects in unusual amounts at the growing bottleneck in the busy blood pipeline. The "helpers" continue to send signals that cause more of the blood's clotting agents to pile on the growing mass.

The result is atherosclerosis: a form of hardening of the arteries caused by fatty plaque growing on and changing the walls inside arteries. These plaque blockages reduce blood flow, especially in arteries feeding the heart. Reduced blood flow, in turn, starves whole areas of the heart muscle, resulting in heart pain (angina) or even heart attacks. Plaque blockages also cause blood clots to form, further reducing blood flow. That can happen in many areas of the body besides the heart.

Omega-3 fish oil helps the artery-healing process by making the blood helpers less sticky, and by keeping them from piling up and blocking the artery.

❑ **Fortifies cells.** One part of the fish oil, EPA (eicosapentaenoic acid), gets into the cells that make up the artery walls. The EPA-fortified cells start cranking out their own chemical signals that order sticky, clot-forming platelets to stay away.

"Increasing fish oil in the diet leads to a slight lowering of cholesterol [of the harmful LDL type], and it sometimes reduces high blood pressure as well," reports Dr. Alexander Leaf, writing in *Your Good Health,* a publication of Harvard Medical School.

Other studies reported in *Total Nutrition Guide* (Bantam Books) suggest it helps the joints, cuts down on arthritis discomfort, and reduces the pain of and even prevents migraine headaches.

More recent animal studies reported in *Science News* (134:228) indicate that well-fed mice on high-fat diets that included fish oils rich in omega-3 displayed the following responses:

❑ lived twice as long as normal mice

❑ had half the normal levels of harmful autoimmune responses

(inflammatory diseases like rheumatoid arthritis and lupus, in which antibodies attack the body's own tissues)

❏ showed a complete absence of kidney disease, which normally strikes all these kinds of test animals

❏ had blood cholesterol levels half that in normal mice, even lower than those in another study group of mice that had been fed calorie-restricted, low-fat diets

Researchers are now testing fish oil in people to see what effect it has on several other diseases. These problems being researched include psoriasis, nephritis (inflammation of the kidneys), lupus, arthritis, and some forms of cancers involving the immune system.

Although you can get fish oil supplements (usually sold as omega-3 in capsule form), many physicians say a safer way is to forget the pills and eat fish containing the oils. To get adequate amounts of omega-3 fatty acids, fish oil supplements must be taken in high doses, which can cause several problems, including:

❏ Diarrhea, flatulence (gas) and upset stomach.

❏ The blood can't clot as easily. Increased bleeding time could be very dangerous and in some cases could cause fatal hemorrhaging, reports *The Medical Letter* (29:731). You should avoid fish oil supplements if you are taking blood-thinning drugs or aspirin regularly, if you are planning surgery, or if you have a family history of strokes or hemorrhaging.

❏ You could consume too much vitamin E. High doses of fish oil supplements could cause you to ingest large amounts of vitamin E. In large doses, vitamin E hinders the blood's ability to clot (which adds to the blood-clotting problem) and can cause possibly fatal results, according to a study by Pauling and Enstrom.

❏ Blood sugar levels in diabetics may go up. People with inactive diabetes may discover that the fish oil activates their diabetes, says Harry S. Glauber of the University of California at San Diego. Jan Lipkin of the American Diabetes Association says use of fish oil supplements "makes it harder for patients to control their blood sugar levels." Glauber and the American Diabetes Association recommend that diabetics and people at high risk for developing diabetes should avoid fish oil supplements.

❏ You'll consume high amounts of vitamin A, which can be toxic, reports *The New England Journal of Medicine* (316,10:626).

❑ You could consume toxic amounts of vitamin D, reports the American Diabetes Association.

❑ Cod liver oil should be avoided because it contains cholesterol and can lead to overdoses of vitamins A and D, according to Dr. Nathaniel Shafer of New York Medical College in the *Medical Tribune.*

Fresh or frozen fish that normally live in deep, cold waters contain the highest levels of the two kinds of beneficial fish oil ingredients (EPA and DHA fatty acids). Eating canned fish is not recommended, since the canning process destroys most of the omega-3 oil.

If you don't like fish that much, you can still get some EPA through plant sources, according to *Everyday Health Tips* (Rodale Press). But, most plants generally are lower in omega-3 than the same amounts of fish.

Margarine also is a rich source of omega-3, largely because it's made from soybeans. Unfortunately, it also has more saturated fats than fish or plant sources of omega-3.

Fish oil — how much is enough?

About three grams a day, or a little under one ounce a week, of omega-3 fatty acids — commonly known as "fish oil" — is the best dose size for cutting levels of fat in the blood, say researchers in *The American Journal of Clinical Nutrition* (52,1:120).

In a Dutch study, researchers at Amsterdam's Free University Hospital tested the effects of four different dosages of omega-3 oils on several types of cholesterol and triglycerides, as well as on the germ-killing power of white blood cells. The doses tested ranged from zero to six grams a day. It takes 28 grams to make one ounce.

Triglycerides are a form of fat carried by the blood. Scientists consider high levels of triglycerides to be a risk factor for heart disease. They found that fish oil even in small doses reduces triglycerides and raises the concentration of HDL ("good") cholesterol. The effect was dose-dependent, meaning that the more fish oil taken by the volunteers, the more they benefited.

Up to a point, that is. Above three grams of fish oil per day, the body seems to be unable to use the extra fatty acids in a beneficial way. Feeding the volunteers six grams per day had no more effect than giving them three grams a day, the researchers report.

Fish oil can decrease the blood's ability to form clots. In addition, some people report heartburn and belching as side-effects of taking fish oil capsules.

Check with your doctor before taking any omega-3 supplements.

Fish oil's top 20

Based on an uncooked serving size of 100 grams (approximately three and one-half ounces), the following kinds of fish are highest in total omega-3 fatty acids content.

Fish	Total Fat (in grams)	Omega-3
Atlantic mackerel	13.9	2.6
Chub mackerel	11.5	2.2
King mackerel	13.0	2.2
Lake trout	9.7	2.0
Japanese horse mackerel	7.8	1.9
Pacific herring	13.9	1.8
Atlantic herring	9.0	1.7
Bluefin tuna	6.6	1.6
Albacore tuna	4.9	1.5
Sablefish	15.3	1.5
Chinook salmon	10.4	1.5
Atlantic sturgeon	6.0	1.5
Lake whitefish	6.0	1.5
European anchovy	4.8	1.4
Atlantic salmon	5.4	1.4
Round herring	4.4	1.3
Sockeye salmon	8.6	1.3
Sprat	5.8	1.3
Bluefish	6.5	1.2
Mullet	4.4	1.1

Source: U.S. Department of Agriculture, Human Nutrition Information Service

Best plant sources of omega-3

If you don't like fish, you'll be glad to hear that there are plenty of plant sources of omega-3. Walnuts, soybeans, and many everyday beans are high in omega-3. (You'll notice that some of the choices are high in fat, too.) Check out these plant sources that are high in omega-3 fatty acids. The comparisons are based on a serving size of approximately three and one-half ounces (100 grams).

Food	Total fat (in grams)	Total cholesterol	Total omega-3
Rapeseed oil	100	0	11.1
Walnut oil	100	0	10.4
Wheat germ oil	100	0	6.9
Soybean oil	100	0	6.8
English walnuts	61.9	0	6.8
Black walnuts	56.6	0	3.3
Tomato seed oil	100	0	2.3
Soybeans, sprouted, cooked	4.5	0	2.1
Dry soybeans	21.3	0	1.6
Oat germ	30.7	0	1.4
Leeks, raw	2.1	0	0.7
Radish seeds, sprouted	2.5	0	0.7
Wheat germ	10.9	0	0.7
Common dry beans	1.5	0	0.6
Navy beans	0.8	0	0.3
Pinto beans	0.9	0	0.3

Source: U.S. Department of Agriculture, Human Nutrition Information Service

Other sources (for comparison)

Food	Total fat (grams)	Total cholesterol	Total omega-3
Salad dressing, blue cheese, commercial	52.3	17	3.7
Salad dressing, Italian, commercial brands	48.3	0	3.3
Hard margarine, made with soybeans	80.5	0	3.0
Butter	81.1	2.19	1.2
Shortening, household lard and vegetable oil	100	56	1.1
Cured bacon, raw	57.5	67	0.8
Fresh pork, trimmed	76.7	93	0.7
Whole milk	3.3	14	0.1
Chicken, white meat, no skin	1.7	58	trace

Source: U.S. Department of Agriculture, Human Nutrition Information Service

Fish oil is not just a passing fad

Omega-3 fish oil has definite health benefits for people of all ages, agreed more than 300 researchers at a recent health conference in Washington.

Studies indicate that men who eat two or three helpings of fish a week are 40 percent less likely to die of heart attacks than men who eat no fish, says an article in *The Atlanta Journal* (108,22).

"It is quite apparent that fish had a protective effect against coronary heart disease, as well as against cardiovascular death and death from all causes," says Dr. Therese Dolecek, a nutrition epidemiologist at the Bowman Gray School of Medicine in Winston-Salem, North Carolina.

Other researchers at the conference praised the benefits of omega-3, not only for its role in preventing and treating heart disease, but also for its apparent beneficial effects on cancer, diabetes and psoriasis.

Studies show that omega-3 in infant formula appears to improve vision in premature infants, slows the buildup of platelets and other substances such as cholesterol on blood vessel walls, and helps reduce problems with irregular heart rhythms.

Fish oil and surgery

Recent studies suggest that fish oil taken before and after two very different kinds of surgery can have highly beneficial effects. In one study, fish oil seemed to help keep arteries unclogged after "balloon" surgery. In another, fish oil apparently helped prevent the spread of cancer cells that escaped after operations.

An extremely high intake of fish oil can "dramatically improve" the results of coronary angioplasty, popularly known as "balloon" surgery, according to one new study at the Washington Hospital Center.

Usually about one-third of arteries opened with angioplasty get clogged up again with cholesterol and plaque within six months. But Dr. Mark R. Milner said his research suggests that taking large doses of fish oil for just six months can cut that failure rate in half.

Fish oil seemed to help patients after another kind of surgery, as well. A Harvard Medical School study suggests that highly purified fish oil supplements help prevent the spread of cancer cells that may escape during and after surgical operations to remove cancerous tissue.

Dr. George Blackburn of Harvard, who's also chief of nutrition support at New England Deaconess Hospital, said the fish oil supplements were given to cancer patients a week before surgery. Following surgery, the patients continued taking the fish oil for three to six months. Blackburn noted lower rates of cancer spread, known as metastasis, in those who took fish oil.

Both Dr. Milner and Dr. Blackburn have a very conservative approach to fish oil therapy for all but these two classes of surgery patients.

Milner advised against taking fish oil capsules for any other reason, because, he said, the long-term effects are still unknown. "I never give fish oil supplements to any of my patients unless they are having coronary angioplasty," he said.

In the fish oil study on heart patients, 194 people were randomly assigned to two groups following successful angioplasty. One group took nine fish oil capsules per day for six months after the procedure. Each capsule contained a total of 4.5 grams of omega-3 fatty acids. That's about the daily equivalent of the fish oil in two cans of sardines.

The other group got no fish oil, but patients in both groups were told to eat low-fat, low-cholesterol diets. Both groups received the same post-operative therapy.

Nurses trained in diet therapy called each patient monthly to provide counseling and to evaluate if the patients were sticking to their strict diet.

"Dietary compliance was equally good in both groups of patients," Milner noted. "They really tried to stick with a strict low-cholesterol diet." Patients' cholesterol intake was restricted to 100 milligrams per day, and dietary fat was limited to 25 percent of their total calories.

By the end of six months, 35.4 percent of people who didn't take the fish oil showed signs that their dilated heart arteries had narrowed again. However, the recurrence rate in the fish oil group was only about 19 percent, Milner reported.

During the study, eleven patients stopped taking the high doses of fish oil because of disagreeable, but not dangerous, side effects including flatulence and other mild digestive problems.

Milner said that most patients were willing to tolerate the side effects in order to possibly lower their risk of having a repeat angioplasty or needing bypass surgery.

Coronary angioplasty is less invasive than heart bypass surgery because it does not involve cutting open the chest cavity. Instead, the surgeon cuts into a leg or arm artery and inserts a catheter with a tiny balloon on the tip.

He threads the narrow catheter through the circulatory system until its tip reaches the portion of the heart artery that is narrowed by fatty "plaque." Then the doctor inflates the balloon, squashing the plaque against the artery wall and enlarging the inner diameter of the blood vessel. Several blockages can be opened during the procedure.

Aspirin has proven to be helpful in reducing the numbers of heart attacks that happened during or soon after angioplasty.

But aspirin doesn't seem to make a significant difference in reducing the six-month reclogging rate, known as "restenosis," said Milner, who is assistant professor of medicine at George Washington University.

Milner's findings are similar to the results of a smaller study of 82 patients at the Dallas VA Medical Center, reported in *The New England Journal of Medicine*. Milner said several research teams are doing comparable studies to confirm his results.

Fish oil seems to suppress the inflammatory response that follows an injury, Milner said. In angioplasty, the inner wall of the artery is sometimes injured by the balloon catheter.

If the injured area heals rapidly, excess inflammation, scar tissue and blood clots may combine to clog the artery again. Fish oil seems to slow the unwanted speedy healing process and to prevent the inflammation and scarring. It also seems to reduce the tendency of blood platelets to form clots at the once-clogged site.

The outer membranes of almost all cells contain oils called omega-6 fatty acids. "Overdosing" patients with fish oil high in omega-3 fatty acids alters their cell membranes. Omega-6 fatty acids in the membranes are replaced by omega-3 fatty acids. This change seems to make cell membranes less "reactive," Milner said.

Thus, a person whose cell membrane content is high in omega-3 fatty acids may have white blood cells that are slower to cause inflammation and red blood cells that are slower to form clots, both good effects for heart health.

Food Poisoning

Microwaving may contribute to food poisoning

British researchers believe they may have found a hidden danger in microwaving prepared foods. The amount of salt or sugar in these foods may change the way the foods absorb microwave energy, says a report in *Science News* (137,14:215).

Researchers found that a high salt or sugar content prevents foods from reaching a high enough temperature to kill salmonella and other dangerous bacteria. In fact, microwaving may only heat these bacteria to a temperature that helps them grow rather than kills them.

To avoid food poisoning, researchers agree that you should microwave foods longer and at a lower power than the package recommends. Then let the food sit for a few minutes to make sure dangerous bacteria have been killed.

The microwave is surely one of the greatest conveniences of all time, but recently consumer groups have raised questions about the safety of microwave packaging — those plastic trays, wraps and bags that magically brown and crisp foods.

According to the *Nutrition Action Health Letter* (17,1:5), "microwave ovens can't brown and crisp foods on their own." The "magic" is heat-susceptor packaging, which acts as a "little frying pan," says Food and Drug Administration chemist Les Borodinsky.

That little frying pan is actually thin, gray strips of polyethylene terepthalate (PET) on the bottom of the package. (You can sometimes see the strips if you hold the package up to the light.)

The FDA says PET is safe to use at 300 degrees F, but when PET reaches higher temperatures, it breaks down and releases chemicals into food. In the microwave, PET can reach 500 degrees or higher.

According to the *Health Letter*, heat-susceptor packages often contain a number of chemicals — "all known or suspected carcinogens" — that can be released into the foods. Carcinogens are cancer-causing agents. Some of the chemicals are not actually part of PET, but rather are part of the adhesive strips that hold PET on the package.

The FDA is constantly testing microwavable products, and they've asked manufacturers not to use certain chemicals in food packages, but it never hurts to take some precautions when it comes to the microwave. The *Health Letter* offers these tips to keep your family safe:

❑ Avoid frozen "pizza, french fries, waffles, popcorn, breaded fish, and other food that use heat-susceptor packaging."

❑ Some foods are packaged so that you can cook them in a microwave or conventional oven (the package will have directions for both cooking methods). This type of packaging doesn't contain heat-susceptors but still releases chemicals into food, even when heated in a conventional oven. To avoid this hazard, transfer all such foods from the plastic trays to glass cookware, which is the safest type container to use in the microwave. (At this point, Corning Ware appears safe.)

❑ Don't cover glass containers with plastic. The chemicals that give plastic wraps their "cling" could poison your food if overheated in the microwave. Use glass covers, or, if you must use plastic wrap, don't let it touch the food.

❑ Don't use margarine tubs to reheat leftovers. They'll eventually melt and release chemicals into your food.

Don't poison yourself with potatoes

Beware of eating potatoes that have shriveled brown spots on the skins. Store-bought potatoes with these signs of potato dry-rot may contain harmful levels of a poison produced by a plant fungus, according to a biochemist with the federal government.

Potato poisoning, even at low levels from only one or two potatoes, can cause vomiting, hair loss, a damaged immune system, nervous system problems, coma and even death, according to Anne E. Desjardins of the U.S. Department of Agriculture's Research Service in Peoria, Ill. The finding of danger from potato fungus poisoning is new, she says in *Science News* (135,15:238).

One other study in France also showed dangerous levels of the poison trichothecenes in some ordinary potatoes bought in grocery stores there. Tests for fungus poisons in corn and wheat are common, but until now, nobody has routinely looked for toxins in potatoes, the USDA researcher says.

Just cutting off the obviously rotted part of the potato won't remove all the poison, the researcher says. Even disease-free parts of those potatoes studied contained about 10 percent of the amount of poison found in the rotted parts, says Desjardins. That's still enough to cause sickness.

Even worse — the fungus-produced poison is heat-stable, meaning that normal cooking methods won't remove or lessen the danger.

Gallstones

Rapid weight loss may trigger formation of gallstones

It takes a lot of gall to tell someone who's overweight bad news about losing weight, but …

If you don't eat reqularly or are on a strict diet to shed pounds fast, you have a good chance of developing gallstones, a recent medical study suggests.

Doctors found a big increase in gallstone formation among 51 obese people who participated in an 8-week, quick-weight-loss program, compared with a group of overweight people who didn't diet.

The people on the crash diet had 25 percent more gallstones than the nondieters, according to the report in *Archives of Internal Medicine* (149,8:1750). In all, 13 of the 51 men and women developed the hard, cholesterol-containing stones during the 8-week diet.

Three of them required gallbladder-removal surgery within a few weeks of quitting the diet. A control group of nondieting fat people, on the other hand, showed no abnormal gallbladder developments, the report says.

"A large number of individuals undergoing prolonged calorie restriction and rapid weight loss may be at risk for development of gallstones," the doctors report.

The dieters ranged in age from 27 to 58, and all were more than 30 percent over their ideal weights. They went on a 500-calorie-per-day diet. A normal intake can range from 1,200 to 2,000 calories per day.

Average weight loss was between 36 and 39 pounds per person. The ones who developed gallstones, on average, lost about three pounds more than the ones who remained free of the cholesterol-containing sludge or stones in the gallbladder.

Obesity itself is a big risk for developing gallstones. Out of every 10 greatly overweight people, three to five of them eventually develop the cholesterol stones, the report says.

A study in *The New England Journal of Medicine* (321,9:563) found that "grossly overweight" women are six times more likely to develop gallstones, compared with women whose weight is average for their height.

Even "slightly overweight" women face nearly double the risk of developing gallstones, the *NEJM* report says.

Not all gallstones are formed from cholesterol, and not all of them cause trouble. But when they plug up bile ducts, they trigger pain, swelling, jaundice (yellowing of the skin) and other problems, sometimes requiring surgery. Some drugs and treatments can slow stone formation or dissolve gallstones already formed.

The doctors in the *Archives* study theorize that when you diet too strictly, the gallbladder doesn't have to work very hard. The cholesterol in the bile seems to leap at the chance to lump up and form gallstones. Dieting also reduces the bile acids that normally keep the cholesterol from forming stones.

The doctors still think fat people should lose weight, since obesity is a major health risk for heart disease, high blood pressure, diabetes and gallstones. Using stone-dissolving treatments along with a slowed-down weight loss plan may reduce the risk of gallstone formation, the report says.

If you want to lose weight fast with a low-calorie diet, check with your doctor first about the relative risks involved, the researchers suggest.

Fish oil may help prevent the development of gallstones

Fish oil not only helps reduce heart-disease risk by lowering cholesterol, but it may also help prevent gallstones, says researchers at the Johns Hopkins University School of Medicine in *Science News* (135,21:332).

Gallstones — actually, cholesterol "crystals" — form in the gallbladder, a pouch located near the liver. A substance known as bile flows from the liver through the bile duct to the gallbladder, where it is stored and used for digestion. You could have stones in your gallbladder without knowing it, but if one lodges in the bile duct, you could need surgery.

A main "ingredient" of bile is liquid cholesterol. Researchers don't know how liquid cholesterol hardens into gallstones, but they believe that omega-3 fatty acids found in fish oil halt the process.

Researchers recently tested their theory on prairie dogs. They fed 16 animals high-cholesterol diets; half were given fish-oil supplements. After two weeks, researchers removed the animals' gallbladders. The eight animals given fish oil had no gallstones; the other eight did.

Researchers are hopeful humans will show the same results. They plan more studies.

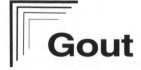

Gout

Bouts with gout

People who are overweight might greatly reduce their chances of suffering from gout by losing weight — but only if they lose weight slowly. Rapid weight loss can actually increase your chances of getting gout.

Gout is a painful type of arthritis which affects your joints. It usually starts in the knee or foot.

A sensible diet that helps you lose weight slowly is much more effective in preventing gout than a crash diet, suggests a report in the *Harvard Medical School Health Letter* (14,6:1).

You also can help prevent gout by avoiding some foods that seem to trigger bouts with gout: anchovies, asparagus, brains, kidney, liver, mincemeats, mushrooms, sardines and sweetbreads. Caffeine and alcohol intake should be limited as well.

Blood pressure medication may cause gout

Diuretics are supposed to drain excess sodium from your body, helping to keep high blood pressure under control. Because they flush the kidneys so effectively, they are known by many people as water pills.

But there are increased reports of elderly women suffering from attacks of gout, a sudden arthritic flare-up of pain in their hands or knees, apparently triggered by the diuretics.

"We are finding this in a population over the age of 70, as opposed to the usual gout sufferer, who is usually about 40," says Dr. Steven R. Weiner in *The Western Journal of Medicine* (150,4:419). "We are seeing women more commonly than men, which is a total reverse," says Weiner.

If you are taking water pills, you may be susceptible to this drug reaction, indicates the report.

Even if you have osteoarthritis, suspect diuretic-caused gout if your hand suddenly becomes very painful in the joints and shows evidence of inflammation, suggests Weiner.

If this happens, don't try to treat yourself or to change your medication on your own. Check with your regular doctor about what needs to be done.

Headaches

Aspirin therapy for migraine headaches

If you're one of the millions of Americans who suffer from migraine headaches, a small daily dose of aspirin may relieve your pain, Boston researchers reported at a recent American Heart Association conference.

In an eight-year study, 22,000 male doctors aged 40 to 84 took either 325 milligrams of aspirin or a placebo without aspirin every day to test how aspirin helps fight heart disease.

During this heart disease study, scientists accidentally discovered that aspirin also helped relieve the doctors' migraine symptoms, such as nausea, light sensitivity and severe pain on one side of the head.

In a follow-up questionnaire, 840 people taking the placebo had migraines, compared with only 672 taking aspirin — a 20 percent difference.

Migraine headaches and their causes are not well understood. However, scientists suspect that one cause may be the platelets in the blood, says *The Journal of the American Medical Association* (264,13:1711).

When a migraine occurs, the platelets get together and release a substance called serotonin. This causes the blood vessels to swell and produce the symptoms that make a migraine nearly unbearable.

The trick is to begin this low dosage program before the migraine and then to continue the treatment during and after the attack to reduce your chances of having another migraine and to keep your migraine from getting worse.

Some people are sensitive or allergic to aspirin. So you should check with your doctor before you start taking aspirin. Your doctor can recommend whether this is a safe and effective treatment for you.

Cool relief for headache pain

If you have frequent headaches, or even migraines, a recent article in *Modern Medicine* (58,4:84) suggests that a cold pack on your head could be your key to relief.

The results of a study done at a headache clinic indicate that using an ice pack in addition to the usual medicine helped most people feel better.

Check with your doctor: 20 or 30 minutes of cold pack treatment could be the remedy you've been looking for.

Re-leaf for headache pain

Using herbal "medicines" to relieve common aches and pains is not just old folklore. Some scientists say that herbs may be just as helpful and useful in treating illnesses as modern medicine.

One such herb, called feverfew, may help cut the number and severity of the migraine headaches you've been experiencing. A digest report in *Science News* (134:106) suggests that taking daily capsules of ground feverfew leaves reduces migraine headache discomfort and also helps relieve the nausea that sometimes accompanies migraine headaches.

However, you should check with your doctor before trying any herbal supplement.

Hearing Loss

Help prevent loss of hearing with vitamin A

If you want to make sure you don't lose your keen sense of hearing, ask yourself if you are getting enough vitamin A in your diet.

Some cases of hearing loss may be linked to a vitamin A deficiency, *The Journal of Nutrition* (120,7:726) reports.

Studies show that a lack of vitamin A in the diet first increases the ear's sensitivity to sound. In other words, your hearing is actually more sensitive during the first stages of deficiency.

However, an increased sensitivity to noise increases the chances of noise-induced hearing loss. The very sensitive ear can be damaged more easily and quickly than a normal ear.

So, the vitamin A deficiency does not actually cause the hearing loss. It simply makes the ear more sensitive to sound — which increases the chances of hearing loss due to noise damage.

If you suspect you may have a problem with your hearing, even if your ears seem supersensitive, talk to your doctor immediately. He can help you determine whether you need more vitamin A in your diet.

Vitamin A is found in many sources. Cod liver oil is loaded with Vitamin A, so much, in fact, that it can be toxic if too much is taken. After cod liver oil, salmon, mackerel, tuna and other fish also contain Vitamin A.

It is good to eat fish for its nutritional content which includes Vitamin A and vitamin D. Vitamin D helps to prevent bone loss and although unproven, may help to strengthen the bones in the ear's hearing mechanism which, if deteriorating with aging, may lead to progressive hearing loss.

Good sources of vitamin A are butter, egg yolks, cod liver oil, liver, yellow vegetables and green, leafy vegetables. Some fruits are also good sources of vitamin A: prunes, pineapples, oranges, limes and cantaloupes.

I beg your pardon

If you're finding yourself having to ask people to repeat themselves more and more often because of a slight hearing loss, you may need to check your diet.

Too much fat in the diet can clog tiny arteries in your ears, say researchers at Mercy Hospital in Rockville Centre, New York. The clogged arteries in your ears may result in a slight loss of hearing.

Heart Problems

What to do if you feel a heart attack's warning signs

You feel a fast fluttering in your chest. You get dizzy and feel close to fainting. You sense your heart racing wildly. You break out in a cold sweat, even if the weather is cool, and you feel some chest pain.

If you feel those symptoms, you may be experiencing the final warning signs of a potentially fatal heart attack. The symptoms can happen when a sick heart short-circuits and blows its rhythm fuses.

The catch-all medical name for this dangerous disturbance to the heart's pumping rhythm is arrhythmia. When the heart loses its rhythm, it loses its ability to pump effectively. When the pump stops working right, blood pressure throughout the body takes a disastrous plunge, and tissues begin starving for oxygen.

Two kinds of arrhythmias are real medical emergencies. One kind is ventricular fibrillation, when the pumping chamber totally loses its sparkplug rhythm and just quivers instead of pumping. The other dangerous kind is ventricular tachycardia, when the heart races wildly to more than 100 beats a minute without being driven by exercise or drugs.

Movies and television dramas routinely show patients with arrhythmia being shocked to restore normal heart electrical activity. The doctor rubs two wired paddles together, snaps, "Stand clear!" and then jolts the patient into "conversion." But what if you have a heart attack and there's nobody around, certainly not with electrical paddles ready to quickly shock your heart back into beating normally? According to *Southern Medical Journal* (82,1:1), there are at least two natural methods you can use — even when alone — to halt your own heart's crazy rhythms.

The methods may keep you conscious and buy you enough time to get medical help.

❐ **Cough CPR** — CPR stands for cardiopulmonary resuscitation. It means getting the heart and lungs back to work transporting oxygen to body cells that can live only a few minutes without oxygen.

Coughing is what you do for yourself. "It has been documented that regularly repeated vigorous coughing can be as effective as classical CPR in providing effective blood flow to critical organs for the heart that has recently ceased to function properly, such as the heart in ventricular fibrillation," says Dr. Carl E. Bartecchi of the Southern Colorado Clinic in Pueblo, Colo.

When you suck in breath just before a cough, you fill the lungs with oxygen, and the blood passing through the lungs carries it to vital organs. "This maneuver can buy time ... and can even be used for one's own cardiac arrest," Dr. Bartecchi says. A shorter version of this method emphasizes one or two "forceful" coughs to squeeze the heart into regular rhythm again. "Forceful coughs have been shown to be capable of terminating ventricular tachycardia and allowing reestablishment of normal cardiac rhythm," Dr. Bartecchi says.

❑ **Thump pacing** — Basically, this means hitting yourself hard with the heel of your hand on the sternum, the bony middle of the chest where the ribs come together over the heart.

The thumping acts like an artificial heart pacemaker and can be kept up "over lengthy periods." "This maneuver is much more effective than its alternatives — external cardiac compressions [classic CPR] or cough CPR," the doctor says. A shorter version emphasizes that "a firm blow to the precordium with the clenched fist can terminate ventricular fibrillation and ventricular tachycardia," Dr. Bartecchi says. "Repeated effectiveness of this maneuver over many years has been reported."

The classic heart attack is the myocardial infarction. That means the blood supply is suddenly cut off to a portion of the heart muscle, usually because of a clot in one of the arteries feeding the heart. But it's the loss of heart rhythm that accompanies the blood cutoff that is most dangerous, even fatal.

In about three out of every four cases of cardiac arrest (when the heart stops regular pumping), the victim experiences ventricular fibrillation. "The lay person should assume ventricular fibrillation in the emergency in which the victim has no pulse," Dr. Bartecchi says, "and he should direct the treatment toward that more common and potentially reversible [happening]."

If you see a person suffer heart difficulties or suddenly collapse, here's what Dr. Bartecchi says you can do to save a life.

- ❑ If the victim is conscious, get him to begin deep, hard, vigorous coughing. The coughing can stop the rhythm disturbance or at least maintain consciousness. Get him to keep coughing while medical help is being called.

- ❑ If you recognize a full cardiac arrest within one minute of its happening, try the thump version. Feel the rib cage at its bottom center, go up about two inches and hit that central bony area over the heart. Deliver a sharp blow with the bottom or heel of your clenched fist. In effect, use your fist like a hammer to the heart.

❑ Check for a pulse. If you don't feel one, try another, harder blow. If the pulse seems present only when you thump the victim's heart, keep up the thumping.

(**Note**: Caution should be used in striking blows to the chest of a possible heart attack victim. A blow that is too sharp could break a rib and puncture a lung. We recommend that you discuss the risks versus the benefits of this procedure with your own physician and get his approval before using it.)

❑ If the victim fails to respond to the thumping, use classic CPR techniques, the doctor says. Thumping should be used only immediately after the heart stops its normal rhythm, Dr. Bartecchi says. If you don't know how long the person has been unconscious or in rhythm distress, you should only use classic CPR methods, not the thumping methods, the doctor says.

The key is speed — coughing and thumping work best in the first minute after the heart loses its rhythm. In all cases, seek immediate, professional medical help. If you don't know how to administer CPR, contact your nearest Red Cross office to learn CPR techniques.

Dr. Bartecchi wrote a book on the natural rescue methods described above: *Emergency Cardiac Maneuvers — a Rescuer's Handbook*, which was published in 1988. The publisher is Essential Medical Information Systems Inc. in Amityville, N.Y.

Aspirin every other day reduces risk of first heart attack

In the United States alone, heart attacks strike over 1.5 million people each year, killing about half of them. Taking a 325-milligram aspirin tablet every other day can sharply reduce the risk of first heart attacks in healthy men, especially those over age 50, according to a major medical study published in *The New England Journal of Medicine* (321,3:129).

The aspirin therapy resulted in a 47 percent reduction in risk of a first heart attack among 22,000 male doctors, says the final report of the Physician's Health Study, which was sponsored by the National Institutes of Health. Daily aspirin in doses from 160 to 325 milligrams, when prescribed by a physician, currently is FDA-approved to help prevent second heart attacks and recurring unstable angina. Buffered aspirin was used in the study, but regular aspirin or enteric (coated) aspirin would also be effective, the researchers say. However, acetaminophen (like Tylenol) does not have the same effect.

The researchers tested several different doses of aspirin and found that one aspirin every second day was the most effective. An aspirin every day (for people without previous heart problems) did not increase its protective effect, but did increase unwanted side effects like stomach bleeding and indigestion.

It is important to remember that in healthy people and heart patients, aspirin therapy does not treat the plaque buildup and artery disease that causes heart attacks. Aspirin only reduces the blood's ability to clot.

Aspirin should not be used as a substitute for other prevention therapies for heart attacks, cautions FDA commissioner Dr. Frank E. Young. All known ways of fighting artery disease — like not smoking, reducing fat intake, lowering high blood pressure and exercising — should be carefully followed, the report says.

Dr. Lawrence Cohen from Yale University School of Medicine, a member of the research committee overseeing the study, is optimistic about the report. But Dr. Cohen cautions that using aspirin to prevent heart attacks must be a decision made between doctor and patient.

Aspirin acts like a blood thinner, reducing its ability to clot. That could pose serious problems for people who already are taking blood-thinning medicine, have bleeding ulcers or have recently undergone surgery.

In an *NEJM* editorial (321,3:183), the journal says, "Aspirin should be used cautiously, if at all, in patients with diabetic retinopathy or poorly controlled hypertension."

Beta-carotene helps cut heart problems in half

Taking a 50-milligram dose of beta-carotene every other day for six years seemed to help slow artery clogging in male doctors who already had heart disease, according to *Science News* (138,20:308).

Compared with men who took a placebo (fake pills), the beta-carotene group had half as many "major cardiovascular events," such as heart attack or stroke, during the long-term study, according to another report of the Harvard Medical School findings in *Medical Tribune* (31,24:2).

Researchers took into account that the men in the study were also taking aspirin on alternate days. The 333 randomly selected participants were drawn from the much larger Physicians' Health Study, which studied the effect of aspirin on heart disease. The doctors can't say for sure that people without heart disease who aren't taking aspirin would benefit from taking beta-carotene.

Scientists guess that beta-carotene hinders the formation of the harmful low-density lipoprotein (LDL) cholesterol. LDL cholesterol is known as "bad" cholesterol because of the damage it sometimes does to arteries.

Once linked with oxygen in the bloodstream, the harmful LDL cholesterol damages artery walls, leading to plaque buildup. Like sticky putty in a pipe, the plaque deposits choke off blood flow in arteries, resulting in heart attacks and strokes. Beta-carotene, they speculate, derails that process in some way.

The 50 milligrams of beta-carotene taken daily by the members of the study group is about four times the amount in a half cup of carrots. The daily study supplement was well within the "safe" range, the SN report noted. However, it's best to check with your doctor before taking supplements of beta-carotene or any other nutrient.

Magnesium cuts risk of heart disease

Good news: If the drinking water in your area is considered "hard," that could be good for your health! Hard water is rich in magnesium, and magnesium is a mineral that helps your nerves and muscles function properly.

Better news: Scientists now realize that magnesium also plays a beneficial role in preventing heart disease. A new study described in Science News (137,14:214) suggests that magnesium teams up with a low-cholesterol diet to discourage atherosclerosis, or the buildup of fat deposits on the walls of coronary arteries.

Researchers believe that a good supply of magnesium in your diet discourages the production of cells that form the fatty deposits on artery walls.

Scientists also suggest that a diet that is too low in magnesium can cause your body to draw magnesium from your muscles. This reduces the amount of magnesium in the muscles that is necessary to keep the muscles working properly.

Unfortunately, magnesium alone will not prevent or cure atherosclerosis. Eating a low-cholesterol diet is still your best protection against this form of heart disease. However, you can strengthen your defenses by including high-magnesium foods in your menus.

Boost your body's supply of magnesium by eating more green vegetables, nuts, whole grains and shellfish — all good natural sources of this essential mineral. And as you protect your heart, you will also help your other muscles function smoothly. Remember, check with your doctor before using vitamin supplements to increase your supply of magnesium.

Graze your way to a healthier heart

Snacking during the day, sometimes called "grazing," may be better for your heart than eating three square meals a day, Canadian researchers report in *The New England Journal of Medicine* (321,14:929).

But that doesn't mean you can eat just potato chips and ice cream — or simply snack between meals.

To get the benefits, you must eat small, nutritious meals throughout the day, researchers say, and your calorie count must not increase. Researchers believe snacking works by controlling the production of certain chemicals in the body.

Insulin, a hormone released by the pancreas, helps the body produce cholesterol. How much insulin the pancreas releases into the bloodstream depends on the size of the meals you eat. Snackers may have lower cholesterol levels because they eat smaller amounts of food at once, and the pancreas produces less insulin in response. Less insulin usually means less cholesterol. Eating more meals throughout the day and adding more fiber to your diet may be keys to keeping your cholesterol levels under control.

During the snacking study, seven men aged 31 to 51 ate three meals a day for two weeks or 17 snacks a day for two weeks and then switched to the other diet. The snackers' insulin levels dropped by 28 percent during the study. Their total cholesterol levels were 8.5 percent lower than men eating three meals a day.

Based on the results of this study, researchers believe that nutritious nibbling throughout the day may help you lower cholesterol levels and fight heart disease.

Low-fat diet fights heart disease

Lower your cholesterol without cutting back on calories? Eat meat, and lower harmful LDL cholesterol at the same time? It sounds improbable, but the results of a recent study suggest that it is possible, even for people with heart disease.

According to a study in *The Wall Street Journal*, one way to fight heart disease is with simple, effective changes in your diet. To demonstrate this, researchers watched a group of men with proven coronary heart disease over a two-year period.

The men in the study didn't cut back on the number of calories they ate, and they didn't lose weight. Instead, they lowered the amount of fat in their diets by substituting protein calories for fat calories.

By changing the kinds of foods they ate, these men reduced the amount of fat in their diet to an average of 27.5 percent of their total calorie intake. As a result, no new fat deposits formed on the walls of their coronary arteries, and their blood levels of LDL cholesterol went down.

On the other hand, the men who allowed their fat intake to exceed 30 percent of their total calories developed new fatty deposits on the walls of their arteries, risking more heart trouble in the future.

These dramatic results should encourage people, especially those with coronary heart disease, to change their diets to help fight heart disease. As a goal, the National Cholesterol Education program recommends that you lower your fat calories to less than 30 percent of your total caloric intake. To start with, choose lean meats instead of fatty meats and use low-fat dairy products instead of those with a high-fat content.

Switching to low-fat foods may not seem that important on a daily basis, but this simple change can make a big difference to your heart.

'Miracle' clove reduces rate of heart attacks

For a long time, it seemed that garlic was popular with everybody except vampires and scientists. For centuries, garlic has enjoyed great fame and popularity as a "miracle, cure-all" clove. But scientists and researchers often dismissed the subject as simply another example of "primitive" folklore — until now, that is.

Now, researchers are beginning to investigate the actual "powers" of garlic, and they like what they're finding. Garlic seems to reduce the rate of heart attacks. Garlic eaters had 32 percent fewer second heart attacks and 45 percent fewer deaths from heart attacks than nongarlic eaters, reports *Science News* (138,10:157).

Garlic might interfere with the body's bad habit of over-producing cholesterol and other blood-clotting agents that contribute to heart disease, says *Science News*.

Olive oil gives double-barreled protection for your heart

Studies show that olive oil provides double-barreled protection for your heart, reports *Medical Tribune* (31,20:15).

Olive oil is rich in monounsaturated fatty acids, and these fatty acids can have two positive effects on your health.

❑ Lowers cholesterol. Your doctor has been telling you to avoid saturated and hydrogenated fats (usually hardened fats, such as cooking lard) because they can raise your cholesterol. However, olive oil is rich in unsaturated fats that can actually lower your LDL cholesterol level.

❑ Reduces risk of atherosclerosis. This disease begins as "scratches" on the inside of your arteries. This is similar to rubbing coarse sandpaper on the inside of a plastic pipe. These "scratches" are a good place for cholesterol to attach and build up.

The scratches can be caused by a chemical change (oxidation) in the LDL cholesterol in your blood. The olive oil helps stop the chemical change in the LDL. So, olive oil reduces the chance of "scratches" forming and lowers your risk of heart disease.

Insulin and heart disease

High levels of insulin in the blood may be a silent heart-disease risk factor for 25 percent of the trim and otherwise healthy people in the United States, according to a report in *Science News* (136,12:184).

This was confirmed by a report recently presented to the American Diabetes Association by Dr. Annick Fontbonne, a researcher at the French National Institute of Health and Medical Research, who stated, "Our studies indicate that the earliest marker of a higher risk of coronary heart disease mortality is an elevation of stimulated plasma insulin level."

Scientists believe that a long-term excess of insulin "silently damages the cardiovascular system," although how remains a mystery. "Some speculate that high insulin levels may directly damage the artery wall, leading to a buildup of fat that narrows the vessel."

People who have too much insulin in their blood have a problem called insulin resistance. It occurs when the pancreas produces enough insulin — a hormone that directs cells to take up glucose (sugar) from the blood — but the body does not respond well. Blood sugar levels rise, and the pancreas then churns out more insulin to meet the body's demand.

Type-II diabetes (also called non-insulin-dependent diabetes) results from high blood sugar levels. It affects 10 million Americans — generally, overweight people over age 40. People with type-II diabetes are "two to four times as likely as nondiabetics to develop heart disease," according to the report.

Not all insulin-resistant people are diabetic. Dr. Gerald M. Reaven of Stanford University School of Medicine has researched insulin resistance for more than 20 years. He has identified what he calls "syndrome X" — the heart-disease risk factors that insulin-resistant — but otherwise healthy — people have. The risk factors are the following:

- **High blood pressure**

- **High triglycerides (a form of fat in the bloodstream)**

- **Decreased high-density-lipoprotein (HDL) cholesterol**

- **High cholesterol**

Although Type-I (insulin-dependent) diabetics have a definite heart-disease risk, Dr. Reaven is having a difficult time convincing diabetes specialists that people who are insulin-resistant — whether diabetic or not — are at risk as well.

The syndrome X theory is controversial, yet may explain why people in countries such as India and Pakistan have lower cholesterol levels but greater incidence of heart disease than people in other countries.

Many researchers believe syndrome X is hereditary, but further research will try to determine whether environmental factors, such as obesity, trigger it.

Studies in France and Italy have confirmed the syndrome X theory, which has also been put to the test at the Pittsburgh School of Medicine.

At Pittsburgh, researchers studied "489 healthy, white, premenopausal women aged 42 to 52" and found "an increasing risk of heart disease as blood levels of insulin rise."

The women had an average total cholesterol level of 185, considered normal. "Women with the highest blood insulin levels proved the most likely to have high blood pressure, elevated triglycerides and decreased HDL cholesterol values," according to the report.

Insulin levels increased as body mass (weight in kilograms divided by height in meters) increased, but the "study doesn't offer any hints as to which came first, the increased body weight or higher insulin levels," reports *Medical World News* (30,16:14)."

Other studies have identified insulin levels as a heart-disease risk factor for men. In a report recently presented to the American Diabetes Association, Israeli researcher Michaela Modan stated, "Tests for insulin resistance could be an even earlier indicator of coronary heart disease risk than cholesterol and other blood lipid evaluations."

Dr. Modan suggests that finding a simple test for insulin resistance might pave the way for mass screening of people for this "red flag" indicator of heart disease.

The technique Dr. Modan used was an oral glucose tolerance test. The test involved taking repeated blood samples over a two-hour period. This "crude method" is effective, but is not simple enough for mass screenings, she says.

An added caution: Hypertension (high blood pressure) is an independent risk factor for heart disease, but it presents a three-fold greater risk when it occurs in the presence of hyperinsulinemia.

In fat people, weight loss and physical activity usually can help reduce or eliminate hyperinsulinemia.

Ear crease could be early warning sign of fatal heart attack

A diagonal crease across your earlobe at a 45-degree downward angle toward your shoulder may be an early warning sign of a potentially fatal heart attack, according to reports in *Modern Medicine* (57,10:126) and *British Heart Journal* (611,4:361).

In one study, researchers found telltale ear creases in both fat and skinny people who died from sudden heart attacks, so weight wasn't a factor. The common denominator was sudden death, often in people who apparently didn't know how sick they were.

Researchers randomly selected 303 people whose cause of death was unknown before autopsy. They found diagonal ear creases in 72 percent of the deceased men and 67 percent of the deceased women.

Men with diagonal ear creases were 55 percent more likely to die of heart disease than men without ear creases. The risk was even greater for nondiabetic women (1.74 times more likely to die of heart disease). Interestingly, ear creases did not predict death from heart disease in diabetic women.

People generally don't get ear creases until after age 50, the reports say. Fatness apparently does not influence whether people have ear creases, researchers say, because both fat and thin people have them in roughly equal numbers.

However, people with heart disease seem to develop the creases, regardless of their age, they add. The alarming thing was the link between ear creases and unexpected death. Many people in this study had died suddenly from heart attacks, but had no history of heart disease, the researchers say.

Earlobe creases alone were a greater predictor of sudden death from heart attack than known risk factors, such as previous heart disease, the studies report. That fact has led researchers to speculate that some doctors may be missing severe heart disease cases among some middle-aged and elderly people.

Help yourself by checking your ears for diagonal creases. If there is a crease, tell your doctor about the crease and about these studies. The idea is to catch unsuspected heart disease so you can get appropriate treatment.

Breathless? You may be at risk for a heart attack

If you are a middle-aged man who is frequently out of breath, you may be a prime candidate for a heart attack, suggests a report in *Modern Medicine* (57,9:139).

In a British study, nearly four out of every 10 men who had breathlessness but no signs of heart disease at their initial screening exam developed angina, suffered a heart attack or died within five years, according to the report.

By contrast, only one out of every 12 men without breathlessness at screening developed angina or other heart problems in the next five years.

Angina is severe pain in the chest and arms brought on by blocked heart arteries. It indicates serious, even potentially fatal, heart disease.

"A strong association was also found between breathlessness and silent electrocardiographic evidence of [coronary artery disease], even in men with no other evidence of [the disease] at screening," say the authors of a report from the British Regional Heart Study, a study involving 7,735 British men 40 to 59 years old.

The likelihood of eventual heart disease seemed to be linked directly to the severity of the breathlessness, the report says. In other words, the more out of breath you are, the more likely you are to come down with heart problems.

Check with your doctor if even minor exertion causes you to puff and pant for breath. The doctor may recommend immediate steps you can take to begin lowering your heart attack risk, including changing to a healthier diet and getting into better physical shape.

Bigger isn't better

The old saying "he has a big heart" may have more meaning than it once did. Scientists have found that an enlarged heart may be hazardous to your health and could result in sudden death, even when other heart disease is absent.

This condition is known as left ventricular hypertrophy (LVH) and is often a result of years of high blood pressure, says a report in the *Cardiovascular Research Report* (34:2). Taking measures to prevent or to lower high blood pressure decreases the risk of developing LVH.

Which is worse — a fat stomach or fat hips?

A fat stomach, commonly known as a "spare tire" or a "beer belly," is more dangerous to your health than fat hips or legs.

Abdominal (or stomach) obesity is linked with an increased risk of stroke in men and heart failure in both sexes, according to researchers from Boston University who studied a group of 4,500 adults for 20 years as part of the Framingham Study. "As the ratio of abdominal girth to height increases, so does the risk of developing cardiovascular disease," said Dr. Joseph Stokes III, professor of medicine at Boston University.

"Just looking at overall weight didn't predict which people would develop cardiovascular disease or die," Stokes explained. "Abdominal obesity was a stronger predictor." Heart failure was the complication most strongly associated with abdominal obesity, according to Stokes. For each 2.5 inches of fat, another 10 to 12 people per 1,000 developed heart failure.

The thickness of the skin fold under the shoulder blade, an estimator of upper body fat, appears to be another independent indicator of risk, noted William B. Kannel, another researcher involved in the Framingham Heart Study.

At this point, researchers can only theorize why they believe excess stomach fat is more damaging than other fat. Some think that since the blood flows through this fatty tissue directly to the liver, the organ that secretes and removes cholesterol from the blood, the fat causes more heart problems.

Others suggest that the fat cells in the stomach may be regulated in a different way from those in the buttocks and thighs.

Poor dental health may be a risk factor for heart disease

According to new research from Finland, poor dental health may be a risk factor for developing heart disease, the *British Medical Journal* (298,6676:779) reports. In two separate studies, people with heart disease "had worse dental health than controls" even when other risk factors for heart disease were excluded, Dr. Kimmo Mattila explains in the journal.

The results were adjusted for age, sex, economic background, high blood pressure, cholesterol levels, smoking, diabetes and resistance to insulin, all factors known to be heart-disease risks.

"Little is known about the long-term effects of chronic low grade bacterial infections" that are associated with cavities and gum disease, says the journal. The authors suggest that poisons produced by these bacteria in the mouth may have a harmful effect on the heart.

However, one risk factor that could not be excluded was lifestyle. The researchers speculate that an unhealthy lifestyle could lead to both heart disease and dental infections. If people aren't concerned about their health, they might ignore their teeth as well as their hearts, Mattila suggests. A poor diet also could affect both the heart and dental health, according to the study.

Doctors and dentists in Helsinki began the studies because "only half to three quarters" of coronary heart disease can be attributed to the known risk factors. "Thus, important risk factors seem not yet to have been identified," says Dr. Mattila.

Other studies have shown some relationship among acute viral infections, bacteria and heart disease, they report. However, no studies have pinpointed the links. Although the researchers don't draw any cause-and-effect conclusions, they recommend more studies to determine the effect that poor dental health has on heart disease.

Don't rest up — get up!

Rest is no longer the recommended treatment for people who have had chronic heart failure. Doctors are now encouraging heart patients to exercise.

In a recent study, stable chronic heart failure patients who rode an exercise bike for 20 minutes, five days a week, showed improvement in exercise tolerance, peak oxygen use, heart rate and in symptoms of breathlessness, fatigue and general well-being, says a digest report in *Medical Abstracts* (10,2:3).

People who have had heart failure should talk to their doctor about the benefits of exercise. Your doctor can help plan an exercise program designed especially to meet your needs.

Estrogen therapy fights heart disease?

Should women take estrogen replacements after menopause? Some experts believe they should because estrogen replacement therapy helps reduce a woman's risk of heart disease, says a recent report in *The Western Journal of Medicine* (152,4:408).

Premenopausal women have a lower rate of heart disease than men. Apparently, estrogen helps decrease total cholesterol levels and LDL levels in the blood. Estrogen also increases HDL levels. In effect, the estrogen protects women from heart disease.

However, after menopause, women lose this advantage because they stop producing estrogen. When a woman produces less estrogen because of the onset of menopause or because of a surgical removal of her ovaries, her body no longer fights cholesterol buildup naturally.

Obviously, this places her at a greater risk for heart disease. This causes a woman's risk of heart disease to increase at the same rate as a man's. However, a woman can continue to benefit from the positive effects of estrogen if she replaces the estrogen that her body no longer produces.

According to a study reported in *Medical World News* (31,9:10), women who used estrogen replacement therapy were 40 percent less likely to die of heart attack than nonusers. Estrogen users also had a 50 percent lower risk of stroke than nonusers.

Yet estrogen replacement therapy is not for everyone. Women who still have a uterus must be especially careful. Because of a risk of cancer and other diseases, these women must take progestin replacements along with the estrogen replacements.

Progestin has the opposite effect on blood cholesterol levels than the estrogen does. Progestin raises the LDL levels and lowers the HDL levels, which increases the risk of heart disease.

However, some researchers have recently reported that even a small positive effect of estrogen replacement therapy would outweigh any increased risk of death from endometrial or breast cancer, according to a report in *Geriatrics* (45,5:84).

These researchers report that a 50-year-old white American woman has a 31 percent risk of developing heart disease and only a nine percent risk of breast cancer and a three percent risk of endometrial cancer.

Since a very high number of women die from heart disease, these studies suggest that all women should consider estrogen therapy unless they have other risk factors. The combined effects of progestin and estrogen therapies on blood cholesterol depends on the kind of progestin used. Some forms of progestin do not affect the blood as much as other forms.

Your doctor can recommend which type of progestin and estrogen replacement therapies to use to obtain the best results and the greatest protection from heart problems.

Allergy-causing histamine may have role in heart problems

Histamine, most commonly associated with allergies, may also play a role in the development of atherosclerosis — "hardening of arteries" — that can lead to heart attacks and stroke.

Atherosclerosis is a dangerous accumulation of fat, calcium and other materials, known as plaque, on the inside walls of vital arteries. Plaque on the artery walls causes the blood vessel to lose its flexibility, commonly known as "hardening of the arteries." Then, as the blood vessel becomes narrower and narrower, the volume of blood it can carry is reduced.

Ultimately, the plaque may break up and release its loose pieces, which can block the free flow of blood to the heart muscle or brain and trigger a heart attack or stroke.

Pathologist James B. Atkinson and a team of researchers at Vanderbilt University in Nashville are investigating the relationship between athero-sclerosis and histamine.

Histamine is a chemical involved in allergic reactions. It's contained in mast cells that are related to the immune system. For example, when a wasp bite triggers an allergic reaction, mast cells release the natural bodily substance histamine, which causes redness and swelling around the bite.

Sneezing in people who are allergic to many airborne particles, like ragweed pollen or dust, is caused by histamine in the body. Histamine can also cause blood vessels to constrict and cause an increased heart rate.

Atkinson and his colleagues have suspected that the mast cell also starts an allergic-type reaction in the walls of the arteries that may cause atherosclerosis. As plaque builds up in the arteries, the number of mast cells and the amount of histamine in the arteries is increased, they report.

"We're looking at patients aged 15 to 34 and we're studying changes in the coronary arteries and aorta that may lead to advanced atherosclerosis," says Atkinson. Coronary arteries bring oxygen-rich blood to the heart muscle. The aorta is the trunk artery that takes blood out of the heart to the body.

Add fish to your diet to help prevent fatal heart attacks

Eating fish at least twice a week might prolong your life, according to a new study in *The Lancet* (2,8666:757). Even people with advanced heart disease could benefit, the two-year study suggests. During a two-year study, 2,000 men who had suffered their first heart attacks received advice about fat, fish and fiber intake. Those men who ate fatty fish — such as mackerel, herring, salmon and trout — or took fish oil supplements reduced their chances of dying from another heart attack by nearly one-third.

Although eating fish didn't cut the number of new heart attacks, it seemed to cut the number of fatal attacks, the study indicates.

Heartburn

Can 'harmless' heartburn harm your heart?

For years, doctors have cautioned us not to mistake the warning symptoms of a heart attack for what they considered "harmless" heartburn.

Now, new studies suggest that heartburn itself might represent a real threat to your heart's health. That burning or gnawing pain below the breastbone is triggered when stomach acid backs up into your esophagus, the food tube between the mouth and stomach. We call it heartburn. Doctors call it gastroesophageal reflux.

A University of Maryland doctor reports that such acid backups can actually slow down the heartbeat by 20 beats a minute in otherwise healthy people. Slowing down the heart rate could be dangerous for people with heart disease and previous heart attacks, says a report in *Geriatrics* (45,7:22).

Because of the risk involved with a slowed-down heart, doctors should be "aggressive" in treating reflux, especially among the elderly and people with heart-rhythm problems, says the report.

If you have heart disease and suffer regular episodes of heartburn, ask your doctor about this report in *Geriatrics*. That acid backup into the esophagus might also trigger unexplained coughing and even asthma, says an editorial in *The Lancet* (336,8710:282). About one out of every 10 chronic coughers could get relief by getting treatment for acid reflux, or heartburn, the article suggests. A super-fine acid spray from the stomach possibly irritates lung and esophagus tissues, causing wheezing and asthmatic breathing spasms.

How to help heartburn

"Up to 36 percent of healthy persons report at least one episode of heartburn per month, and 7 percent of these report daily heartburn," according to *Modern Medicine* (57,4:92).

Repeated attacks of heartburn are known medically as gastroesophageal reflux disease (GERD). GERD is caused when stomach acid "backs up" from the stomach into the esophagus, or food pipe, and causes the familiar discomfort we call heartburn. Actual symptoms can range from a burning sensation to sharp stabs of pain.

Heartburn can be ignited by one or more "triggers" acting alone or in combination with each other. Here are several:

- **Problems with the lower esophageal sphincter (or LES), a small flap that helps stop acid from backing up. The LES can become relaxed and lose effectiveness.**

- **Pressure on the stomach.**

- **Delayed emptying of the stomach.**

- **Hiatal hernia.**

- **The content of the material backing up from the stomach.**

Since GERD can be a serious medical problem, recurring heartburn should be brought to the attention of your doctor, Dr. John Goff suggests in *Modern Medicine.*

Some common GERD symptoms include the following:

- **Stomach burning, pain or discomfort below the breastbone.**

- **Regurgitation for no apparent reason or when you bend over.**

- **The sudden filling of your mouth with salty fluid, known as water brash.**

- **Painful or difficult swallowing.**

- **Unusual chest pain not associated with the heart.**

However, even if GERD is diagnosed, there are many simple steps you can take to help alleviate reflux problems, Goff says.

❒ Raise the head of your bed by at least six to eight inches. This should create enough difference in the level of your head and your stomach so that the acid cannot flow up out of your stomach. Researchers in England have found that a 9-inch "lift" to the head of the bed provides great relief for nighttime heartburn, says a report in *The Lancet* (2,8569:1200).

❒ Do not eat for two to three hours before bedtime. During the day, do not lie down if you are bothered by indigestion. Lying down usually makes the problem worse. Sitting up or standing helps the stomach acids remain in the stomach.

❒ Avoid caffeine, fat, chocolate and alcohol. Peppermint, aspirin, tea, fried foods, citrus fruits and juices, onion or garlic can also aggravate indigestion and should be avoided or used only in moderation.

❐ If you are taking a prescription drug that is known to aggravate reflux, talk to your doctor about possibly switching to a different drug.

❐ Reduce or eliminate all types of tobacco use.

❐ Take banana powder.

❐ Lose weight, especially around your waist.

❐ Don't wear tight clothes, girdles or belts.

❐ Eat slowly and avoid chewing gum to reduce the amount of air you swallow.

❐ Suck on lozenges (but not the peppermint-flavored ones). Increasing the flow of saliva by using lozenges can decrease heartburn symptoms.

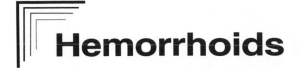

Hemorrhoids

When you should never read

If you read during a leisurely bathroom break, you are likely to develop painful hemorrhoids, says a study reported in *The Lancet* (1,8628:54).

"We found that patients with hemorrhoids tend to spend longer defecating and also are more likely to read and strain while defecating than are patients without hemorrhoids," the researchers said.

While this subject may strike some as indelicate, an attack of hemorrhoids is one of the most common conditions suffered by Americans. Many millions of dollars are spent every year on over-the-counter remedies, visits to doctors and more drastic surgical solutions.

The study suggests that many sufferers may bring the problem on themselves, mostly through poor bowel habits.

Infections

Swimmer's ear can spoil summer fun

Imagine you're at the beach. The weather is perfect, and you've been swimming every day. Then one of your grandchildren complains that her ear feels itchy and sore. When you touch the ear or she moves her jaw from side to side, the pain is worse. It's likely that she has a bacterial infection called otitis externa, or swimmer's ear, and she'll have to stay out of the water until it's cleared up.

Swimmer's ear can happen to anyone, but it happens most often to people who get moisture in their ears during water activities. When water stays in your ears, it breaks down the protective covering in the ear canal, and sets up the perfect conditions for bacteria to grow. People get swimmer's ear for other reasons, too. Some people's ears are formed so that debris and water accumulate in the outer ear canal, encouraging bacterial growth. Also, people who have certain skin conditions tend to get swimmer's ear more often.

U.S. Pharmacist (15,5:73) reports that swimmer's ear can usually be cured in the early stages with nonprescription ear drops containing alcohol and acetic acid. If a more serious infection develops, you will need to see your doctor for treatment and antibiotic ear drops.

However, if you keep the outer ear as dry as possible, you will probably be able to avoid swimmer's ear, even if you swim frequently. Never clean or dry your ears with cotton-tipped applicators. They may push debris deeper into the ear or damage the lining of your outer ear canal, making it easier for bacteria to grow.

To get the water out of your ears after water sports, shake your head vigorously or tilt your head to the side and jump up and down. You can also fan your ears or blow them dry with a hair dryer set on a very low temperature. Finally, use a trick practiced by competitive swimmers: After every swim, put three to six drops of an alcohol-acetic solution into each ear. You can buy these drops at your drugstore without a prescription.

Life-threatening blood infection from deer ticks

Another dangerous disease from the deer tick — this time it's a life-threatening blood infection called babesiosis.

A 63-year-old Wisconsin woman was sick for a month with fever, chills, headaches, extreme tiredness and jaundice. Jaundice is a yellowing of the skin caused by a liver problem. Earlier, she had been treated for Lyme disease. Doctors believe she was bitten by a tick that had earlier bitten an animal infected with babesiosis.

The same tick bite that caused the Lyme disease also might have carried the Babesia germ as well, says Dr. Vincent Iacopino in *Archives of Internal Medicine* (150,7:1527). Because of a long incubation period, it took many months for the babesiosis to make her sick.

The woman required breathing help from a ventilator until she received intense treatment with an antibiotic, quinine and a nearly complete exchange of blood by transfusions. Babesiosis has been rare in the United States, but this report says more cases may show up in the northern Midwest.

Deer ticks are about the size of a pencil point, making them hard to see. Prevent tick bites by wearing clothing that covers you completely. Apply insect repellent before going outside, and take a shower immediately after returning from woods or areas where wild animals might have been.

Lung infection triggered by chopping wood

Can you catch pneumonia from cutting firewood?

A man and his dog both did, reports the *Annals of Internal Medicine* (113,3:252). The 53-year-old Minnesota man spent a day felling a rotten elm tree and cutting it up with a chain saw while his mixed black Labrador played nearby. Two weeks later, man and dog came down with histoplasmosis, a lung infection triggered by spores of a yeast that grows on rotting wood. Both got well after taking antibiotics.

Avoid or wear a special breathing mask in these places: rotting wood close to streams or lakes, chicken coops, starling roosts, caves, attics and cellars, and any place littered with bird or bat droppings, says the article.

Use caution in public restrooms

You were right to be concerned about the hygiene of public toilet seats, according to new research from the University of Arizona. Normal flushing splatters virus-infected water from the bowl onto the seat, handle and surrounding area, says a report in *American Family Physician* (39,6:20). A microbiologist proved the germ splatter by using time-lapse photography, the report says.

What's the worst area for viruses? The middle stall is used most often, thus receiving the most splatters, the report says.

Kidney Problems

Everyday painkiller may seriously harm kidneys

Long-term use of acetaminophen, a widely used painkiller, has been linked to serious kidney damage, according to researchers in North Carolina. Acetaminophen is the main painkilling ingredient in such over-the-counter medications as Tylenol, Datril, Panadol and Anacin-3.

"We found an increased risk associated with daily use of acetaminophen," says the study in *The New England Journal of Medicine* (320,19:1238). The researchers compared the effects on the kidneys of long-term use of acetaminophen, aspirin and another kind of painkiller called phenacetin. Kidney damage was linked to regular use of acetaminophen and phenacetin, but not to aspirin. Phenacetin is no longer in use because of its association with kidney disease and bladder cancer.

The risk of kidney disease increased with the number of pills containing acetaminophen taken each day, but the risk did not increase with years of use after five years, says head researcher Dale P. Sandler.

Caffeine taken with the painkiller increased the kidney damage risk, too. Caffeine is a standard ingredient in many analgesic preparations.

Combination products are also risky. "Regular use of acetaminophen-aspirin combinations, especially when taken jointly with caffeine," was strongly associated with kidney damage, according to *The New England Journal of Medicine* (320,19:1269). For a variety of reasons, the National Institutes of Health recommend against products that combine two or more analgesics.

Kidney disease caused by painkillers can be severe and can lead to the need for dialysis or a kidney transplant. Thirteen percent of people needing dialysis in Australia and 16.8 percent of patients requiring dialysis or transplants in West Germany suffered the kidney damage as a direct result of long-term use of painkillers, the report says. "Acetaminophen has been available in the United States without a prescription since 1955, but aspirin substitutes did not become popular until the early 1970s," says the study.

Many cold, allergy and sinus medications also include acetaminophen as one of the active ingredients. Be sure to read the ingredients listed on the label or box of a product before buying it.

Arthritis drugs cause severe kidney damage

Commonly prescribed arthritis medicines known as NSAIDs cause reversible kidney failure in some elderly people, reports Dr. Jerry H. Gurwitz in *The Journal of the American Medical Association* (264,4:471).

The NSAIDs (nonsteroidal anti-inflammatory drugs) fight pain and inflammation in arthritis conditions. But people in their 70s, 80s and 90s seem to face a high risk of developing a condition called azotemia from heavy doses of NSAIDs.

In azotemia, the kidneys falter and unhealthy levels of nitrogen waste products like urea get into the bloodstream. Take away the high doses of NSAIDs, says the article, and most people get better within two weeks.

However, you should always check with your doctor before you stop taking medications.

If you have bad kidneys, less protein is better

A low-protein diet can reduce the chances of further kidney damage for diabetics and other people with kidney diseases, researchers report in *The Lancet* (2,8677:1411).

For years doctors have advised diabetics to eat the same amount of protein as healthy people. But now they're saying that too much protein could stimulate heavy blood flow into the kidneys, making them work harder. This extra strain on the kidneys could be dangerous.

You have a better chance of avoiding kidney damage if you follow a low-protein diet in the early stages of a kidney disease, researchers say. Low-protein diets can't stop kidney damage in the late or final stages of a serious kidney disease.

In a British study of 19 people with kidney disease, a low-protein diet reduced stress on the kidneys and slowed kidney damage.

Similarly, an 18-month Australian study of 64 diabetics showed that restricting protein intake delays kidney damage. Half of the group ate their regular diet, while the other half ate a protein-restricted diet. Nine of 33 people on the regular diet developed kidney failure, compared with only two of 31 people on the protein-restricted diet.

Although a low-protein diet seems to be the best way to protect kidneys from further damage, be very careful about changing your diet. A drastic change may do more harm than good.

Your doctor or nutritionist can help you plan a safe and healthy diet to suit your nutritional needs and give you the best possible results.

Liver Disease

Lose weight to help keep your liver in good health

If you're at least 11 percent over your ideal weight, you may be headed for liver disease, researchers report in *Science News* (135,21:332). Thirty-nine people who enrolled in a New York City study were.

Researchers put those 39 people on a diet and exercise program. Eighteen months later, 17 people had lost 10 percent of their body weight and showed no signs of liver disease. Those who couldn't stick to the program or gained weight continued to have liver problems.

You could call the liver the chemical factory of the body. It's the largest gland in the body, and it stores bile, a substance which helps digest food.

The liver also filters wastes and toxins from the blood, such as drugs, bacteria and food additives. It stores vitamins and minerals such as iron, which is important for the production of healthy red blood cells. When the liver stops working, the body is in trouble. Unfortunately, liver disease often produces no symptoms, so it is hard to diagnose.

One of the earliest symptoms is jaundice, which causes the skin to turn yellow. Jaundice results when the liver fails to filter certain substances from the blood — a sign that the liver system is breaking down.

If you are overweight, you may want to check with your doctor about starting a safe and healthy diet and exercise program to help reduce your risk of liver disease. After all, the best way to fight liver disease is to prevent it.

Megadoses of slow-release niacin could damage your liver

Slow-release forms of niacin in large doses could damage your liver, warn two recent reports in *The Journal of the American Medical Association* (264,2:181 and 264,2:241).

Doctors have known for a long time that megadoses of niacin, also known as vitamin B3, can cause liver failure. But until now, some had believed that people needing large doses of niacin might be better off taking the sustained-release tablets, the kind that dissolve slowly in the body and feed out small levels of the vitamin over many hours.

According to the report in *JAMA*, four people developed serious liver damage after taking the slow-release niacin instead of the crystalline form.

Two of them changed from the prescribed crystalline kind to the slow-release kind — one 62-year-old man on his own initiative and a 47-year-old man on a pharmacist's recommendation. In a third case, a doctor prescribed slow-release niacin for a 50-year-old woman. All three had been receiving doctor-prescribed treatment of high-dose niacin to lower their high cholesterol levels. They had been taking between 1,500 milligrams and 4,000 milligrams of niacin daily under doctors' supervision. The fourth said he had been taking one 500-milligram slow-release niacin tablet as a daily supplement for two months without checking with a doctor.

The Recommended Dietary Allowance for niacin is 15 milligrams per day for men over 50, and 13 milligrams daily for women over 50. Normally, doctors prescribe the crystalline form of niacin, known as nicotinic acid (no relation whatsoever to the drug nicotine found in tobacco).

Niacin in high doses — sometimes 100 or more times the RDA — is very effective in lowering excessive levels of cholesterol in the blood. The problem is that such high-dose niacin can cause liver damage and other unpleasant side effects, such as skin flushing, especially of the face, and widespread itching.

The slow-release form cuts down on the flushing and itching. But, apparently, it's more dangerous to the liver, even in lower doses and over shorter periods of time. Slow-release niacin tablets are available without prescription in many health food stores and pharmacies.

Such cases point out again the wisdom of checking first with your doctor (and of checking up after your doctor) before taking supplements of any kind. Be especially cautious about taking megadoses of vitamins and minerals that are far beyond recommended daily needs. Some megadoses can be dangerous, even deadly.

Alcohol and painkiller combo can damage liver

If you drink four or five highballs every day, don't take Tylenol for your resulting headache. If you have an alcohol problem, taking the painkiller acetaminophen could deliver a knock-out blow to your liver, warns a report in the *Southern Medical Journal* (83,9:1047).

Acetaminophen is a common over-the-counter pain reliever found in Tylenol, Anacin-3, Contac and more than 80 other brand-name pain relievers and cold and sinus medicines. Doctors commonly warn people about taking too much acetaminophen — an overdose could result in deadly liver damage.

In a new wrinkle, researchers warn that taking acetaminophen in amounts only slightly over the suggested dose could be deadly for people suffering from chronic alcoholism.

The danger lies in the combined effect of chronic alcoholism and acetaminophen. The combination actually can poison the liver. This condition is usually treatable, but it occasionally results in death.

People who drink moderate to large amounts of alcohol on a regular basis should ask their doctors about which over-the-counter pain reliever is most safe and effective for them.

Soybean extract reverses liver disease

Years of heavy alcohol consumption often result in severe liver damage called cirrhosis of the liver. Until now, cirrhosis has been untreatable.

But 12 hard-drinking baboons in New York might point the way to preventing and even reversing the deadly disease, according to *Science News* (138,22:340).

The doctors in the New York study fed the baboons the alcohol equivalent of eight cans of beer a day. Along with the alcohol, some animals received a diet supplemented daily with three tablespoons of soybean lecithin. Others ate just regular baboon foods, without the lecithin. Most of those fed alcohol without lecithin developed severe scarring of the liver, including two cases of cirrhosis. But the eight-beers-a-day group that got the daily lecithin developed almost no scarring, even after eight years of hard drinking, the *SN* report says.

To clinch the case for lecithin, researchers kept on feeding alcohol to three of the baboons but withheld all lecithin. Within two years, all three animals had developed cirrhosis of the liver.

Another researcher reports that lecithin even heals liver tissue scarred by alcohol. That might mean a reversal of early cirrhosis damage, the report says.

Animal tests don't always translate into human benefits. Researchers caution that people who drink too much alcohol should cut back or stop drinking, rather than seek some "magic pill" to allow them to continue their substance abuse.

If you suffer from cirrhosis of the liver, check with your doctor before taking lecithin or supplements of any kind.

Medicine Use and Drug Reactions

Name brand or generic —
there's more at stake than cost alone

Many pharmacists will routinely give you the generic brand of a drug rather than the prescribed "name brand" because the generic brand is usually less expensive. However, the few pennies you save might not be worth the trouble you can get in return.

Some researchers believe that some generic substitute drugs are not as effective as the prescribed brand-name drugs and could even cause severe problems. *The Journal of the American Medical Association* (263,18:2459) reports a recent case in which a 28-year-old man had been taking a drug to help his pancreas function correctly. He had been taking the drug for approximately 25 years with no reported side effects or problems.

One month, his pharmacist replaced the prescribed drug with a generic brand of that drug, and the man immediately began having problems. He telephoned his doctor about the problems that had developed, and his doctor changed the drug back to the original kind. The man's negative side effects disappeared within one week, and he had no more complaints thereafter.

Usually, generic drugs perform exactly as the prescribed medications do, and people have no problems with negative side effects.

However, if you suddenly develop unexplained side effects after switching to a generic drug, ask your doctor or pharmacist to determine if the generic drug is causing the problem. Careful, though — don't stop taking your medicine without checking with your doctor first.

Store your medicine safely

The Food and Drug Administration recommends storing your medications in a cool, dry place — not the bathroom. One drug in particular, carbamazepine (brand name Tegretol), which is taken to prevent epileptic seizures, can "lose one-third of its effectiveness if it is stored in humid conditions," such as a bathroom, the FDA says. Poor storage may explain why some epileptic patients complain that carbamazepine sometimes doesn't work for them.

Store all medications at room temperature unless otherwise directed by your doctor or pharmacist. Refrigerating drugs can change the way they work, endangering your health, says a digest in *Bottom Line* (9,13:4). Ask your doctor or pharmacist if it's safe to put your medication in the fridge.

When medications do more harm than good

Medications can literally be lifesavers in their ability to improve an elderly person's health. However, some medications can also seriously compromise or endanger someone's health through their bad side effects.

Bad side effects are especially common among elderly people. Due to the bodily changes that accompany aging, a healthy dose of many medications for a younger person may be too strong for an older person. For example, a 10-milligram dose of Valium for a 35-year-old man might just relax his muscles. That same dose of Valium in a 75-year-old woman would relax her muscles so much that she could lose all muscle coordination and be unable to get around, warns *FDA Consumer* (24,9:24). Or, some kinds of medications that cause few or no side effects in younger people often cause a wide variety of side effects in the older population.

For instance, a simple anti-inflammatory drug could help ease the pain of aching joints without any adverse side effects in a young athlete. That same anti-inflammatory drug in an older person could help relieve the pain and stiffness of arthritis. However, it could also cause gastrointestinal irritation, ruin the appetite, and interfere with proper digestion.

In fact, two of the most common adverse side effects of many oral medications are digestion problems and nutritional disturbances. Some drugs prevent vitamins and minerals from being absorbed into the body properly. Other drugs interfere with your enjoyment of food by causing dry mouth or decreasing the sense of taste, reports *Geriatric Nursing* (11,6:301). Diarrhea and constipation, as well as depression and dementia (mental confusion), are other common side effects of many medications.

A very common problem that many elderly people face is that of drug interactions. Most elderly people take more than one kind of medication. Occasionally, these different drugs react to each other and cause negative side effects when they meet in the bloodstream or digestive system.

Sometimes, improper use of the medications causes negative drug side effects. Many people do not fully understand the proper way to use the medication. Using some drugs at the wrong time or with the wrong kinds of food or drink can produce side effects that could be easily avoided.

If you think you are experiencing some negative side effects from one or more of your medications, talk to your doctor immediately. If you are taking prescription drugs, do not stop taking the drugs without first consulting with your physician. The negative effects of stopping drug therapy can be much more dangerous, or even life-threatening, than any of the negative side effects you're experiencing.

Here's a list of questions that may be helpful to ask the doctor:

- **What is the drug I'm taking?**
- **What is the drug supposed to do?**
- **What are the possible side effects?**
- **Is the drug habit-forming?**
- **Should I take the drug with food or without food?**
- **At what times of the day should I take the drug?**
- **Should I avoid any activities while taking the drug, such as driving or exercising?**

If you are experiencing negative side effects from one or more over-the-counter drugs, the wisest course of action is to talk with your local pharmacist. He can suggest some other over-the-counter drugs that will perform the same service without the negative side effects. Or, he may suggest a nondrug form of therapy for dealing with your situation.

To ensure the safest and most effective use of your medications, see the following table of some "Dos" and "Don'ts" of drug therapy.

Dos and Don'ts of medicine use

Dos

❐ Call your doctor immediately if you notice any new symptoms or side effects, such as confusion, sleeplessness, incontinence or impotence.

❐ Store your medicines properly. This usually means storing them in a cool, dry place. Some medicine should be stored in the refrigerator. The bathroom is usually not the best place to store drugs. Bathrooms are warm, damp places, and some drugs may lose their potency if exposed to moisture.

❒ Always read the labels and other information and instructions provided with the prescription.

❒ Always throw away old or expired medicines. Make sure you flush them down the toilet instead of throwing them into the trash can.

❒ Be sure to take the exact amount prescribed.

*Don't*s

❒ Do not take medicine in the dark. Always turn on the light and make sure you are taking the right medicine.

❒ Never stop taking a drug suddenly without checking with your doctor — even if you feel better.

❒ Do not take drugs prescribed for someone else or give your drug to anyone else.

❒ Don't transfer a drug from its original bottle to another.

❒ Never drink alcoholic beverages while you're taking your medication unless your doctor says it's OK. Mixing alcohol with medicine can be dangerous. Of the hundreds of medicines commonly prescribed, many contain at least one substance that reacts badly with alcohol.

Drugs that interfere with nutrition

❒ **Aspirin:** Interferes with levels of folic acid and ascorbic acid in the blood, and causes a deficiency of iron.

❒ **Laxatives:** Interfere with the absorption of calcium in the body.

❒ **Penicillin:** Reduces the amount of potassium in the body by increasing the amount of potassium released in the urine.

❒ **Mineral oil:** Interferes with the absorption of vitamins such as vitamins A, D and E.

❒ **Antacids that contain aluminum:** Reduce absorption of fluoride and phosphorus in the body, and reduce the amount of calcium by increasing the amount of calcium lost in the urine.

❒ **Antacids with aluminum or magnesium:** Lower the absorption of phosphorus in the body by increasing the amount of phosphorus lost in the urine.

❏ **Antacids with sodium-bicarbonate:** Result in bloating due to water retention and sodium retention.

❏ **Tetracyclines:** Inhibit the absorption of vitamins such as iron, calcium, magnesium and zinc.

❏ **Corticosteroids:** Inhibit absorption of phosphorus and calcium and raise the body's need for other vitamins, such as vitamin D, folic acid and ascorbic acid.

Beware of mixing drugs

If you take a number of medications and suffer from agitation, confusion, delirium and dry mouth, you may be overdosing yourself, according to *Drug Therapy* (19,11:45). For example, if you take three medications — two prescription and one over-the-counter — that happen to produce the same side effects, the side effects will be tripled. Always tell your doctor about every medication you take, and ask your pharmacist whether prescription drugs can be used with over-the-counter drugs.

'Take only as directed ...'

How closely you follow the directions on your medicine bottles will determine how effective your medicines will be. For example, food can either help or hurt the effectiveness of a drug.

Medications that should be taken with food are obviously most effective when taken with food. When taken on an empty stomach, the medications don't work as well. And medications that should not be taken with food lose some of their effectiveness if taken on a full stomach, reports *The Lancet* (335,8689:597). If you have questions about when or how to take your medicine, be sure to contact your doctor or pharmacist immediately.

Commonly prescribed sedatives contribute to falling accidents

One of the most commonly prescribed sedatives may play a major role in causing older people to fall, leading to more broken hips, says a study in *The Journal of the American Medical Association* (262,23:3303).

The culprit is the tranquilizer ingredient benzodiazepine. It or closely related drugs are found in many preparations including Valium, Xanax,

Tranxene, Ativan, Serax, Centrax, Paxipam, Librium and Libritabs, Limbitrol and Menrium brands.

In the study, people over 65 who used the long-acting benzodiazepine faced a risk of broken hip nearly double that of people who took other kinds of tranquilizers, according to the *JAMA* report.

"For older patients, a serious consequence of [using] ... benzodiazepines may be an increased risk of falling and fall-related fractures," say the researchers. They recommend that doctors avoid prescribing this tranquilizer and sleeping pill for people over 65, the report says. If you are taking this medication, talk with your doctor before changing or discontinuing use of the drug.

Driving under the influence of ... antihistamines?

Taking a common, over-the-counter antihistamine might affect you in the same way as drinking several quick shots of liquor, two independent studies suggest. The kinds of antihistamines that cause sleepiness also can knock precious seconds off your reaction time while driving an automobile, says a report in *Medical World News* (31,11:19).

In one test, two hours after taking a pill containing diphenhydramine, men reacted to traffic hazards half as quickly as when they took a fake pill. Their slowed reactions were about the same as drivers with 0.10 percent blood alcohol levels. A driver with that level of blood alcohol is considered legally drunk in most states. Diphenhydramine also is the active ingredient in several nonprescription sleeping pills.

Another test used the antihistamine triprolidine. Driver impairment was equivalent to a drinking driver with 0.06 percent blood alcohol, enough to get you in trouble with the law in many states.

Most over-the-counter antihistamines contain package warnings against driving while using the medicines, but more than six out of 10 people ignore the instructions, the report says.

People vary in their responses to so-called sedative-type antihistamines, so a blanket prohibition against driving after taking a sneezing-sniffling pill probably is "inappropriate," the report concludes.

Most newer types of antihistamines don't cause sleepiness, and people in tests don't show any driving impairment while taking them, the report says.

Products containing sedative-type antihistamines

The following products contain sleep-inducing antihistamines (this is not a complete list):

- Diphenhydramine
- Alka-Seltzer Plus Night-Time Cold Medicine
- Excedrin PM tablets and capsules
- Benadryl syrup, tablets, spray and capsules
- Miles Nervine Nighttime Sleep-Aid
- Nytol tablets
- Sleep-eze 3 tablets
- Sleepinal Night-time Sleep Aid capsules
- Sominex tablets and liquid
- Sominex Pain Relief formula
- Unisom Dual Relief Nighttime Sleep Aid/Analgesic
- Triprolidine
- Actidil syrup and tablets
- Actifed capsules, syrup and tablets
- Actifed Plus caplets and tablets
- Actifed 12-Hour capsules

Source: *Physicians' Desk Reference for Nonprescription Drugs*

Your antidepressant may be depressing your blood pressure

If your doctor has prescribed medication to ease depression, take note: Some antidepressants may do more harm than good if you have a heart condition. This warning comes from researchers at the Mayo Clinic in Rochester, Minn., who say doctors should fully evaluate a person's health before prescribing an antidepressant.

The most common side effect of antidepressants is low blood pressure, which in the elderly may lead to stroke and heart attack and sometimes results in death. Side effects may be more harmful in the elderly because they often take many different medications which may interact with one another. Elderly people are also more sensitive to certain drugs, so dosage is important. Here are a few common antidepressants and their side effects:

❏ **Imipramine**: Low blood pressure, erratic heart rhythm, increased heart rate, heart block (the heart works at less than capacity).

❏ **Maprotiline**: Heart block, low blood pressure, nerve disorders, seizures.

❏ **Trazodone**: Low blood pressure, irregular heart beat.

Generally, antidepressants are safe and effective. If you take an antidepressant and have had side effects, or are concerned about them, talk to your doctor.

When your heart can't keep its beat, this drug may throw your rhythm off more

Could the heart medication you've been taking to prevent dangerous irregular heartbeats actually be doing the opposite? Could it be creating irregular heartbeats and increasing your risk of sudden death? Many researchers think so.

According to a recent news release from the American Heart Association, "anti-arrhythmic drugs, rather than protecting against life-threatening irregular heartbeats, may actually worsen some patient's conditions and possibly increase the risk of sudden death." Apparently, anti-arrhythmic drugs prevent one kind of life-threatening irregular heartbeat (arrhythmia), but they cause a different kind of irregular heartbeat that may cause sudden death. Most doctors prescribe anti-arrhythmic drugs for people with congestive heart failure in an effort to cut the high death rate among these patients.

This practice could be changing now. "A lot of people are taking anti-arrhythmic drugs who don't need them," says Dr. Milton Packer in *Circulation*, an American Heart Association journal.

Doctors are beginning to think that this drug therapy should be limited to patients with serious arrhythmias that cause significant symptoms or are life-threatening. In these serious cases, the benefits of the drug may outweigh the risks.

If you are taking anti-arrhythmic drugs, you may want to ask your doctor to reevaluate your need for them in light of the new studies. But do not stop taking these medications on your own. Stopping the drug therapy without checking with your doctor could be just as dangerous.

Heart medication caution

A type of drug commonly prescribed to treat high blood pressure may cause a persistent, dry cough in some people, warns a report in *Emergency Medicine* (22,4:8). The culprits: angiotensin-converting enzyme inhibitors (ACE inhibitors), which help improve blood flow.

A mild cough is nothing to worry about, but some people cough so severely that it causes other serious problems, such as urinary incontinence and rectal and vaginal muscle strain. If you take an ACE inhibitor and have an unexplained cough without a sore throat or a fever, check with your doctor to see if your medication is at fault.

Bee stings and beta-blockers: a dangerous combination?

A British doctor blames his heart medication for causing a simple wasp sting to endanger his life. The doctor was stung on the head while shifting some logs in his garden, according to his report in *The Lancet* (2,8663:619). Although he had never before experienced an allergic reaction, within 30 seconds itchy patches erupted on his hands and around his waist and hips. Within three minutes, his tongue and lips had swollen, and hives had broken out all over his body.

By the time his wife was able to get him into a car five minutes later and drive him to the hospital, the doctor was going into allergic shock with a dangerous drop in blood pressure. Emergency room doctors gave him hydrocortisone and antihistamines to stop the potentially fatal shock reaction, and he recovered nicely.

The doctor believes the allergic reaction to the wasp sting was greatly aggravated by his prescription heart drug, a beta-blocker called atenolol. He had been taking the drug for two years, following a heart attack.

Beta-blockers are a class of heart drugs that act on the heart to make it reduce the rate and force of its contractions, thus cutting down on the heart's workload. Some beta-blockers are being tried in other ways, too, notably to treat some psychiatric illnesses.

"In giving advice — apart from the obvious warnings to avoid bees, wasps, yellow jackets and hornets — doctors might think of mentioning the need for urgent hospital attendance should a person on beta-blockers be stung," Dr. D.L. Pedersen writes. The doctor says he now carries a bee sting kit with appropriate medicine in his golf bag.

Flying high or nose dive — it's all in the medication

One common medicine for high blood pressure seems to cause a nose dive in people's quality of life, while another kind seems to give people a nice boost, reports an *Associated Press* story.

People taking the prescription beta-blocker propranolol reported that it seemed to worsen their sex lives, emotions, work and sleep habits. But people taking the calcium channel blocker nicardipine said they noticed improvements in all those areas. Beta-blockers and calcium channel blockers work about equally well in controlling high blood pressure, said Dr. Lars G. Ekelund at the 13th meeting of the International Society of Hypertension in Montreal.

Another strike against beta-blockers: This class of drug increases LDL ("bad") cholesterol and lowers HDL, the "good" form. That raises people's risk of heart disease, the report says.

Check the scale, then check the medicine cabinet

Before you start blaming yourself for an unexpected weight gain, maybe you should check your medicine cabinet.

A study reported in the *British Medical Journal* (300,6729:902) suggests that weight gain may be a side effect of long-term use of propranolol, a beta-blocker used for heart problems.

According to *BMJ*, the medicinal weight gain was seen in both men and women involved in a 40-month study, and the weight gain wasn't limited to any age group. Although the weight increase was moderate, it was in addition to any other weight differences due to aging or overeating.

Because some people suffer physically or emotionally from even a slight increase in weight, the news that medication can cause a further gain is important.

Weight gain is never a simple problem. Why one person can eat anything and remain thin, while another person counts calories and still gains has always been difficult to answer. Obviously metabolism plays an important part, but to further complicate the matter, certain medications bring about undeserved gain. These pounds seem especially hard to control since eating and exercise habits aren't to blame.

Your doctor will advise you if it's important to your health to take propranolol. Always follow his advice — just be aware that a gradual increase in weight may accompany the medical benefits of the drug.

Diuretic drug plus dieting can be fatal

A woman lost 22 pounds and her life, probably because she combined a popular low-protein diet with diuretic drugs to lose weight, all without her doctor's knowledge, says a report in *The Lancet* (2,8662:572). The 59-year-old woman was found dead in bed seven weeks after going on the "Cambridge diet," says Dr. C.E. Connolly.

She had lost about 22 pounds, down to 185, during the six weeks she stayed on the low-protein diet. She skipped a week, and died a day after resuming the diet. "She had complained of headache and dizziness for a few days before her death, but did not go to see her doctor," according to the report.

Officials discovered the woman had been taking diuretics on and off for several years. She apparently was under the impression that the "water pills" would help her lose weight. She probably died when her heart rhythms went haywire, the doctor says.

Several people on low-protein diets have died in recent years. Drastic, "crash" dieting and too much of a diuretic can cause big disruptions in the body's normal electrolyte balance. Low-protein diets can starve the heart muscle itself, Dr. Connolly says. Both problems can lead to jumbled heart rhythms and death.

Makers of the Cambridge diet products warn in literature sent to doctors that diuretics should be avoided while on the diet, the report says.

Lessons to be learned: Don't go on a crash diet without checking with your doctor. And don't "self-medicate" with drugs that may have dangerous side effects and interactions with other drugs or food.

'Water pills' may disrupt heart rhythms

If you take thiazide diuretics — "water pills" — to control your mild or moderate high blood pressure, your heart may be starving for two vital minerals, warns a report in *American Family Physician* (40,5:256).

Long-term use of thiazide medicines may drain potassium and magnesium along with the excess water from your tissues, the report says.

Shortages of those two nutrients can cause the heart to misfire, resulting in increased numbers of what's known as ventricular premature complexes.

When that happens, the heart muscle quivers between beats — something called arrhythmias. The misfires increase with exercise, the report says. Bad heart rhythms make the heart beat less efficiently, overworking a muscle already strained by high blood pressure.

A string of such bad rhythms could completely disrupt the normal beating, in effect, stopping the heart. That's what happens to victims of electrical shock — the jolt of current knocks the heart's normal electrical pulses out of kilter.

Doctors often prescribe potassium supplements for their patients taking thiazide medicines. But they just as often neglect to recommend more magnesium, the report says.

"In addition to potassium supplementation, magnesium supplementation should also be considered in patients who receive thiazide diuretics," the report warns. Check with your doctor before taking or changing medicines.

Serious side effects of some arthritis drugs

Heavy doses of several common arthritis drugs can cause severe side effects, a medical report warns.

The side effects include ulcers, stomach bleeding, ringing in the ears, lightheadedness, slurred speech, difficulty with concentration, confusion, memory loss, hallucinations, paralysis and even death, according to *Geriatrics* (44,4: 95).

The drugs are NSAIDs (nonsteriodal anti-inflammatory drugs), including aspirin and ibuprofen. They are used to treat arthritis, menstrual cramps and general pain.

Another issue of *Geriatrics* (45,4:18) reports that more than one-third of all hospital admissions for bleeding ulcers in British hospitals were directly linked to these arthritis drugs — especially in people over age 60.

People with arthritis who need to take high doses of NSAIDs over many months or years are at highest risk of suffering from dangerous side effects, the medical journal says.

The elderly are at an increased risk because their liver and kidneys do not work as well. When kidneys get sluggish with age, the body doesn't clear out the drugs as quickly, leading to more serious side effects than experienced by younger people. Elderly people may also have worse side effects because they take many different drugs. As a group, the elderly are seven times more likely than the general population to experience adverse drug reactions, the report says.

Studies show that up to four percent of patients on continuous therapy with NSAIDs may have serious gastrointestinal reactions, like peptic ulcers and stomach bleeding. These dangerous side effects can occur without warning symptoms and can lead to death, reports Marie R. Griffen in the *Annals of Internal Medicine* (109:359).

According to the FDA, studies indicate that one out of 100 patients treated for three to six months suffers some of these serious effects at some time during the treatment. For every 100 patients treated with NSAIDs for one year, two to four will experience ulcers and stomach bleeding.

Dr. James F. Fries, Associate Professor of Medicine at Stanford University Medical Center in California, warns that all people who have experienced previous upper abdominal pain and anyone taking antacids or certain digestive medications are probably in a high risk category for GI (gastrointestinal) disturbances. Smokers and people taking corticosteroids also need to be alert to signs of GI disturbances.

Irritability, disorientation and exhaustion have also been linked to NSAIDs, *Geriatrics* reports.

Another arthritis fighter, gold compounds, have severe side effects, too. They can cause skin rashes, diarrhea and even severe central nervous system problems like delirium, cranial nerve palsy, tremor, pain syndrome and paralysis.

If you notice any of these side effects, contact your doctor immediately. Many times the dose or drug can be changed, and the side effect eliminated. However, don't stop taking or change the dose of any drug without consulting your doctor first.

Ibuprofen: friend or foe?

Millions of Americans rely on nonprescription pain killers to help with arthritis pain and other ongoing physical problems. The group of medicines most often recommended are nonsteroidal anti-inflammatory drugs (NSAIDs).

Ibuprofen is one of the most effective and widely used NSAIDs, but according to a study conducted at the Johns Hopkins University School of Medicine, it isn't a panacea.

The Johns Hopkins researchers conducted the study because they wanted to learn more about the effects of NSAIDs on the kidneys, reports the *Annals of Internal Medicine* (112,8:568. A group of twelve women, ranging in age from 28 to 75, were given 800 milligrams of ibuprofen three times daily for eleven days.

Their renal function was then closely monitored for signs of renal failure. Kidney function in these women was considered "stable" if adequate amounts of prostaglandins, an ingredient necessary for the regulation of healthy renal activity, were present.

Prostaglandins play a critical role in people over 60 years old, or in anyone with circulatory problems, such as kidney failure or liver disease.

Through urine analysis, the researchers found that ibuprofen suppressed the prostaglandin levels below those considered healthy. When prostaglandin levels are low, ibuprofen-induced, severe renal failure can occur. In most cases, renal failure brought on by ibuprofen is reversible once the constant doses are discontinued. But the message here seems to suggest moderation in your intake before a problem can occur.

Remember to work closely with your doctor, especially if you suspect any change in the way your pain-reliever is affecting your general health.

Anti-baldness drug can cause pain and burning

Four men tried a prescription hair grower, minoxidil, to fight their baldness. In addition to hair, though, they got severe cases of pain and burning sensations in the shoulders, pelvic girdle, arms and legs, reports a letter to the editor in the *Annals of Internal Medicine* (113,3:256).

Minoxidil was the only medicine they were taking. They applied it to their scalps twice a week for two to 14 months. In addition to the days and nights of severe pain (called polymyalgia), some of them suffered loss of taste, loss of appetite, weight loss, chest pains and fatigue. Doctors took them off the hair-growing medicine, and all their symptoms disappeared, the report says.

Glaucoma eye drops may react with other prescribed medications

Are you suffering from light-headedness, nausea, vomiting, memory loss, blurry vision and fatigue, and your doctor doesn't know why? If you have glaucoma, your eye drops could be the culprit, according to a report in the *Annals of Internal Medicine* (112,2:120).

Headache, tremors, disorientation, bowel distress, and lower heart rate and blood pressure are just some of the side effects that have been linked with glaucoma medications. If you have any of these side effects accompanying your eye problems, see your doctor right away.

Most people with glaucoma are elderly, and they may be taking other medications to treat a host of medical problems. Although most glaucoma medications are made to reduce pressure in the eye itself, some of the drug can be absorbed into the body through the tear ducts, interacting with other medications you may be taking.

To reduce the amount of glaucoma medicine that is absorbed by your body, apply gentle pressure on your tear ducts. Experts recommend that you lie down while putting in eye drops and apply only one drop at a time.

After putting in eye drops, hold a soft tissue to your tear ducts in the inside corners of your eyes for five minutes.

The best thing you can do to prevent drug side effects is to let all your doctors know what medications you take. That includes over-the-counter medicines and even vitamin and mineral supplements. Your eye doctor and family physician probably don't talk with each other about your health and about the medications you're taking, so it's up to you to keep them informed.

Glaucoma drug causes taste disturbances

If you're taking the drug acetazolamide to help manage your glaucoma and you've noticed that things don't taste like they used to, you are probably suffering from an adverse drug side effect.

Apparently, the drug acetazolamide can cause a taste disturbance that can occur as quickly as six hours after taking the first dose and last for as long as 24 hours after the last dose, reports *The Lancet* (336,8724:1190).

This little-known side effect could be serious in an indirect way. If you are suffering from taste disturbances, you may begin neglecting your meals because the food doesn't taste right. This could lead to nutritional problems and vitamin deficiencies.

If you are experiencing changes in your sense of taste, do not stop taking the drug. Instead, speak to your doctor. He may be able to prescribe another drug that will help manage your glaucoma and not interfere with your sense of taste and your eating habits.

Antibiotic blamed for fatal reaction

A 75-year-old man being treated for bronchitis developed severe blood vessel inflammations and hemorrhages and died after taking the prescription antibiotic known as ofloxacin.

The man was in the hospital being treated for heart failure when he came down with a lung infection. After he had taken 200 milligrams of ofloxacin twice a day for five days specifically for the bronchitis, the trouble started, according to the report in the *British Medical Journal* (299,6700:685). He developed a typical drug rash, and numerous blisters and bleeding areas popped up in his mouth and on his hands and feet, the report says. Doctors found blood in his urine and bowel movements. Despite intensive care, he died within two weeks of starting the antibiotic.

Typical reactions from the fluorinated quinolone drug usually show up as nausea, diarrhea, headache and restlessness, the *BMJ* report says.

"Ofloxacin was probably an important factor in this case," say the attending physicians. "We suggest that because of this, the drug should be used only when other, better-known agents are ineffective."

Mouth Problems

Are there hidden dangers in your mouth?

Those silver fillings in your teeth contain one of the most poisonous "heavy" metals known, and some dentists are beginning to worry about the long-term risks, cautions an article in *The Atlanta Journal*.

The potential danger is this: Although silver is relatively harmless, the fillings are not 100 percent silver.

The fillings are made of silver "amalgam," a mixture that is about 50 percent mercury. The chemical and physical processes that produce amalgam are supposed to keep mercury locked into the tooth and away from your tissues.

However, a small but growing number of scientists believe that mercury in tooth fillings can "leak" into the tissues in the mouth in dangerous amounts and then spread to other parts of the body.

"Fillings release small amounts of mercury into the body, particularly when the amalgam is new," cautions Dr. Miroslav Marek, a researcher at the Georgia Institute of Technology.

"It is quite clear that the highest amount of mercury is released during and immediately following the actual filling of the cavity," he warns. "There is a question about what happens during those peaks of exposure, as the body absorbs the mercury and distributes it to various organs."

In addition to the immediate danger associated with new fillings, there is also a concern about mercury being released over longer periods of time.

The filling is covered with a layer of tin — part of the amalgam material — which prevents the mercury from "leaking" into the tissues in the mouth, Dr. Marek explains.

However, this film of tin can be damaged or destroyed over time by chewing and other abrasive actions. When the protective layer of tin is damaged, mercury can escape, he argues.

Autopsy studies in Sweden and California show that mercury levels in the brain appear to be linked to the number of silver amalgam fillings in the mouth, the report in the *Journal* states.

Researchers are also finding that when mercury does "leak" from fillings, it accumulates in the highest levels in the liver and kidneys.

Some of the side effects of mercury poisoning include insomnia, slurred speech, brain damage, deafness, blindness and muscle tremors.

The alternatives to amalgam fillings are gold, porcelain, and plastic-quartz-mix fillings.

These materials cost more and aren't as easy to work with as amalgam.

The jury is still out on whether "leaky" fillings pose a measurable danger to significant numbers of people.

In the meantime, if you have unexplained symptoms that match those of mercury poisoning, ask your doctor about tests and treatments available. Some symptoms of mercury poisoning are increased salivation, stomach cramps and kidney problems.

Suffering from dry mouth?

Dry mouth could be caused from using snuff or chewing tobacco.

People who use smokeless tobacco have a lot of saliva when they are using the tobacco. But they have a lower-than-normal amount of saliva in their mouths when they are not using it.

Researchers from Emory University believe that the increased dryness may lead to more plaque on the teeth, which can cause tooth decay, says a report in *News Tips From Emory University*.

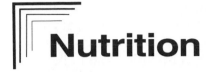

Nutrition

Build a 'foundation diet' for good health

You may think it's too late to change your eating habits, but that is not so. Changing your eating habits today will go a long way toward promoting good health tomorrow, regardless of your age.

Take these tips from nutritionist Nancy Clark, who outlines a "foundation diet" in *Senior Patient* (1,5:95). She encourages you to eat more of these good foods:

❐ **Dairy products** — Even if you're watching cholesterol, don't eliminate dairy foods entirely, she advises. Choose nonfat (rather than low-fat) products, which have all the vitamins and minerals you need without the fat. You should have three servings of dairy products each day. With lunch, try a cup of nonfat yogurt with fruit or add powdered milk to mashed potatoes. A hefty scoop of cottage cheese has only 130 milligrams of calcium but a whopping 20 grams of protein (equivalent to a quarter-pound hamburger before it's cooked).

❐ **Fruits** — Orange and grapefruit juices are more nutritious than other fruit juices, such as apple, grape and cranberry — and they're lower in calories, too. A six-ounce glass of orange juice will provide your daily requirement of vitamin C. But eating the whole fruit is better than drinking a glass of juice, according to the nutritionist. Bananas are potassium-rich and have only about 100 calories — a good afternoon snack. Spread peanut butter on top for extra protein.

❐ **Vegetables** — Choose dark, colorful vegetables — romaine lettuce, spinach, green peppers, broccoli and carrots. One carrot — whether cooked or grated into a salad — will provide the recommended daily allowance of vitamin A, the report says. Celery, cucumbers, onions and radishes have a greater "crunch factor" but aren't as nutritious. Another way to get your RDA of vitamin C is to eat "one stalk of cooked broccoli, half a green pepper, two medium tomatoes or a spinach salad." Avoid canned or processed tomatoes, which are high in sodium. Tomato juice and sauce are fine and "are as nutritious as fresh tomatoes." Winter squash is high in vitamin A and potassium.

Potatoes are nutrient-rich (potassium, fiber and vitamin C) and can be prepared in many ways. Potatoes are not fattening; what you put on them is. Avoid butter, sour cream and gravies. Instead, "mash" a baked potato with a butter substitute or a little skim milk.

Don't overcook vegetables. They will retain more nutrients if they're microwaved or steamed rather than boiled.

Don't use soap to wash your vegetables before eating, warn government health officials. Soap leaves unseen residues on your vegetables, which can cause intestinal problems, says Myron Johnsrud of the U.S. Department of Agriculture. Best way to clean your vegetables: Rinse thoroughly under plain running water, says USDA.

❐ **Starches** — Generally, darker breads are more nutritious than refined white breads. Whole-wheat, bran and rye breads are fiber-rich. Try a slice with a thin spread of peanut butter. Freeze bread to keep it fresh; it takes only a few minutes for slices to thaw. Bran cereals are good sources of fiber and iron and help lower cholesterol. "Look for the words 'enriched' or 'fortified' on the labels," the nutritionist suggests. To get a healthy start in the morning, try bran cereal with skim milk, a banana and a glass of orange juice.

❐ **Meat and fish** — Nutritionists recommend two weekly servings of fish, which keeps your heart healthy and is easy to prepare. "Put the fish in a shallow pan, add a little water, cover and cook over medium heat for about five minutes until it flakes easily when pierced with a fork," Nancy Clark says. Choose extra-lean ground beef and turkey — good sources of protein, vitamins, iron and zinc. Limit beef to three four-ounce servings a week. Commercially prepared turkey usually has more fat and calories than turkey prepared at home.

❐ **Treats** — "Fig newtons, raisin squares, animal crackers and gingersnaps are acceptable treats because they're lower in saturated fats than most desserts and offer slightly more nutritional value than chocolate chip cookies," says the report.

Low-fat diet helps strengthen immune system

Are people who eat high-fat diets more likely to become ill? Yes, say University of Massachusetts researchers in *The American Journal of Clinical Nutrition* (50,4:861). A low-fat diet, combined with regular exercise, can help you build up your resistance to illness and disease, they add.

They studied 17 healthy, male nonsmokers 21 to 39 years old who were not overweight. After analyzing their diets, researchers advised them how to eat less fat. After eating a low-fat diet for three months, the men were found to have built up a large supply of natural killer cells. Natural killer cells form an important part of the body's immune system. These specialized "warrior" cells attack and kill cancer and tumor cells.

In addition to improving immunity, the low-fat diet helped the men control their weight. They ate fewer calories and exercised regularly. Those two factors directly affect the buildup of killer cells, researchers say. Scientists have known for some time that poor diet directly affects our ability to fight disease.

Some researchers suggest that diseases such as cancer may be linked to a "defective immune system." In everyday terms, "defective immune system" means the same thing as lowered resistance.

The Massachusetts researchers are quick to point out that their study was small, not large enough to prove anything. In addition, they say, a low-fat diet affects only natural killer cells, not the entire immune system.

Larger studies are needed to see whether women, cancer patients and the elderly would gain immunity from low-fat diets.

Raw vegetables help guard against cholesterol buildup

Four ounces of raw broccoli contains twice as much vitamin C as four ounces of orange juice made from frozen concentrate.

If the broccoli is really fresh — just-picked broccoli has a bluish-green color — it contains nearly 40 percent more than stalks that have been in the store for a few days.

But freeze the broccoli, or steam it, blanch it, boil it, or cook it in any way, and it loses half its vitamin C content, says a report in *Science News* (137,23:367).

Some research indicates that vitamin C serves as a powerful guard against buildups of cholesterol on artery walls. That protects against hardening of the arteries and lowers the risks of heart attacks and strokes.

Other protective substances in broccoli, cabbage and related cruciferous vegetables also lose their potency when hit by cooking heat.

Cooked vegetables are good for you, the report reaffirms. But the best deal is to eat veggies raw and as fresh as you can get them.

When eating vegetables can be dangerous

"Eat your veggies!" may be very bad advice for a few people. In fact, for a small group of people, eating vegetables regularly could literally shorten their lives!

A few people have a rare genetic disorder called phytosterolemia. This condition causes a person to absorb a large amount of plant sterols (vegetable fats) from regular vegetables.

Someone with phytosterolemia has a high level of sterols in the blood and a large number of fatty deposits under the skin, resulting in little tumor-like growths on the eyelids, buttocks and other places. Such a person also has a higher risk of developing hardened arteries and blocked blood vessels, says an article in *Diet and Health*, a publication of the National Research Council.

People with this genetic disorder "therefore should greatly limit their intake of plant sterols," the article says.

Oat bran extract

Lower your blood cholesterol level by eating ice cream! A fantasy, you say? U.S. Department of Agriculture scientists say they have come up with a new process that extracts the fat-fighting part of oat bran and turns it into a creamy substance that could be used to replace many kinds of fats in foods, including ice cream.

Called oatrim, the white, tasteless flour is loaded with beta-glucans, the part of oat bran that researchers believe lowers cholesterol levels. Researchers treat oat bran with enzymes to produce either a flour or a powder.

In animal tests, oatrim slashed cholesterol by 18 percent. Even better, it hits hardest at LDL cholesterol, the "bad" form, while it seems to slightly increase HDL or "good" cholesterol, says a report in *The Wall Street Journal* (215,79:B1).

Adding about an ounce of oatrim to an instant breakfast drink gives you more cholesterol-lowering beta-glucans than three ounces of pure oat bran, the report says.

Use moderation in eating oat bran

He must have thought, if a little oat bran is good, a lot is better. That's why a 75-year-old man ended up in a Connecticut hospital with nausea, abdominal pain, frequent vomiting and a week without bowel movements, according to a report in *The New England Journal of Medicine* (320,17:1148).

Surgeons opened up his lower intestine and found a 2-foot-long plug of "vegetable matter" that completely blocked his small bowel. They removed the mass, and three weeks later the man went home.

Doctors discovered that a week before he had to check into the hospital, the man had begun eating 60 grams (a little over two ounces) a day of oat bran in the form of oat bran muffins.

Six years before that, the man had part of his intestine removed because of diverticulitis. Some inside scars from that operation, along with the "excessively high dose" of oat bran and the suddenness of the high dose without any gradual increase, probably caused the man's problem, the doctors speculate. "We suggest that caution be exercised in the prescription of large doses of bran for the patient who has had abdominal surgery," the doctors advise.

A daily maximum intake of 10 to 25 grams (under a half-ounce up to just under one ounce) would be better, the report says. There should also be a gradual "breaking-in" period, starting with low doses of bran, before building up to the maximum, the doctors say.

The benefits of rice bran

Oat bran and wheat bran aren't the only brans you should be eating. New studies have shown that rice bran is more effective than wheat bran in providing bulk and protecting against colon cancer. Like oat bran, rice bran is also effective in lowering total cholesterol.

Rice bran is "nutritious, has a light, slightly sweet taste, is a good source of protein and iron, and yet is low in calories and sodium," says Doug Babcock in *Cereal Foods World* (32,8:538). "Rice products are hypoallergenic and easily digestible." Rice is also cholesterol-free and "contains only a trace of fat," explains Cornell University's *Consumer News*. "Rice is an excellent source of complex carbohydrates and provides thiamine, niacin, riboflavin, iron, calcium, fiber, phosphorus and protein," *Consumer News* continued.

The nutrients in rice are concentrated in the bran layers of the rice kernel. Brown rice contains the bran layers while white rice doesn't, so brown rice has the most food value.

Until recently, you could only get rice bran by eating brown rice. Now, stabilized rice bran is available separately and can be added to your daily diet.

Researchers at the Royal Hallamshire Hospital in Sheffield, England, recently compared rice bran and wheat bran. "The results of this study indicate that rice bran is an efficient stool bulking agent," said J. Tomlin, who led the research team for the report in *European Journal of Clinical Nutrition* (42:857).

Even though volunteers ate only a slightly larger amount of rice bran than wheat bran, "it increased stool mass and frequency by over twice the increase caused by wheat bran." The more bulk created in the stool and the faster the waste can be moved from the intestines, the lower the incidence of colon cancer.

Rice bran is a type of dietary fiber, commonly known as roughage, that decreases the risk of colon cancer because it helps move waste products through the intestines rapidly. The less contact that cancer-causing substances have with the lining of the intestines, the better.

In a separate study in Japan reported in *Journal of Nutritional Science Vitaminology* (32:581), researchers compared a brown rice diet to a diet of polished rice, where the bran was removed. "The results suggest that rice fiber produced an increase in fecal weight, which is assumed to be effective in preventing colonic disease in advanced countries," the researchers concluded.

Your fiber intake should be at least 30 grams each day and should include a variety of fiber types, according to the National Cancer Institute. "Dietitians recommend a high-fiber diet for patients with cardiovascular problems, obesity and diabetes, diverticulitis, and gastrointestinal problems or diseases," according to Babcock.

Another benefit of rice bran is that it can lower levels of total cholesterol, low density lipoprotein (LDL) and very low density lipoprotein, while raising the amount of the good cholesterol — high density lipoprotein (HDL), according to a study in *Lipids* (21:715).

Research at the U.S. Department of Agriculture (USDA) in Albany, California, shows that rice bran lowers total cholesterol as well as oat bran, reports *Science News* (134,20:308).

"Preliminary results show a balanced diet, including 10 percent dietary fiber from defatted rice bran, reduces cholesterol in hamsters by more than 25 percent."

In diabetics, rice helped lower cholesterol levels when it replaced potatoes. "When rice was the major carbohydrate source the very low density lipoprotein triglycerides decreased," *The American Journal of Clinical Nutrition* (39:598) reports.

A third major benefit of rice bran is that it helps lower the incidence of calcium-containing urinary stones by decreasing the amount of calcium excreted in the urine, reports the *Journal of Urology* (132:1140) and the *British Journal of Urology* (58:592).

"In almost all patients, rice bran caused a significant decrease in urinary calcium excretion," wrote Dr. Ohkawa in the *Journal of Urology*. "Evidence of stones has decreased clearly among patients treated with rice bran for one to three years. ... We suggest that ... rice bran treatment should be effective for prevention of recurrent urinary stone disease."

For health's sake, take coarse approach to baking

Using coarse flour for routine baking may lower your risk of getting high blood pressure, hardening of the arteries, gallstones, obesity and diseases of the colon, even colon cancer, a new report says. That baking suggestion is from three doctors at the Bristol Royal Infirmary in England, as reported in the *British Medical Journal* (298,6688:1616).

Part of the healthful effect of coarsely ground flour may be that it escapes complete digestion in the stomach and upper intestines, the doctors say.

"Overefficient digestion of starch" may give rise to excess levels of insulin in the blood and to problems with the colon, the lower end of the digestive tract, the report suggests. Some cases of high blood pressure may be triggered by problems with insulin levels.

Like rough dietary fiber, undigested coarse flour could beneficially affect the colon and insulin levels, the doctors say. The doctors tested this theory on 20 patients who either suffered from non-insulin-dependent diabetes or had undergone colon surgery to treat ulcerative colitis.

"In both groups, the meal containing bread made from coarse flour resulted in lower plasma glucose and insulin concentrations than that containing bread made from fine flour. Unabsorbed starch was 42 percent higher after the meal made from coarse flour," the report says.

Therefore, diabetics may achieve better control of blood sugar levels by eating lots of breads baked from coarse flour, and the risk of some colonic diseases, including cancer, might be reduced if coarse flour is eaten regularly and combined with other less completely digested starchy foods, the doctors conclude.

Here's how the doctors measure whether flour is coarse: Nearly half the flour won't pass through a sieve with holes one millimeter wide, and at least 80 percent of the flour won't pass through holes of 140 micrometers diameter.

Unsaturated fats: How do you know if they are 'good' or 'bad'?

Forget saturated and unsaturated fats. From now on, think of fats this way: There's good fat and there's bad fat. But, you argue, my doctor has been stressing the importance of eating unsaturated fats and steering clear of saturated fats.

Well, now there's a new twist to the story, says *The New England Journal of Medicine* (323,7:439). Usually, unsaturated fats are better for you than saturated fats. But now you need to watch which kinds of unsaturated fats you eat.

The kinds of unsaturated fats that you now need to avoid are known as "trans" fatty acids — the "bad" fats. These trans fatty acids are formed by a process called "hydrogenation."

During the hydrogenation process, regular unsaturated fatty acids ("good" fats) are changed into a different form. Instead of being in liquid form at room temperature, they are changed into solid form. (This is kind of like ice and water — the same substance in two different forms.) The new, solid form of these unsaturated fatty acids is referred to as "trans" or "hydrogenated," and they are used in baking products such as margarines and shortenings. (Margarine, because it contains some of the "good" unsaturated fatty acids, may still be slightly better for you than butter.)

Trans fatty acids ("bad" fats) raise levels of LDL serum cholesterol and lower the levels of HDL serum cholesterol. This produces the highest — and the unhealthiest — ratio of total cholesterol to HDL cholesterol. And that high ratio is a huge risk factor for coronary heart disease.

In the typical American diet, two to four percent of the calories come from these dangerous "bad" fatty acids. Researchers suggest that it would be a good idea for people who have an increased risk of atherosclerosis to avoid a high intake of "bad" fatty acids.

One way to avoid a high intake of "bad" fatty acids is to read labels very carefully. Avoid partially or completely hydrogenated fats. Regular unsaturated fatty acids ("good" fats) that haven't been hydrogenated at all are your best bet. Try to use liquid vegetable oils instead of hardened vegetable oils. Choose soft margarines over stick margarines and butter. And, as always, try to keep your total fat intake below 30 percent of your daily intake of calories.

'Fat' reading: lessons in labels

Puzzled about how much fat is contained in the foods you buy? In calculating the fat content of the products you buy, don't let the labels fool you. Hamburger that is labeled "75 percent lean" is really 25 percent fat.

If a label says the product provides 25 percent of your recommended daily allowance, you will need four servings to get 100 percent, a report in the *Archives of Internal Medicine* (149,6:1253) points out.

Although the FDA has passed new, strict laws regulating food labeling, you still have to keep your wits about you to make wise choices.

"Products highlight the fact that they are '97 percent fat free, only 3 percent fat,' when indeed they are 50 percent to 65 percent fat by content. "The label refers to the fat percentage by weight. Milk that carries the label '2 percent low-fat milk' is in fact 33 percent fat by content and is not particularly low in fat," says the *Archives* report.

Oat-bran muffins must be healthful, right? Not necessarily. Eggs are the primary ingredient of many store-bought muffins, followed by soy oil, honey and molasses. This type of muffin has 12 grams of fat.

Although granola bars look good, they're loaded with fat and calories. Low-fat frozen yogurt is a better choice than Tofutti, which has twice the fat of ice cream. For a low-fat snack, try air-popped corn — but not too much salt, and hold the butter!

Why yogurt's good for you

Remember when only dieters ate yogurt? The many brands of yogurt on the supermarket shelves and the frozen yogurt stores that have popped up across the country are signs that times — and tastes — have changed. Yogurt is in.

The popularity of yogurt is more than a fad. It's based on years of medical research that suggests that fermented milk products like yogurt can help keep people in good health.

Yogurt is a good source of calcium, especially for people who can't drink milk because they have trouble digesting lactose (a milk sugar). Yogurt contains less lactose than milk, which makes it easier to digest. Easily digestible calcium is important in preventing osteoporosis, a bone loss disease that afflicts some middle-aged and elderly women.

Fermented milk products are beneficial in treating other conditions, too, says a report in *The American Journal of Clinical Nutrition* (49,4:675).

Indigestion, high levels of cholesterol in the blood, bowel irregularity, high blood pressure and even food poisoning have been known to yield to a diet that includes fermented milk.

Although researchers don't know the exact reasons for the benefits, they speculate that the bacteria used in fermenting milk changes the bacteria already inside the stomach and intestines. Those changes may help the body absorb nutrients and produce enzymes needed for proper digestion of milk proteins, among other functions.

Fermented milk is identified by the bacteria it contains, and not all types are equally beneficial. Look on the yogurt's list of ingredients to see what it contains. Thermophilus milk, for example, is effective in reducing lactose intolerance, but buttermilk is not. Acidophilus milk has laxative effects in older patients.

Acidophilus milk also has slowed growth of tumors in mice. Other studies have shown that it eliminated some forms of digestive tract infections. Drinking fermented milk also helps to ease travelers' diarrhea.

Yogurt bacteria, injected directly into mouse tumors, made the growths shrink, the report says. Researchers believe that the bacteria stimulate the immune system into action, because the animals tested survived more than one bout with cancer.

Yogurt — probably the most popular form of fermented milk — also is a good source of protein, riboflavin (vitamin B2) and folic acid (one of the B-vitamins).

A four-ounce serving has 115 calories, about one-half that of premium ice cream, and contains a teaspoon of fat. "Light" yogurt has fewer calories and less fat. Frozen yogurt has about the same amount of sugar, calcium, calories and protein as the equivalent amount of ice milk, but less fat.

For most folks, fermented milk like yogurt may be a good, natural way to raise overall immunity levels and fight some kinds of digestive problems.

Eat less to live longer

Saying "no thanks" to seconds at the dinner table may actually help prolong your life, Texas researchers report in *Geriatrics* (44,12:87).

Reducing calories while still eating healthy, well-balanced meals prolonged the lives of healthy rats in their study, but did not stunt growth, researchers said. Even animals with heart and kidney problems lived longer and developed tumors later in life than rats on unrestricted diets.

Other benefits of a disciplined diet include healthier bones and improved immunity, they added.

Would humans reap similar benefits? Scientists have known for some time that diet, growth and aging are related, but animal studies such as this are the first step in understanding how diet may prolong human life.

Researchers have several theories. This study suggests that digesting three well-balanced meals a day constitutes an "eight-hour workday" for your body. Eating more than you need means your cells must work overtime to digest the extra food.

"Tired" cells weaken with age and can't fight disease and illness effectively. In a nutshell, the less you eat, the less work for your body.

What you eat may also be a significant factor in prolonging life, researchers said. Chemicals in certain foods cause a "red alert" in your body, meaning that it must work double-overtime to digest them.

Further studies will look at what foods cause this response in the body. In the meantime, eating less seems to have many more positive benefits than always eating until you're stuffed.

Some herbal teas are toxic

If you enjoy brewing herbal teas, or even growing and mixing your own, take note. Some herbal teas, especially those that are home-grown, are toxic and can lead to liver, digestive and nervous-system disorders, according to a report in *American Family Physician* (39,5:153).

"Most commercial herbal teas are considered safe," says Dr. Paul M. Ridker, author of the report. However, "Lewis Carroll's account of Alice's tea party, during which the participants became 'mad as a hatter' and 'dry as a bone,' aptly describes the effects of some herbal teas," says the doctor.

Herbal remedies were widely used by 19th-century physicians to treat a host of ailments. As modern medicine developed, "folkloric" remedies fell by the wayside, although the public's interest in herbs did not. Understandably, today's physicians are not as well-versed in herbal toxicities, but they are catching up, Dr. Ridker says.

Many people enjoy growing their own herbs for teas and cooking, and for the most part, herbs are safe to use. But mark the following herbal teas as potentially dangerous and possibly unsafe to drink:

❐ **Comfrey, groundsel, gordolobo, sassafras, T'u-San-Chi and tansy ragwort** — These teas have sometimes caused liver failure, which is "among the most worrisome complications of herbal tea exposure," according to Dr. Ridker.

   The danger of comfrey tea is confirmed in a report in *The Lancet* (1,8639:657). Teas made from the comfrey plant have been marketed in many countries in the past as "natural" remedies for everything from arthritis to infections. At least four different toxic alkaloids have been identified in common comfrey, prickly comfrey and Russian comfrey. The poisons attack the liver, sometimes causing hepatic veno-occlusive disease, a form of worsening portal hypertension. Portal hypertension is a kind of high blood pressure involving the liver, and can lead to liver failure and death. In addition, the comfrey poisons are linked to higher rates of cancer and lung tumors in animal tests.

"Comfrey products are marketed as herbal teas, herb root powders, and as capsules: Their continued availability must be questioned," *The Lancet* report warned. Canada already has attempted to ban the sale of some comfrey products. The report concluded that the number of comfrey-tea-related poisonings may be "grossly underestimated."

❑ **Senna, pokeroot and buckthorn** — These teas may cause diarrhea, hypotension (low blood pressure) and dehydration.

❑ **Lobelia, burdock, thorn apple and jimson weed** — These teas may cause delirium, disorientation, blurred vision, dry mouth and dilated pupils.

❑ **Melilot, woodruff and tonka bean** — These teas contain coumarin, which causes an anticoagulant (anti-clotting) effect. They are especially dangerous for people already taking anticoagulant medication or large doses of aspirin.

Mint, raspberry, blackberry, rose hips and citrus peel teas are beneficial and are not harmful.

Sometimes otherwise harmless teas are contaminated with dangerous additional plants. Researchers have identified foxglove, squill, lily of the valley, yellow oleander and common oleander as contaminates of some herbal teas. These substances may mimic the effects of cardiac glycosides, which are found in heart-stimulating medications such as digitalis (which, incidentally, is another name for foxglove).

According to Dr. Ridker, "Labels warning of potentially dangerous side effects of tea constituents are currently not required, and inadvertent exposure to toxic ingredients in herbal teas is likely to continue." The Canadian Health Protection Branch (similar to the U.S. Food and Drug Administration) began regulating herbs in March 1989, and controversy has been brewing ever since, according to *Herbalgram* (20:14).

The Canadian agency singled out herbs because they are not a food or a drug. They fall somewhere in between and were not previously regulated. The Canadian regulations divide plants into two classifications. The first class is herbs that cannot be sold as food; in effect, they are banned substances. The second class is herbs that must be sold with labels warning about toxicity.

Opponents charge that the Canadian Health Protection Branch (HPB) has not been consistent in regulating foods used for medicinal purposes. Prunes, for example, are known for their laxative effects but are not regulated, and coffee does not have labels cautioning consumers about its diuretic effects.

The HPB may have bitten off more than it can chew in trying to regulate foods that contain carcinogens, cancer-causing agents. It banned sassafras, for instance, as a carcinogen-containing plant. Opponents argue that "99 percent of the known carcinogens are of natural origin."

Danger from a Japanese dish

Doctors operating on the 24-year-old college student thought the patient had appendicitis. He had been hospitalized with pain and tenderness in the lower right part of his abdomen. But when they opened him up, they found everything normal and healthy.

Normal, that is, until the surgeon — about to sew up the incision — was shocked to see a bright red worm an inch and a half long crawl out of the man's intestinal cavity onto a surgical cloth near the wound.

The patient recovered nicely, but the worm died, doctors report in *The New England Journal of Medicine* (320,17:1124).

It turns out the young man had eaten a dish that's become popular in this country recently — sushi, a meal of raw fish long associated with Japan. He ate it the night before at a friend's house, according to an Associated Press report.

Cooking would kill any fish parasites like the eustrongylides, the worm found in the man's innards. But since some Oriental fish dishes like sushi and sashimi are normally served raw or nearly raw, some internal fish parasites may come along for a live ride into a human digestive tract.

Once inside, such nematodes and other parasites can live long enough to cause severe lower abdominal pain. Occasionally, some worms can pierce the digestive tract and enter into the peritoneal cavity, causing more serious problems, including the risk of infection.

The report says that such parasites can show up in both salt and freshwater fish. Commercial fish that may be infected include mackerel, herring, rockfish, salmon and cod. Pacific fish are more likely to have the parasites than Atlantic catches.

Avoid the problem by fully cooking all fish that you eat, the journal recommends.

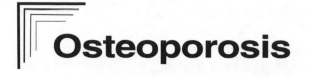

Osteoporosis

High risk factors for osteoporosis (brittle-bone disease)

- Being female

- Being Caucasian

- Family history of osteoporosis or hip fractures

- Slender build

- Being inactive

- Low muscle mass

- Early menopause

- Being past menopause

- Fair or translucent skin

- Cigarette smoking

- Low calcium intake

- High alcohol consumption

- Drinking lots of soft drinks

- Consuming large amounts of caffeine

- High protein diet

- Taking thyroid hormones

- Long-term treatment with steroids for arthritis, asthma or other diseases

- Having anorexia nervosa, a serious loss of appetite

Sources: *Modern Medicine* (57,3:114) and *The Encyclopedia of Top Secret Ways to Defeat Old Age* (FC&A Publishing)

Take steps to prevent osteoporosis

The best way to manage the loss of bone mass known as osteoporosis is to prevent it from developing. Since osteoporosis develops silently over many years, proper diet and exercise throughout your life are extremely important.

Osteoporosis causes the stooped posture and distinctive "dowager's hump" in elderly women. It's also responsible for many of the hip, leg and arm fractures suffered by many older people.

Follow these steps for bone-loss prevention:

❒ Adequate calcium. The daily diet should include foods that are high in calcium like dairy products (including milk, cheese and yogurt), dark-green, leafy vegetables (like collards, turnip greens, spinach and broccoli), salmon, sardines, oysters and tofu.

❒ Adequate vitamin D. Vitamin-fortified milk, cereals, saltwater fish, liver and daily sunshine are good sources of this vitamin.

❒ Adequate manganese. Manganese is an important mineral found in whole-grain products, fruits (especially bananas), vegetables (especially legumes), eggs, liver and other organ meats.

❒ Adequate exercise. Walking, jogging, dancing, bicycling, aerobics, rowing, hiking, rope jumping, tennis and other exercise in which the bones have to support body weight help promote bone growth.

❒ With your doctor, consider estrogen replacement therapy during menopause. When estrogen replacement therapy is started right after women stop menstruating, hip and wrist fractures can be reduced as much as 60 percent.

❒ Avoid smoking, alcoholic beverages, drinks containing caffeine, soft drinks, meat and high protein foods.

Sources: National Institutes of Health and *Stand Tall* by Notelovitz and Ware

How caffeine affects your bones

Everyone loses some bone mass as part of the aging process, especially after the age of 40. But for some, it becomes a much more serious problem than for others.

Here's some news about what you can do to protect your bones and to avoid the dangers of osteoporosis.

First, the abnormal amount of bone loss, known as osteoporosis, is the result of calcium in the bones being drawn out into the blood and excreted in the urine. The bones become brittle, the amount of bone mass is reduced, and the strength of the remaining bone is weakened.

The condition can cause loss of height or a humped back, especially in women past menopause, and usually is first diagnosed because of a fracture of the hip, wrist or spinal vertebrae.

Several studies have shown that coffee causes bone loss. But new research has confirmed that it is the caffeine in coffee that causes calcium loss. Put simply, the more caffeine you drink, the more calcium is driven out of your bones.

At Mt. Saint Vincent University in Halifax, Nova Scotia, researcher Susan Whiting tested different properties of coffee in animals to determine exactly what causes the loss of calcium. Whiting demonstrated that it is the caffeine in coffee, not the diuretic effect, that takes calcium from the body.

Other researchers suggest that people who drink two to three cups of caffeinated coffee daily, or five to six cups of caffeinated tea daily, have almost a 70 percent greater risk of osteoporosis than those people who do not drink caffeine, reports *Science News* (138,16:253).

And people who drink three to four cups of coffee daily or six to seven cups of tea daily seem to have an 82 percent increased risk of osteoporosis compared with people who do not drink caffeinated beverages.

In another study, Dr. Linda K. Massey reported that caffeinated-coffee drinkers lose twice as much calcium as people who drink decaffeinated coffee. In her work at Washington State University, Massey found that caffeine causes calcium to be excreted in urine.

Since many coffee drinkers are not getting enough calcium to begin with, drinking coffee containing caffeine is making their problem worse, Massey believes. If you must drink coffee, use decaffeinated coffee with lots of milk. The additional milk will help replace some of the calcium that the body needs, reports *Prevention* (39:5).

Smoking linked to bone loss

Researchers at Argonne National Laboratory in Illinois report yet another link between osteoporosis and smoking. They discovered that high levels of the poisonous element cadmium promotes bone loss in both animal and laboratory tests. Cadmium is found in cigarette tobacco. "Bone loss was greatest at cadmium levels roughly equivalent to those found in smokers' blood," states a report in *Medical World News* (30,3:18).

Too much salt causes body to lose calcium

Too much salt in the diet may increase a woman's chances of suffering osteoporosis after menopause, Canadian researchers report in *The American Journal of Clinical Nutrition* (50,5:1088). They studied 17 women aged 52 to 72 who ate their usual diet and were then given salt supplements.

Excess salt causes the body to rid itself of calcium through urination, researchers say.

Many postmenopausal women do not get enough calcium to begin with. If salt intake is low, women susceptible to osteoporosis might need less calcium after menopause, a New Zealand team of researchers concludes in the *British Medical Journal* (299,6703:834). Thus, if you eat less salt, you might enjoy better bone health, the study suggests.

Ten women over age 65 volunteered for the study. They alternated their regular diet with low-salt and high-salt diets for periods of 10 days. Women had the least loss of calcium when they were on the low-salt diet and the most when they followed the high-salt diet.

Osteoporosis linked to thyroid medication

A medication commonly prescribed for women — thyroid hormones — poses bone loss dangers for premenopausal women, according to a recent study at the University of Massachusetts Medical School in Worchester. The data showed that women on long-term therapy with thyroid hormones experienced losses of hip bone mass. They also may face increased risk of hip fractures later in life.

The study of 31 women (all premenopausal) compared their bone densities after five years of thyroid treatment with those of 31 women of similar ages and weights who had not received thyroid hormones. While both groups showed little decrease in lumbar spine densities, the hip bone densities in the thyroid group showed decreases ranging from 10 to 13 percent, as reported in *Science News* (133:359).

The researchers suggest that doctors should more carefully tailor hormone doses to individual needs and monitor thyroid levels diligently.

They say that thyroid doses often are higher than "normal" levels, and such high doses should be given only when absolutely necessary, such as when a woman has been previously treated for thyroid cancer.

Osteoporosis affects men as well as women

Osteoporosis — the brittle-bone disease — is nondiscriminatory after all, affecting both women and men, new research suggests.

Latest finding: Men in later life lose about 2.3 percent of spinal bone every year, reports a study in *Annals of Internal Medicine* (112,1:29). After age 30, men lose about 1 percent per year of bone mass in the wrists and hands. And the rate of bone loss in the hands and wrists gets worse as men get older.

Until now, most researchers thought osteoporosis affected mainly women past menopause.

Unfortunately, this study suggested that taking calcium supplements later in life seemed not to stop or even to slow the rate of bone loss in men. "We found a substantial rate of bone loss, despite a generous calcium intake," the study reports.

Young and old need calcium for strong bones

To get the best protection against osteoporosis, you should make sure you get recommended amounts of calcium in your diet beginning early in life, a new study revealed in *The Journal of the American Medical Association* (260:3150).

Women who maintained high-calcium diets throughout their lives, as children, adolescents and reproductive women, have the highest bone density, according to the study.

"Swallowing calcium pills at 50 years of age probably is not going to make your bones thicker," one researcher said. But calcium probably will help older women maintain their present bone thickness.

"In our analysis, the only group in which a protective effect of calcium could be observed was in women who reported both a high milk consumption during periods of growth and development, as well as currently," the report concluded.

Dr. Robert P. Heany, of Creighton University in Omaha, Nebraska, notes the importance of calcium in two major stages of life:

> • **It helps develop bone mass during the first 30 years of life.**
>
> • **Then it maintains bone mass during the remaining years of life.**

As you get older, your body doesn't use calcium as efficiently as when you were young. Menopausal women may need even more calcium than younger women because their estrogen loss puts them at greater risk of developing osteoporosis.

Damage from osteoporosis is usually permanent. The most common treatments include heat, drugs for the pain, a back brace and rest.

Rest, combined with moderate exercise like walking, helps keep the muscles in shape to support the weak bone structure. Since damage from osteoporosis is difficult to repair, prevention should be a lifelong goal.

Vitamin D helps fight crippling bone loss

If you have passed menopause and want to protect yourself from osteoporosis, be careful not to neglect your vitamin D. According to a report in *The New England Journal of Medicine* (321,26:1777), vitamin D is an important weapon in fighting crippling bone loss.

Without proper amounts of vitamin D, your body cannot regulate the level of parathyroid hormones that it makes. Parathyroid hormones can speed up bone loss by interfering with the body's absorption of calcium.

It's true that calcium is a major building block of strong bones, but you can't eat enough foods rich in calcium to make up for a diet low in vitamin D. When vitamin D levels drop, too many parathyroid hormones are produced. When this happens, the body loses its ability to absorb the extra calcium.

In other words, you may be eating a lot of calcium, but your body can't use it because you don't have enough vitamin D.

Researchers stress the importance of getting enough vitamin D in the diet, especially when exposure to sunlight is limited. Your body produces vitamin D naturally in sunlight, so sunlight helps the body keep parathyroid hormones below dangerous levels.

Vitamin D supplements during winter months help maintain hormone levels that would ordinarily vary from summer to winter. Without the advantage of vitamin D supplements, many women experience seasonal bone loss.

Drug and vitamin therapy may reverse effects of osteoporosis

A combination of calcium, vitamin D and the drug etidronate seems to reverse the effects of osteoporosis.

The New England Journal of Medicine (323,2:73) reported a seven-city study involving 423 women who were past menopause and had spinal fractures caused by osteoporosis.

After two years, the group receiving etidronate along with calcium and vitamin D recorded a 5 percent gain in dense, new bone in the spine. A group receiving only calcium and vitamin D lost bone mass. The number of new spinal fractures in the etidronate group was half that of the others.

An earlier study in Denmark also used the same combination and had about the same results, says *NEJM* (322,18:1265).

Etidronate is a drug that suppresses formation of osteoclasts. Osteoclasts are scavenger cells whose job is to destroy old bone cells.

In osteoporosis, the bone-eating cells destroy more strong bone than the body can replace, leading to soft, porous bones and increased fractures, says *Science News* (138,2:22).

Study shows it's never too late to reduce the risk of osteoporosis

Regular exercise like walking, jogging or climbing stairs, combined with adequate calcium intake, can help reduce the risk of osteoporosis in women past the age of menopause, reports the *Annals of Internal Medicine* (108,6:824).

Researchers studied a group of women between 55 and 70 years of age. The women exercised three times a week for 50 to 60 minutes each session.

Each woman also took 1,500 milligrams of calcium daily. "The response to exercise was positive for at least 22 months" (the length of the study), explained Gail Dalsky, the researcher who led the study at Washington University School of Medicine in St. Louis. The density of the bones actually increased, she said.

However, when the women stopped or cut back on the regular exercise, the bone density returned to its pre-exercise condition, even with calcium supplementation. The study suggests that regular exercise may fight bone loss in women over 50. Dalsky stressed that exercise should supplement, not replace, other known treatments for osteoporosis like estrogen-replacement therapy and additional calcium.

"Exercise can usually be safely added to such therapies, but it can't be substituted for them," Dalsky says in another report of her study in *The Physician and Sportsmedicine* (17,2:48).

Other studies have also shown that weight-bearing exercise helps the bones to grow stronger and more dense. Weight-bearing exercise is physical activity in which the bones have to support body weight, including aerobics, dancing, walking, jogging, hiking, rope jumping or tennis.

Weight-bearing exercise may be combined with other types of exercise like swimming, bicycling and rowing to provide a variety of activities that will keep the exercise sessions interesting.

Until now, doctors did not know if exercise after menopause would just stop the bones from deteriorating farther, or if it would actually help to increase the density of the bones.

Ask your dentist about the risk of developing brittle-bone disease

Swedish researchers are urging dentists to be on the lookout for warning signs of osteoporosis.

Recent studies reported in the *British Medical Journal* (300,6730:1024) have shown that the fewer teeth women have, the greater their chances of developing brittle-bone disease.

Women should ask their dentists to be alert for two warning signs — loss of teeth and gum disease (problems with the tissues around the teeth).

If these conditions are present, women should consult their doctors about osteoporosis risks.

Fluoride fails to prevent osteoporosis

Thinner, weaker bones trouble many women in the years after menopause. In other countries, doctors have widely recommended sodium fluoride as a treatment for this condition.

But, according to the *Mayo Clinic Health Letter* (8,4:5), new bone growth stimulated by sodium fluoride is so weak that it actually fractures more easily.

The best way to strengthen your bones is to exercise regularly and eat a diet rich in calcium-containing foods like dark-green vegetables, dairy products and canned salmon or sardines.

Smoking and drinking too much alcohol can also increase your risk of developing osteoporosis.

Pet-related Illnesses

Is your pet making you sick?

Pets are part of the American way of life. A wagging tail or a loving purr means unconditional love to millions of avid pet owners across the country.

Pets supposedly keep people with heart disease living longer, help psychiatric patients be more self-sufficient and help children develop social skills. But according to a report in *FDA Consumer* (24,3:28), some pets have more to offer than devotion.

"Zoonoses" is a modern term for an age-old problem. It identifies diseases capable of being passed from animals to humans. The ancient Greeks realized the connection between rabies and dogs, and flea-infested rodents transmitted the bubonic plague to all Europe.

Now, thanks to improved technology, most animal-transmitted diseases are documented and studied. Once identified, most zoonoses can either be prevented or treated.

The best way to avoid problems with zoonoses is to simply be aware of the dangers.

❏ **Toxicare Canis**, also known as roundworm, is a parasite carried by nursing dogs and their puppies. Some estimates say that virtually every puppy has roundworm. In fact, the dog roundworm is so well-established that roundworm-free puppies can only be found in litters where several generations have been raised in isolation.

Since children and puppies just naturally go together, children are prime candidates for roundworm. Coming in contact with soil contaminated with the feces of an infected dog spreads the disease. When a human becomes infected, he experiences fever, headache, cough and poor appetite.

Your veterinarian can advise you on the best steps to take for your dog or puppies to help keep roundworm from being a health problem.

❏ **Toxoplasmosis**, a feline-related disease, is capable of living in many different animals. The one-celled animal, Toxoplasma gondii, is a parasite found in cat feces or dirt contaminated with cat feces. The cat is infected while doing what cats do best — killing and eating small rodents.

Human infection actually comes through a chain of events ending at the dinner table. When infected cats deposit their feces in pastures where cows and sheep graze, the livestock become infected. When the meat from these animals is eaten raw or undercooked, the parasite is passed on to people.

You can also be infected when you clean your cat's litter box.

Symptoms of toxoplasmosis infection in humans can include fever, headache, swollen lymph glands, cough, sore throat, nasal congestion, loss of appetite and skin rash. Many people have immune systems strong enough to fight off the infection, but some people need to be especially careful of contamination.

Anyone with immune system defects or anyone receiving immunosuppressive therapy needs special care to keep the disease from becoming particularly dangerous. Expectant women, especially in their first trimester, should never clean a cat's litter box or eat raw or rare meat, since toxoplasmosis can cause miscarriage, premature births or blindness in unborn children.

❒ **Ringworm** is not really a parasite, but a skin disease caused by a fungus. A variety of animals, including dogs, cows and horses, can carry the disease to humans. But the most likely culprit is your long-haired kitten. The ringworm fungus infects the hair of the cat and is passed on when someone pets the kitty.

In humans, the fungus usually appears on exposed parts of the body or scalp as an inflamed, scaly lesion. Your doctor can make a definite diagnosis using an ultraviolet light known as Wood's lamp. If the suspected fungus is indeed ringworm, the infected hairs will appear green under the light. Most doctors prescribe an iodine-based soap for humans infected with ringworm.

❒ **Psittacosis**, also known as parrot fever, is a bacterial disease affecting the bird families. Pigeons, ducks, turkeys, chickens and parrots are the best known carriers of parrot fever, although there are 130 species of domestic and wild birds that carry the bacteria.

The disease is usually transmitted to humans through contact with the feces or dust from the feathers of parrots or parakeets. People with parrot fever usually suffer from respiratory problems, such as cough and chest pain. They can also have fever, chills, vomiting and muscular pain.

An infected bird may have poor eating habits or droopy feathers, but sometimes they exhibit no symptoms at all. The best precaution is to wear a surgical or dust mask and rubber gloves while cleaning your bird's cage.

If you have reason to suspect you have the disease, a blood test can determine for sure if you have psittacosis. Fortunately, antibiotics are effective in treating both humans and birds.

❒ **Lyme disease**, named after the town of Old Lyme, Conn., was identified in the mid-1970s. However, the disease hasn't been confined to the Northeast.

Deer ticks are the carriers of Lyme disease. These tiny ticks, no larger than a pinhead, attach themselves to white-tailed deer, field mice and other wild animals whose bodies contain the bacteria known as Borrelia burgdorferi. After becoming infected with the host's blood, the tick moves on to other animals or humans and infects them.

Deer ticks can attach themselves directly to you, or they can enter your home on your dog. Checking your dog for ticks after a day in the woods is always advisable. Since deer ticks are so small, they can be "rolled-away" with roller-type lint removers if they aren't already attached.

Doctors use a blood test to help diagnose Lyme disease. Symptoms of Lyme disease are vague and numerous, but generally the first sign is a bull's-eye rash. Some people experience flu-like symptoms in the joints, chronic fatigue, dizziness, shortness of breath and a rash. Antibiotics in the early stages are absolutely necessary to prevent more serious problems (such as arthritis and cardiac/nervous disorders) that have been associated with untreated Lyme disease.

❐ **Rocky Mountain Spotted Fever** is primarily carried by the American dog tick. The infected tick that carries the disease can be found in the woods or on your dog.

Since the tick carrying Rocky Mountain Spotted Fever is much larger than the deer tick, it is much easier to locate — on your dog and on you.

Wearing long sleeves, pants and a hat when walking in heavily wooded areas will give you a measure of protection against any tick that wants to latch on. Always check yourself and your dog for any "hitchhikers" immediately after your outing.

Symptoms of Rocky Mountain Spotted Fever are similar to those of other illnesses and include headache, fever and skin rash. Early diagnosis and antibiotic treatment are necessary to prevent serious consequences.

❐ **Rabies** is a virus transmitted by an infected animal. Left unattended, rabies is deadly. If you are bitten by an animal (wild or tame) that is possibly rabid, cleanse the wound immediately with a strong stream of water and soap or detergent, followed by a solution of alcohol or iodine. Then, and most important, see a doctor immediately. A series of rabies shots could save your life.

❐ **Cat Scratch Fever** is an infection from a cat scratch or bite. No one really understands what causes a particular scratch or bite to become infected. The sore is slow to heal, and after several months, your lymph nodes may swell and become tender and painful. This disease is uncomfortable, but seldom serious. If your lymph nodes stay swollen and the scratch won't heal after three weeks, you should see a physician to determine if medication is needed.

Another problem for pet owners is that common infections are passed from human to pet to human. Dr. Isadore Rosenfeld, clinical professor of medicine in the cardiology division of New York Hospital-Cornell Medical Center, sites an example where a family with children might be plagued constantly with sore throats.

When throat cultures are done, the results show strep throat, which is treated immediately with medication. The children are cured, but within a few weeks everyone is sick again. Finally, someone thinks to check the throat of the family dog and finds the dog has been the carrier of the bacteria all along.

Salmonella, a bacteria that causes mild to severe inflammation of the stomach and intestines, diarrhea and vomiting, can be passed from animals to humans. It's a serious matter for very young children, the elderly or anyone with an impaired immune system. Dogs and birds can carry salmonella, but turtles pose a special risk.

In fact, in 1975, the FDA found "pet-sized" turtles to be such a health problem that they banned the sale of any turtle with a shell length less than four inches. Turtles aren't a great choice for a pet, and those in the wild are just as likely to have salmonella as the pet store varieties.

Proper pet selection and care

Although risks are involved, most pet owners agree that the good times outweigh the bad. To reduce the chance of pet-related illnesses, follow these tips:

❑ Always choose a healthy pet — avoid dull coats, drooping feathers, or lifeless, always sleepy animals. If in doubt about the behavior of certain species, check with your vet.

❑ Look at the cages or pens where your would-be pet is living prior to living with you. How clean are the surroundings? If you are buying from a pet store, are you satisfied with the appearance of the other animals they sell? Chances are, if the rabbits aren't in good shape, the parrots probably won't be either.

❑ Arrange for a vet to check over your new family member as soon as possible. Certain animals need vaccines, and others need care that only a veterinarian could advise.

❑ Once the pet becomes your responsibility, you would be wise to follow a schedule of inoculations and routine checkups for parasites.

❏ Keep all cages and pens clean and free from bacteria by removing droppings and solid waste as soon as possible. Don't use pet waste as fertilizer — you could be spreading disease.

❏ Check for ticks and mites often, especially in the summer months.

❏ Never feed raw meat to your pets.

❏ Teach children never to pet or handle sick or strange animals. A good handwashing should be routine procedure after handling any animal.

❏ Keep your child's sandbox covered to discourage neighborhood cats from using it as a litter box.

Premenstrual Syndrome

Relief from PMS

Try following these suggestions to relieve the monthly terrors of PMS (premenstrual syndrome):

☐ Vitamin B6 (pyridoxine) should be taken daily in premenstrual times. It helps relieve fluid retention, weight gain, arthritis associated with female hormone deficiency, and symptoms of depression.

☐ Supplements of the amino acid DLPA (d, l, phenylalanine) provide amazing relief to chronic PMS sufferers, according to current research. This amino acid has been found to be the substance in chocolate that causes many people to crave chocolate. For maximum effectiveness, supplements should be taken daily at mealtimes for several weeks.

☐ Avoid coffee and caffeine. The more coffee you drink, the more severe your PMS symptoms usually become, says a report in the *American Journal of Public Health* (75,11:1135). Women with the most severe PMS problems were found to drink four or more cups of coffee daily. Despite this discovery, many over-the-counter products for PMS contain caffeine. So remember to read the labels.

Seasonal Affective Disorder

Beat SADness and depression with light therapy

You've got the blues. You're craving starches, gaining weight, sleeping longer. You crave sunshine and want to hibernate.

You may have seasonal affective disorder, commonly called SAD. It affects 5 million Americans every year, according to a recent report in *Postgraduate Medicine* (86,5:309).

SAD — four times more common in men than women — is depression triggered by winter's short, dark days. A lack of sunshine apparently throws some people into deep depression, which usually lifts in spring. SAD can occur in summer but is most common in winter.

Where you live may influence your chances of suffering winter depression, reports *Science News* (136,15:198).

In a survey of patients visiting doctor's offices in Florida, Maryland, New York and New Hampshire, only 1.4 percent of Floridians reported SAD symptoms, compared with nearly 10 percent of New Hampshire residents. Florida's sunny climate probably explains the difference, researchers said. Another study showed that 9 percent of Alaskans suffer through winter depression.

You don't have to move south to beat winter depression. A megadose of artificial light for one to two hours in the morning should do it, says the *Postgraduate Medicine* report.

You'll need a light box (which you can buy) that produces light five times brighter than office light.

You should read or work about three feet from the light source and "glance at the lights a few times each minute," the study says. If you feel eyestrain or headache, sit farther away from the box, the report says.

You should notice some improvement in your mood after four days, the researchers say.

After two weeks, you can reduce the exposure to two or three times a week, but you should continue the "treatment" until winter ends, the doctors say.

Obviously, check with your doctor before trying this technique yourself. Light therapy readjusts your circadian rhythm, or 24-hour sleep-wake cycle. The circadian rhythm responds to light, telling the body when it's time to sleep and time to wake up.

The internal clock also regulates other functions, such as body temperature, which is highest at bedtime to protect the body from cold during sleep, according to a report in *Medical Tribune* (30,26:1).

During the winter when the days are short and often cloudy, your circadian rhythm may "fall behind," causing you to sleep as much as 16 hours a day.

A megadose of artificial light in the morning helps "jump start" your internal clock and readjust it to winter's dark days.

Light therapy helps not only SAD sufferers, but shift workers, frequent travelers suffering from jet lag and elderly people with sleep disturbances, according to the *Medical Tribune* report.

As you get older, your internal clock will change naturally, but light therapy can help you adjust to your changing sleep patterns.

Are you SAD? Here's a list of symptoms

- **Regularly occurring fall and winter depression which disappears in spring.**

- **Increased appetite, weight gain and carbohydrate cravings.**

- **Excessive desire to sleep.**

- **For women, more severe premenstrual symptoms.**

- **A bout of severe depression not caused by another psychiatric disorder or by an event (change in job or marital or financial status, for example) that would affect mood.**

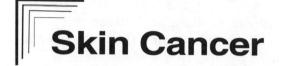

Skin Cancer

How to calculate your skin cancer risk

More people than ever are developing new cases of melanoma, a skin tumor or mole, and more people than ever are dying of the rapidly spreading skin cancer. Skin moles have long been considered a major signal of a high risk of skin cancer.

The more moles on a person's body, the greater the cancer risk, doctors have believed. Doctors have relied upon counts of moles on the arms or the whole body to gauge a person's risk.

Now we are told that the people at greatest risk for melanoma are those with many skin moles on one particular area of the body — their lower legs, according to a new study published in the *Journal of the National Cancer Institute* (81,12:948). In fact, if you have 10 or more moles of any type below your knees, you face four times the risk of melanoma as a person who has 10 or more moles on the arms, the study says.

People with 12 or more moles on their lower legs were twice as likely to develop melanoma as people with 27 or more arm moles, the study says.

Even small numbers of leg moles had a higher prediction rate for cancer than the same number of arm moles. "The relative risk associated with one to nine lower [leg] moles was twice that associated with one to nine arm moles," the researchers report. They counted both raised and flat types of moles to get the clinical figures.

Researcher and dermatologist Martin A. Weinstock wasn't sure why moles on the lower legs were such a powerful marker for increased rates of skin cancer. But he noted that having a concentration of moles in a particular spot on the body didn't necessarily mean that skin cancer would crop up in or near that spot. Instead, a skin cancer was just as likely to develop somewhere else on the body, away from a cluster of moles.

The study also shifted blame for skin cancer away from the moles themselves. "This study suggests it's not the moles themselves that cause melanoma," states a report in *Science News* (136,2:30). "Rather, [Weinstock] says, they serve as a sentinel of who stands in especially high risk."

One problem for mole counters, even medical experts, is accurately identifying the several different kinds of moles.

Three skin specialists report in the *British Medical Journal* (298,6690:16) that even experienced doctors may miss or misdiagnose half of all cancerous and noncancerous moles. Their report indicates that in only half the cases did all three doctors agree in their diagnoses of colored (pigmented) moles, including cancerous types.

One kind of mole — dysplastic naevus — is an especially high-risk signal for skin cancer. The three British doctors say that, as a group, they identified these moles correctly only 51 percent of the time. "Only 20 [51 percent] out of 39 dysplastic naevi were identified correctly by all [three] observers, whereas 24 [harmless] lesions were thought to be dysplastic on clinical grounds."

Such remarkable honesty on the part of experienced skin specialists lets you know that it may be wise to seek more than one doctor's opinion if you have a question about your moles.

Risk factors for skin cancer

Although anyone can develop skin cancer, some people are more susceptible than others.

You should be especially careful about protecting yourself or loved ones from the harmful effects of the sun if you have one or more of the following skin-cancer risk factors, warns The Skin Cancer Foundation:

- **Fair skin and/or freckles**
- **Blond, red or light-brown hair**
- **Blue, green or gray eyes**
- **A tendency to tan little or not at all**
- **A tendency to burn before tanning**
- **A family history of skin cancer**
- **Residence in a warm, sunny climate**
- **Long periods of daily sun exposure or short periods of intense exposure**
- **A large number of moles**

What your nails can tell you about your risk of skin cancer and other diseases

If you see a widening band of color running up and down your fingernail, you might need to see a doctor right away, according to a professor of medicine at the University of Mississippi Medical Center. That colored band could be an early signal of a rapidly spreading skin cancer, the doctor says in *Modern Medicine* (57,5:57).

Two practicing physicians suggest in the medical journal that you may want to become better acquainted with your fingernails and toenails. Those lowly parts may serve as important early warning signs for several serious ailments, including liver and kidney failure, heart and blood vessel disorders, poisonings, various painful inflammations of the joints and muscles and a deadly form of skin cancer called melanoma.

"Melanoma does appear in the nail unit," according to Dr. Ralph Daniel III, clinical associate professor of dermatology at the Jackson, Miss., school. "If you see a widening brownish or blackish band running up and down the nail, especially in a person of middle age or older, a biopsy may be indicated."

Daniel suggests that you get your nails carefully examined by a doctor every time you have a physical examination. "Lines or changes in nail coloration may indicate disease or exposure to toxic substances in the home or workplace," the *Modern Medicine* report says. Pits and beads on nails may also provide clues to the presence of rheumatoid arthritis and two kinds of muscular inflammations called fibromyalgia and myofascial syndromes.

In one study, out of 150 patients suffering from myofascial syndrome, 122 had nail pits and 76 had nail beads. Of 93 patients with fibromyalgia, 80 had nail pits and 45 had beads on their nail surfaces, according to Dr. Kip L. Kemple of Portland, Ore.

In addition, 25 out of 30 patients with rheumatoid arthritis also had beads on their nails, "a surprising association," according to the report in *Modern Medicine*.

Other nail signs include the following:

❐ **Double white horizontal lines** — may be sign of liver disease or poor nutrition.

❐ **Spoon nails** — the nail surface forms a cup or depression. May be sign of iron deficiency or anemia.

❐ **Yellow nails** — hard, yellow nails may be sign of chronic lung disease like emphysema or chronic bronchitis, or it could be sinus trouble.

❑ **Half-brown, half-normal nails** — could be sign of serious kidney trouble if the nail half nearest the knuckle is normal but the half toward the end of the nails is brownish.

❑ **Club nails** — the opposite of spoon nails, the nail is raised abnormally high with steep side curves. May be signal of heart failure, lung disease or thyroid problems.

❑ **Dark specks on the nail bed** — known as splinter hemorrhages, these could be harmless. But beware if the specks cluster at the nail end nearest the knuckle and show up in several nails at once. These could be early signs of a bacterial infection of a heart valve, a serious condition that needs to be treated with antibiotics.

❑ **Soft nails** — normally harmless. Occasionally, it could indicate an overactive thyroid gland.

❑ **Brittle nails** — usually caused by detergents or nail polish remover. Once in a while, it's a sign of an underactive thyroid gland.

Although he's done only preliminary statistical work on the association between nails and bodily diseases, Dr. Kemple says the nail signs may be a marker for whole groups of "systemic biologic disturbances."

At each physical, Dr. Daniel says, the nails should be examined in a good light.

The toes should be relaxed and any nail polishes or coatings should be removed before the exam, the doctor says. "To localize any discoloration, shine a penlight up through the finger or toe," Daniel recommends.

Why sunscreens don't always work

Allergies, photosensitivity or improper application may make sunscreens ineffective and increase the risk of skin cancer, aging spots, wrinkles, redness, rash or skin irritation.

Benzophenone, a chemical used in high-protection sunscreens, may cause allergic dermatitis in sensitive people, dermatologist Elizabeth Knobler reports in *Modern Medicine* (57,3:49). Redness and itching can occur either when the skin is exposed to the sun or just from contact with benzophenone.

"Because sunscreen formulations may vary from year to year (even though product names remain the same)," Dr. Knobler recommends reading the product label and avoiding sunscreens containing benzophenone.

If you have photosensitivity, an exaggerated reaction to sunlight, sunscreen will help, but your best bet is to avoid exposure to the sun. Photosensitivity can be caused by using certain drugs, cosmetics or perfumes, according to *Patient Care* (6:15).

Redness, swelling, hives and itching are symptoms of photosensitivity. If your skin is photosensitive, it reacts to the sun more quickly and more severely than normal skin.

Some of the drugs that can lead to photosensitivity are Retin-A, thiazide diuretics ("water pills" used in treating high blood pressure), tetracycline, anti-diabetics, psoralens, oral contraceptives, anti-psychotics, anti-depressants, antihistamines, anti-bacterials, anti-cancer drugs and corticosteroids. Coal tar products, coal tar dyes, musk fragrances and some other perfumes can also cause photosensitivity, according to *Patient Care*.

If you're taking these drugs or using coal tar products, avoid or limit your exposure to sun. When exposure is unavoidable, use the strongest possible sunscreen.

Even eating certain foods can make you sensitive to the sun. Limes, celery, lemons, parsley and some oranges can cause photosensitivity, Dr. Jonathan Held reports in the *American Family Physician* (39,4:143). You can get a severe skin irritation if you expose your skin to these foods, then to the sun. The irritation may take the form of redness, itching and rash. Redness and blistering usually appear about 48 hours after exposure to the sun, Held warns. Grocery workers are especially vulnerable to this type of skin irritation. They should be careful to avoid direct contact with limes, celery, lemons, parsley and bergamot oranges.

Sunscreens can actually be harmful to some people who have a photosensitive reaction to the sun caused by a particular form of ultraviolet light known as ultraviolet A. The reaction is known as polymorphic light eruption. According to *The Lancet* (1,8635:429), "between 14 percent and 28 percent of the adult female population" suffers some form of this skin reaction.

Since most sunscreens only protect against the ultraviolet B rays, the researchers warn that using a sunscreen is dangerous for these sensitive people.

The sunscreen will block the ultraviolet B rays but actually will allow more exposure to ultraviolet A rays. People with ultraviolet A sensitivity will have even more redness and itching if they sunbathe with sunscreen.

"Patients with polymorphic light eruption ... should be advised to sunbathe without sunscreens but only for a short time," says *The Lancet*.

Sunscreens containing PABA (para-aminobenzoic acid) or alcohol can also cause irritation in sensitive people. To avoid an unwanted allergic reaction, apply your sunscreen to a small area of skin and watch for any unusual irritation. Try this test at least 24 hours before using the sunscreen on your whole body.

Even if you do not have an allergic or photosensitive reaction, you need to be "sun smart" to reduce your risk of skin cancer, wrinkles and age spots.

Use a sunscreen of at least 15 SPF (sun protection factor) daily, especially on your nose, hands and face.

The SPF reading tells you how much extra protection you have from the ultraviolet rays. For example, an SPF of 15 means you have 15 times more protection than without the sunscreen.

Use a thick application of sunscreen. The *U.S. Pharmacist* explains that a sunscreen must be applied thickly — at the same thickness that the sunscreen was tested at — for it to be as effective as its rating number.

"To achieve a good protection from the sun, a layer thickness of 2 milligrams per square centimeter is often recommended," the journal says. However, a recent study found that most people only applied half that amount — reducing their sunscreen protection level by half.

Avoid artificial tanning methods. No matter what fashion dictates, untanned skin is healthier than the "tanned" look — learn to accept that.

Sun exposure guidelines

☐ Use a sunscreen with a SPF (sun protection factor) of at least 15.

☐ Follow the label directions.

☐ Test the sunscreen on a small patch of skin to see if any irritation occurs.

☐ Apply sunscreen 30 minutes before exposure to the sun. Remember that even on cloudy days, up to 80 percent of the sun's radiation reaches the ground.

☐ Apply sunscreen to clean, dry skin.

☐ Apply it evenly and thickly over your entire body — remembering your lips, ears, hands, forearms and the back of the neck, all of which are high exposure areas.

☐ Reapply sunscreen after swimming or sweating.

☐ Avoid direct sunlight between 10 a.m. and 3 p.m.

☐ Remember that ultraviolet rays can penetrate through loosely woven or wet clothes. Wear sunscreen under your clothes when necessary.

❏ Be especially careful at higher altitudes, or when you are close to the equator because the sun's rays are stronger there.

❏ Watch for any changes in your skin — new raised growths, itchy patches, sores that won't heal, changes in moles or new colored areas — and report them to your doctor immediately.

Sources: *The Skin Cancer Foundation, U.S. Pharmacist* (14,4:27) and *Natural Remedies for Super Perfect Health* (FC&A Publishing)

Vitamin product prevents skin cancer

We know that the best way to prevent skin cancer is to avoid exposure to ultraviolet (UV) rays from the sun and in places like tanning booths. But some people at high risk may need to take further preventive action, doctors at Boston University School of Medicine report.

Five people with a rare skin disorder (xeroderma pigmentosum) that causes cancer took high doses of Accutane for two years. Researchers found that it completely prevented the development of skin cancer, according to *The New England Journal of Medicine* (318:25).

Accutane (generic name isotretinoin) is a strong, toxic derivative of vitamin A that is used to treat severe cases of disfiguring acne. It causes birth defects in pregnant women and is considered a drug of "last resort" in acne patients because of its serious side effects. The researchers believe that if Accutane can prevent skin cancer, even in such a small study, some less toxic form of vitamin A may be found that also can prevent cancer. The search is under way.

The good news for light-skinned people or those with a family history of skin cancer is that the vitamin A-derivative approach is not just a treatment. The treatment actually prevented skin cancer among high-risk people.

Don't take too much vitamin A. Megadoses of vitamin A can produce poisonous side effects.

Skin Problems

Get relief from irritating dry skin

Are you bothered with dry, chapped or itching skin? If so, you're not alone. Xerosis, or dry skin, is one of the most common complaints among the elderly, reports *Geriatrics* (45,10:57).

Nearly everyone over 70 has dry skin, says a report in *U.S. Pharmacist* (15,1:20). And eight out of every 10 people over age 60 have dry skin between November and March.

Dry skin is often the result of aging — oil and sweat glands no longer function as well as they should, and so they fail to keep the skin as moist as before. However, there are several other factors that could cause dry skin.

Often the skin loses its moisture due to very dry air inside heated or air-conditioned buildings. The dry air causes the skin to lose water faster than the body can replace it.

Dry skin can also be caused by rubbing and scratching, especially by itchy wool clothes. Symptoms of dry skin include redness, roughness, itching, scaling and chapping. Lips also can become cracked and irritated.

Many people believe that moisturizing lotions alone can put the wet back into dry skin. So they apply lotions several times a day, but they still have dry skin. Putting lotion on dry skin can actually aggravate the situation.

Others think that dry skin can be treated with long baths. So they soak in a bath, but they can't get rid of the dry skin. Taking a long bath without applying any lotion afterwards also can aggravate the condition.

The best treatment for dry skin is to replace the lost moisture and then protect the skin from losing more water, using the "soak-grease" method:

(1) Soak in water for 5 to 10 minutes.

(2) Gently blot the skin dry (do not rub).

(3) Then apply a thin coat of lotion, cream or oil.

Soaking in water replaces the lost water in the skin, and then the lotion prevents the moisture from leaving the skin. Apply the lotion while the skin is still moist.

You can also fight dry skin by drinking at least six to eight glasses of clear liquid, preferably water, each day. "Clear liquids" do not include caffeinated or alcoholic drinks, which may cause you to lose more water from the skin.

Use a humidifier or vaporizer to add moisture to the air at home or at work. This helps protect your skin from drying out.

If you try the soak-grease method, drink lots of liquids, use a humidifier and still have dry skin, see your doctor. Unexplained dry skin can be a side effect of a more serious illness like diabetes mellitus and should be discussed with your doctor.

Skin problems can be very aggravating, but following a few simple steps usually will help clear up the problems right away. If your skin problems continue after trying these home remedies, talk with your doctor. He can determine the next best course of action to help restore your skin to its healthy state.

Tips to relieve dry skin

☐ Try to avoid rubbing or scratching your skin if it itches. If itching becomes unbearable, talk to your pharmacist or doctor.

☐ Don't wear woolen or other rough clothing. If you do wear these items, wear a cotton shirt, blouse or garment underneath.

☐ Cover your skin when outside in the winter to protect it from the wind and chilling air.

☐ Wear rubber gloves when washing dishes or other work that involves putting your hands or arms in soapy water.

☐ Drink at least 6 to 8 glasses of water or clear liquid each day. Limit your intake of caffeinated or alcoholic drinks.

☐ Don't apply cosmetics or perfumed products over areas of dry or itching skin.

☐ If your home heating system doesn't have a humidifier system built in, use portable vaporizers or humidifiers to help add moisture to the air. Your pharmacist can help you select suitable units.

☐ Use warm, not hot, water for bathing and cleansing your skin. Don't use strong soaps or detergents, and don't add bubble bath to the water.

☐ Use a soft cloth or sponge to cleanse your skin. Don't use rough cloth or brushes.

☐ After you bathe, pat your skin dry; don't rub it with a towel. Then, apply a thin layer of lotion or oil.

☐ Avoid frequent bathing. Don't take saunas or steam baths, and don't soak in hot tubs.

☐ Be careful getting into or out of a tub if you have used bath oil in the water. The tub's surface may become slippery.

Source: *U.S. Pharmacist* (15,1:22)

What to do about hard, thick skin

Are certain areas of your skin hard and thick? You may have lichen simples chronicus. It's a common skin irritation of the elderly.

This condition involves a thickening and hardening of the skin caused by persistent rubbing and irritation. The most frequent sites of this skin problem are the arms, lower legs and back of the neck. The most effective treatment for lichen simples chronicus is a strong hydrocortisone cream.

People who suffer from this skin condition must understand the "itch-and-scratch" cycle. The more you scratch, the more you injure the skin. The skin starts to heal, but healing skin itches. So, you scratch, and injure the skin again. To stop the cycle, you must stop scratching. The cortisone cream will help control the itching.

Contact dermatitis: a touchy subject

When you get a rash that itches, burns and stings, chances are you have contact dermatitis. That means you are allergic or sensitive to something that has touched your skin. The key to curing the dermatitis is to find the source of irritation and avoid it, but that may be easier said than done.

Most contact dermatitis is caused by an allergic reaction. A chemical that irritates the skin either on the first exposure or after repeated contact can cause nonallergic contact dermatitis, too.

Although it is common, contact dermatitis is hard to diagnose because there are so many possible sources. Nickel-based jewelry, detergents, dish-washing soaps, deodorants, cosmetics, hair-care products and some rubber products ... all of these can cause inflammation. You can even develop contact dermatitis from breathing in an airborne pollutant.

To complicate the situation, you can actually have allergic and nonallergic reactions at the same time. Sometimes even the medicine you use for a skin infection will cause contact dermatitis, making your problems worse.

In the face of these odds, how can you go about finding relief from contact dermatitis? Various nonprescription remedies will soothe your discomfort, but the best solution is to identify the source of irritation. If you can avoid it, your contact dermatitis will probably go away.

If you cannot locate the source, or your dermatitis gets worse, talk to your pharmacist about how to use the treatments for contact dermatitis safely. You may be able to get relief by using oral antihistamines, wet dressings and anti-itch baths such as colloidal oatmeal.

According to *U.S. Pharmacist* (15,5:13), hydrocortisone cream is the most effective remedy for contact dermatitis. If you use a hydrocortisone remedy for seven days without getting relief from your rash, you should stop using hydrocortisone. Your problem could be more complicated, and you probably need to see a dermatologist to get relief. Although contact dermatitis is common and uncomfortable, it isn't usually serious. However, occasionally it gets bad enough to force a person to change jobs to escape an irritant.

What's causing the itch ... from head to toe

U.S. Pharmacist (15,5:14) has compiled this list of common causes of contact dermatitis:

> • Head — hair-care products, cosmetics, medicated skin creams, plants, face creams, hair spray, nail polish, nickel earrings, perfume, earphones, telephone receivers, lipstick, lip salves, toothpastes, mouthwash, clothing, cologne and jewelry.
>
> • Body — clothing, dress shields, deodorant, depilatories, medicated skin creams, hand lotions, soaps and detergents, rubber gloves and rubber bands, plants, douches, tampons, "jock itch" medicine, contraceptives (creams, rubber diaphragms, condoms) and hemorrhoid products.
>
> • Feet — athlete's foot medicine, stockings, slippers, shoes and shower sandals.

How to avoid run-ins with poisonous plants

If you're heading for the great outdoors this summer, chances are you're also heading for a patch of poison ivy, poison oak or poison sumac.

And whenever the oil from any part of these plants touches you, it can cause an allergic skin reaction that may be red, blistered and oozing, reports *U.S. Pharmacist* (15,5:86).

This rash breaks out gradually and itches intensely for 10 to 14 days. Most people are allergic to these plants, so your best protection is to know what they look like and avoid touching them.

Poison ivy is everywhere ... all over the United States, in fields and forests and your own backyard. You will know it by its shiny pointed leaves that grow in clusters of three. Sometimes it is a bit hard to recognize because it can grow as a plant, bush or vine.

Poison oak is less common. It looks much like poison ivy except that it has hairy leaves that resemble oak leaves.

You won't run into poison sumac unless you are in the swamps of the eastern United States. Look for a bush or a tree with two rows of small pointed leaves opposite each other and a leaflet at the tip.

All three of these poisonous plants have clusters of white shiny berries in the fall.

You can control the poison ivy in your yard by spraying it with herbicide every three weeks. Don't try to burn the plants, because the smoke and fumes can also cause an allergic reaction.

When you come into contact with any of these plants, first take off your clothes and wash the poisonous oil off your skin with soap and water as soon as you can.

Sponging with rubbing alcohol will help remove any remaining oil. Your clothes will need to be washed, too.

If you do break out, you can buy lotions and creams that will soothe the itch and help dry the rash without a prescription at your drugstore. However, if your skin gets severely irritated or you find the rash on your face, you should see your doctor for treatment.

Vitamin D cream for psoriasis

People with the dry, scaly skin disease known as psoriasis may find relief by using a skin cream containing an active form of vitamin D, according to a digest in *American Family Physician* (40,4:301).

In one study, more than three out of four psoriasis sufferers got consistent relief by applying calcitriol in a petroleum jelly base to the scaly areas. Most got better without any side effects from the vitamin. Calcitriol is known medically as vitamin D3.

Psoriasis medicine linked to tanning booth death

A 45-year-old woman who was taking a medicine to treat a skin disease died after being burned in a tanning booth, according to an Associated Press report.

Her medicine — psoralen — makes skin more sensitive to light, especially to ultraviolet rays contained in sunshine and concentrated in tanning booths.

The Indiana woman died of burn complications after using a booth in a beauty salon, the news report says.

The report says she had been taking the medicine as a treatment for psoriasis, a skin condition that causes scaly and often painful sores.

Used with medically supervised doses of ultraviolet light, psoralen has been a standard psoriasis treatment for several years. It also helps fight a type of skin cancer known as cutaneous T-cell lymphoma. Psoralen is derived from a chemical found naturally in figs, celery, limes and parsley.

The report indicates that people taking psoralen should be very cautious about getting too much exposure to light. Exposure that would be OK for most people may be dangerous for those taking psoralen.

Gardeners' alert

If you have the South American lily *Alstroemeria* in your garden, always wear gloves when cutting stems and handling leaves, recommends *Science News* (137:11,174).

Alstroemeria produces a substance, called tuliposide, that caused itchy, scaly hands in 15 of 57 floral workers participating in a Pennsylvania study.

The olive wood itch

Some of the irritants that affect your skin may be in your jewelry box. Avoid olive wood products, especially jewelry made with olive wood.

Many people with sensitive skin will experience an allergic reaction to olive wood, *Cutis* (43,3:202) reports.

Besides jewelry, olive wood is often made into napkin rings, walking sticks, knife handles, musical instruments and crucifixes. All of those can cause redness, itching and swelling upon contact with the skin. The skin reaction usually ends when contact with the olive wood is stopped, the journal report says.

Fast-food flare-up

The skin rashes and acne problems you have today may have been caused by the hamburger and french fries you ate last night.

Many fast-food restaurants serve meals with an iodine content 30 times the Recommended Dietary Allowance for iodine, says *The New England Journal of Medicine* (322,8:558).

The excess iodine can interfere with thyroid functions, causing rashes and acne. To avoid these flare-ups, eat fast-food only occasionally, not every day, the researchers suggest.

A new twist to aspirin pain relief

"Take an aspirin and call me in the morning."

You've heard this phrase a hundred times. But now it has a new twist. Instead of taking an aspirin by mouth, many researchers are telling people to crush an aspirin, mix it with body lotion, and apply it to their skin.

Applying this mixture to your skin seems to provide relief from the intense pain that often comes with shingles, a skin disease caused by a herpes virus, says a report in *Medical Tribune* (31,2:9).

This is the same virus that causes chicken pox in children. People suffering from pain caused by the virus have not been able to find anything to relieve the pain. Until now, that is.

Scientists suggest crushing one 325-milligram aspirin tablet and mixing it in two tablespoons of Vaseline Intensive Care lotion, then applying it to the skin three to four times daily. Apparently, the skin absorbs the aspirin very quickly and easily, so the aspirin gives quick relief from the pain.

Researchers report that a 67-year-old man with Parkinson's disease responded to the aspirin-lotion mixture almost immediately (within 15 minutes).

Before using the lotion, he had been having trouble sleeping due to severe pain in his left shoulder caused by the herpes virus. After three weeks of applying the aspirin-lotion mixture, he was able to sleep peacefully through the night.

Check your skin for warning signs: Stop nutrition problems before they get started

You can watch your skin for signs of nutritional deficiencies that even your doctor might not see, reports Dr. Kenneth Neldner, chairman of the Dermatology Department at Texas Tech University.

Here are signs to watch for:

- **scaly skin**
- **canker sores**
- **wounds that heal slowly**
- **cracks in the corners of the mouth**

Researchers are discovering that even minor nutrition problems show up in the skin, sometimes long before a doctor might see the underlying cause, reports an article in *The Atlanta Journal*.

Here are some common deficiencies and how they show up on your skin:

❑ **Vitamin C shortage** — bleeding gums, soreness in mouth and gums or a rough, scaly rash around hair roots.

❑ **Vitamin B complex deficiency** — cracks and canker sores in the corners of the mouth.

There are other links between nutrition and skin problems, too. Deficiencies in zinc, copper, selenium and vitamins A and E increase the risks of developing various skin cancers.

Psoriasis and eczema are skin problems that might not be caused by nutrient shortages, but sometimes they can be successfully treated by taking fish oil. Fish oil contains fatty acids, which help the body fight inflammation caused by the two skin conditions. Because five out of six medical schools don't even offer a formal course in nutrition for medical students, many doctors don't recognize early signs of nutrition problems, says Dr. Neldner.

Don't try to medicate yourself. If you have some of the possible early warning signs, tell your doctor about this nutritional research and ask that she look at your condition more closely.

Avoid alcohol if you suffer from psoriasis

A high alcohol intake worsens psoriasis, Finnish researchers report in the *British Medical Journal* (300,6727:780).

For two years, they studied 429 men (144 with psoriasis and 285 with other skin diseases) aged 19 to 50 and asked them the following questions:

- **Does drinking increase the risk of psoriasis?**
- **Does drinking worsen psoriasis?**
- **Does psoriasis increase drinking?**

Participants filled out a questionnaire about their drinking habits the year before their skin disease developed and the year before they joined the study. Psoriasis was not associated with any other factor, such as age, social class or marital status, but seemed to be related to alcohol intake and frequency of intoxication, according to the researchers.

Psoriasis sufferers reported that their drinking increased after the disease was diagnosed, and one-third reported that alcohol seemed to worsen their psoriasis. Those who had psoriasis on a greater portion of their bodies tended to drink more as well.

Sleeping Problems

Insomnia — the sleeper's nightmare

We've all probably had a night or two when we just couldn't fall asleep — a minor inconvenience for most of us. But for some people, sleepless nights are a way of life.

The inability to fall asleep, a condition called insomnia, can lead to serious medical problems. One person even died after nine months without sleep.

"After [age] 60, people have more trouble falling asleep, awaken more often, and, once awake, find it more difficult, if not impossible, to drop back to sleep," according to a report in *FDA Consumer* (23,8:13).

Sleep needs vary from person to person. Adults sleep an average of seven and a half hours a night, the report says.

Insomnia has a variety of causes: Anxiety, stress, jet lag or too much caffeine or alcohol cause most sleepless nights. Some medications may cause insomnia as well. Is your sleeplessness serious?

Ask yourself these questions:

❐ Do you always have trouble falling asleep?

❐ Are you still awake a half hour after going to bed?

❐ Do you wake up several times during the night and have trouble falling back to sleep?

❐ Do you wake up early, after sleeping only a few hours?

If you answered yes to those questions, you may have a serious case of insomnia. But don't panic. *FDA Consumer* and *Health Letter* offer several tips to help yourself get a good night's sleep:

❐ Cut down on caffeine intake, especially at night.

❐ Don't nap during the day.

❐ Try a warm bath, reading or eating a light snack just before bedtime.

❐ Stick to a "sleep schedule." Go to bed at the same time every night and don't sleep in on weekends.

❏ Avoid heavy meals before bedtime.

❏ Don't drink that glass of wine before bedtime. Instead of helping you relax, it may have the opposite effect.

❏ Make your bedroom a quiet, restful place and keep it at a comfortable temperature.

❏ Don't exercise near bedtime. (But regular exercise during the day will help you relax at night.)

If you just cannot fall asleep without medication, follow these precautions:

❏ Ask your doctor about specific side effects. If your doctor is not familiar with your history, tell him about all other medications you are currently taking. Some drugs can cause insomnia.

❏ Take the lowest dosage of sleeping medication possible.

❏ Don't have the prescription refilled.

❏ Don't drive, operate machinery or drink alcohol while taking sleeping medication.

If self-help remedies fail, a sleep clinic may be just the thing for you. There are more than 1,000 sleep clinics in the United States alone. Each is manned by teams of experts whose sole purpose is to find out why you can't sleep. Usually, you must stay overnight in the clinic so that the research team can measure your brain activity, breathing and movements.

For a list of accredited sleep centers, write to: American Sleep Disorder Association, 604 Second St., S.W., Rochester, Minn. 55902.

Getting the most out of your rest

Your doctor tells you to get more rest. So you go to bed a little earlier. But you lie awake until the wee hours of the morning. And after you finally fall asleep, you wake up feeling just as tired as you did when you went to bed. Sound familiar? You and millions of other people, particularly older men and women, are not getting as much out of your rest time as you should.

These suggestions found in *Senior Patient* (2,1:57) may help you make your rest time truly restful.

❏ Play soft, relaxing music while you rest or before you go to bed to help you unwind from the day.

❒ Take bedtime medications one or two hours before you go to bed, if your doctor has prescribed them for you.

❒ Take pain relievers and other medications on the schedule that your doctor recommends. Sticking to the schedule helps keep a steady, effective amount of medicine in your body at all times, so you'll be less likely to be awakened by pain or discomfort.

❒ Sleep on a firm mattress for good back support.

❒ Try to avoid caffeine, especially close to bedtime. It interferes with sleep.

❒ Avoid alcohol. It may make you sleepy at bedtime, but it often leaves you wide awake at 2 a.m. or 3 a.m. It can also interfere with medications.

❒ Go to sleep and rise on a regular schedule. And try to sleep at least five to six hours each night.

❒ Exercise enough each day to stay flexible and to keep good muscle tone. It is very easy to "stiffen up" if you don't do some exercise. You and your doctor can plan an effective and fun exercise program to suit your needs.

❒ Take warm baths or use gentle massage to relieve joint or muscle aches and pains.

Following these simple suggestions on a regular, long-term basis will help you get the most out of your rest time. And getting the most out of your rest time will help you make the most out of your day.

A medical reason for your tiredness

If you are tired in the morning and sleepy throughout the day, you might be suffering from sleep apnea (pronounced **ap**-nee-a). Apnea is a medical problem that causes people to stop breathing at least five times during the night for periods of 20 to 40 seconds each time. These periods without breathing decrease the supply of oxygen to the brain, resulting in sleepiness and loss of concentration during waking hours, especially in the evening.

Typical sufferers are middle-aged or older men who are loud snorers and overweight, says a report from the American Lung Association. Many men with sleep apnea also have high blood pressure.

Sleep apnea presents the greatest problem for people who drive, such as truck drivers. Researchers at a sleep-disorder clinic report that the auto-accident rate for people with severe sleep apnea is seven times that of the normal population. Sleep apnea accounts for 38,000 accidents per year in the United States, says a report in the *American Review of Respiratory Disease.*

Even minor, easily controlled sleep disturbances can impair driving ability. But many people fail to tell their doctors about the problem because they fear losing their drivers' licenses.

Perhaps the most common cause of sleep apnea is being fat. Obesity causes an excessive amount of soft tissue to accumulate in the throat, resulting in an obstructed airway, snoring and apnea.

You can help treat the underlying cause of your sleeping disorder by losing weight and quitting smoking, says a report in *British Medical Journal* (298,6678:904).

The most annoying symptom of apnea — for people who live with you, that is — is snoring. To fight snoring, try propping your head up at night.

Or, if you snore only while lying on your back, sew a tennis ball into the back of your pajama top. That will prompt you to roll over onto your side or stomach.

Finally, if you think your problem is beyond your control, see your doctor, who can bring you up to date on the latest medical techniques to treat sleeping disorders. Surgery to correct apnea is a last resort.

If you have a sleep disorder and your physician has advised you not to drive until your condition is controlled, take the advice. If you don't and are involved in an accident, your insurance company may claim that you were driving against medical advice.

Sleep apnea may be underlying cause of some dementia

Some elderly people have a sleep disorder called sleep apnea. Many of them don't know they have this enemy of a good night's rest. Now, researchers are finding that sleep apnea might be the villain behind some cases of mental deterioration that seem like senility, says a report in *Geriatrics* (45,6:16).

The higher the number of episodes of sleep apnea, the poorer some elderly people performed on tests of mental and physical abilities, according to Dr. D.L. Bliwise of the Sleep Disorders Center at Stanford Medical School in California.

These are the same tests given to people to find out if they have Alzheimer's disease or other forms of mental deterioration.

The researcher believes that sleep apnea might be the underlying cause of some cases of mental declines. Treating the apnea might reverse the mental deterioration in some people, Bliwise hopes.

It's not a case of sleeping longer, but of sleeping better. People with sleep apnea tend to snore a lot, and loudly.

More dangerously, they actually stop breathing for periods ranging from a few seconds to more than a minute at a time. It's almost as if they "forget" to breathe. Soft tissue in the breathing passage relaxes and acts like a trapdoor, shutting off the air. That can happen many times a night.

Sometimes they wake up suddenly with a sensation of having lost their breath or of choking without air. Such episodes result in a lighter, "restless" sleep. It's not hard to see how a breathless, restless night could mess up your next day, and even dull your thinking after a while.

If you snore a lot, you might have sleep apnea.

Check with your doctor about the treatments available for this potentially serious disorder.

Skimping on sleep can shorten your life span

Could you be taking eight to ten years off your life by not getting enough sleep at night? Experts are beginning to think so.

Nearly 50 percent of all Americans (five out of every 10 people) short themselves one to two hours of sleep each night. Each night adds up, and by the end of the week, it's as if you missed a whole night of sleep!

The typical 24-hour on-the-go schedule that most Americans keep these days is resulting in a nation of "walking zombies," says a recent report in *The Atlanta Journal* (108,22).

Researchers now are recognizing the consequences of sleepiness: loss of initiative, loss of energy, attention lapses, distractibility and fatigue.

Researchers also report that after five years, people who work night shifts and don't get enough sleep are twice as likely to suffer from heart ailments and gastrointestinal diseases as those who work day shifts and get enough sleep.

"There's even evidence that people getting inadequate sleep shorten their life span by eight to 10 years," reports Dr. James Maas, a researcher from Cornell University.

Here's a simple test to see if you need more sleep: If you need an alarm clock to get up in the morning, or if you feel more than just a minor sag in the middle of the day, you probably need more sleep.

Are doctors mistreating sleep problems, missing major illnesses?

It's a myth that aging itself causes insomnia and other sleep problems, say members of an expert government panel.

In fact, many doctors may be overprescribing sleeping pills while missing more serious, underlying health problems in people over 65, says the report in *Medical World News* (31,8:38).

Poor sleep patterns might even be a cause of death, the report suggests.

If you are over 65 and have trouble sleeping, something is probably wrong with you — something other than just "getting old," points out the University of Rochester's Dr. Robert J. Joynt, chairman of the National Institutes of Health panel.

"Both prescription and nonprescription drugs may actually worsen sleep problems, as they deal with symptoms rather than underlying causes," the report says.

Sleeping pills are sometimes OK as a short-term treatment for sleeplessness caused by stress, anxiety and a few other psychiatric problems, but they should never be used as a long-term solution for sleep problems.

Although sleep clinics are becoming more common, both the general public and doctors still "have a poor understanding of sleep and its disorders," the National Institutes of Health panel says.

"The goal of therapy [for insomnia] should be to identify the underlying cause," the panel says.

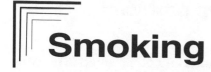

Smoking

You can turn back the clock on heart damage from smoking

You smoke cigarettes, and you're worried about your health. But, you won't stop smoking because you think you've already done the damage to your body, and stopping smoking now won't really do you any good.

Well, the good news is that you can help your body heal if you stop smoking now, even if you have smoked for a long period of time. *The New England Journal of Medicine* (322,4:213) reports that women who quit smoking greatly reduce their chances of suffering from a heart attack.

By the time a woman celebrates her third anniversary as a nonsmoker, her risk of a first heart attack is no greater than if she had never smoked, this study of more than 3,200 women reveals.

This news is true regardless of how heavy a smoker you might have been, how long you smoked, or how old you are.

Women, rather than quitting, usually are more likely to switch to "low-yield" brands, thinking these brands are safer. However, "recent evidence indicates that women who smoke low-yield cigarettes have virtually the same risk of myocardial infarction [heart attack] as women who smoke higher-yield brands," the *NEJM* report states.

Smoking and lung cancer

You've heard the warnings, and you know the equation: Cigarette Smoking = Lung Cancer. But now there's a new addition to that equation. It seems that your lungs are no longer the only thing at risk. Cigarette smoking also can increase your risk of both leukemia and cancer of the bone marrow, reports the *Journal of the National Cancer Institute* (82,23:1832).

As with lung cancer, your risk of getting blood or bone cancer increases with the number of cigarettes you smoke daily and the length of time you've been smoking. The more you smoke and the longer you've been smoking, the greater your risk.

However, there is some good news. Some studies suggest that once a person stops smoking, the body begins a healing process and the chance of cancer decreases. Even if you've smoked for over twenty years, your body can start healing if you quit smoking.

New study tells more
about cigarettes and cancer

It's been suspected for years that it's the high-tar, high-nicotine content in cigarette smoke that causes most of the damage to smokers' lungs. A study in *Preventive Medicine* (18,4:518) adds new weight to that belief.

"Tar [is] the main carcinogenic agent in cigarette smoke," the researchers say. They further charge that lung cancer risk rises in a direct line with tar content in cigarette smoke. In other words, the higher the tar level of the cigarette, the greater the risk of getting lung cancer.

Most American smokers have switched to so-called low-tar brands in recent years, the study says. Most low-tar brands are filter-tipped. One estimate says that when the average male smokes a cigarette, the smoke he inhales contains 13.8 milligrams of tar.

The average woman smoker puffs a cigarette that delivers to her lungs 11.8 milligrams of tar. At that level of tar intake, a 10-cigarette-a-day smoker would be about five times more likely to develop deadly lung cancer than a nonsmoker, according to a risk chart in the new study.

Cigarette smoking is blamed for 85 percent of lung cancer cases in men and for 75 percent of such cases in women, according to the American Cancer Society. Besides lung cancer, the number one cancer killer, smoking has been strongly linked to cancers of the larynx (the voice box), esophagus and bladder.

"Smoking accounts for about 30 percent of all cancer deaths," says *Postgraduate Medicine* (86,2:213). Smokers who puff two or more packs a day die from lung cancer 15 to 25 times more often than nonsmokers, according to the journal report.

Smoking has been called the number one reversible cause of death in the world.

Would you risk a stroke for a smoke?

A new study of twins finds that smoking is a "strong factor" in the development of carotid atherosclerosis, the hardening and narrowing of the large arteries that supply blood to the head.

The study of 49 pairs of identical twins in Finland shows that the association of smoking with carotid atherosclerosis was "highly significant," even after statistically adjusting for age, cholesterol level, blood pressure and other potentially confounding factors, according to the report in *Circulation* (80:10).

In each of the 49 pairs studied, one twin was a nonsmoker or at least never had smoked daily, and the other was a smoker or former smoker. The average lifelong dose of the smoking twins was 20 "package-years" — they had smoked the equivalent of one package every day for 20 years. That contrasts sharply with the twins who were classified as nonsmokers, who had smoked less than five packages (100 cigarettes) in their entire lives.

Because of difficulties in performing well-controlled experiments on human populations, researchers often turn to identical twins who are, in a sense, "natural experiments." Both twins have the same genetic makeup, thus limiting a major variable and giving researchers a better opportunity to study the effects of lifestyle and environmental factors such as smoking.

Using ultrasound in external examinations, the scientists measured "plaques" in the carotid arteries of the twins. Plaque is a fatty deposit attached to a wall of a blood vessel. Studies by others have shown that smoking is associated with development of plaques in the abdominal aorta, in the heart arteries and in major arteries in the legs, say the Finnish researchers.

In the 49 pairs of twins, narrowing of the carotids was found in nine pairs — nine of the smoking twins and two of their nonsmoking co-twins, the researchers report. The total area of artery-narrowing plaques in the carotids was more than three times larger in the smoking twins. The inner layer of the carotid arteries was thicker in the smoking twins, the study says. Both total area and thickness correlated with the dose of smoking — the more one smoked, the worse the plugging effect.

Based on this 12-year study, the researchers concluded, "The smoking twins are at a significantly higher risk of coronary heart disease than their nonsmoking co-twins." For us nontwins, the study demonstrates that smoking greatly raises the risk of plaque plugs in vital neck arteries. Increased plaque, in turn, raises the risk of stroke and hemorrhage due to weakened or blocked arteries.

Cigarette smokers have a three to four times greater risk of stroke than nonsmokers, Australian researchers report in *The Lancet* (2,8664:643).

If you smoke two packs a day, your risk of stroke is twice that of someone the same age who smokes one pack a day. If you live with a smoker, you inhale passive smoke and also are at risk for stroke, researchers said.

There are different types of stroke. Stroke may be caused by bleeding in the brain itself (a cerebral hemorrhage) or a blood clot that travels from the heart to the brain (a cerebral embolism).

Hardening of the arteries in the brain or neck may lead to blockage of major blood vessels supplying the brain. This type of stroke is called a cerebral thrombosis, a major cause of which is smoking.

Researchers examined the relationship between cigarette smoking and stroke. In previous studies, chronic smoking was shown to break down the inner lining of arteries, causing blood to thicken and slow down, but has not been "consistently implicated" as a stroke risk factor.

They studied 844 people — 422 patients suffering their first stroke and 422 residents of the same area who had never had a stroke. The average age of the participants was 65.

In choosing stroke patients for the study, researchers used sophisticated scanning equipment to determine what type of stroke the patient suffered.

Researchers interviewed participants about their previous diet and exercise, medical history, alcohol consumption and smoking habits (what they smoked, how much and how long).

Of the stroke patients, 32 percent were current smokers, 34 percent were former smokers, and 34 percent had never smoked.

Of the subjects who had never had a stroke, 18 percent were current smokers, 32 percent were former smokers, and 49 percent had never smoked, researchers said.

"Smoking, hypertension [high blood pressure], and a history of [heart attack] were significant and independent risk factors, whereas alcohol consumption seemed to have a modest but significant protective effect," the report concluded. The risk of stroke was slightly higher for men than women.

The risk of stroke for smokers was about the same as their risk of heart attack. For those who quit, the risk was still strong after 10 years.

Researchers said that some of the effects of smoking are reversible, but because the stroke risk persists for 10 years or more, they think that smoking has more lasting effects than once believed.

Count years — not puffs — when determining risk of stroke

Who would you think has the greater chance of stroke — someone smoking 40 cigarettes a day for five years, or the person smoking 10 cigarettes a day for 20 years? Be careful of your answer. You could be dead wrong.

The latest study involving cigarette smokers, as reported by the American Heart Association, reveals new danger associated with the number of years smoking.

Dr. Jack Whisnant, a neurologist from the Mayo Clinic in Rochester, Minnesota, says, "This is the first time that the duration of smoking has been found to be more important in influencing the risk of carotid athero-sclerosis than the number of cigarettes smoked over a lifetime."

Temporary loss of vision or temporary paralysis may be the first signs that the carotid artery is in trouble. Once the artery becomes completely blocked, or a blood clot forms, the conditions are right for a stroke.

Dr. Whisnant's study involved 752 men and women who had come to the Mayo Clinic with various symptoms of brain disease and stroke. They took part in a diagnostic technique known as carotid arteriography. The procedure allows doctors to see the inside of the neck arteries, enabling them to better assess the extent of the damage.

Their medical problems and personal habits, including smoking, alcohol intake and exercise, were all taken into account.

It was determined that a 60-year-old man or woman who had spent 40 years smoking was 3.5 times more likely to have disease of the neck artery than a nonsmoker, regardless of the number of cigarettes smoked.

The researchers at Mayo Clinic concluded that the length of time spent smoking contributed to neck artery disease more than the actual number of cigarettes smoked, the person's age, or whether or not the person had diabetes or high blood pressure.

Don't just cut back on the number of cigarettes you smoke each day. According to Dr. Whisnant, this is a "false sense of security." The only healthy option is to completely stop smoking. By limiting your smoking years, you could be lengthening your life.

Indoor tobacco smoke exposure may triple women's cancer risks

Smoking is hazardous not only to the smoker. Just being in the same room with tobacco smoke may be dangerous to nonsmokers, especially women, according to two recent scientific studies.

Nonsmoking women who have been exposed to "sidestream" or "passive" tobacco smoke run increased risks of developing both cancer of the cervix and breast cancer, the studies suggest.

Sidestream smoke, passive smoking and involuntary smoking are all terms that mean the same thing, according to the U.S. Government's Office on Smoking and Health.

The terms refer to the tobacco smoke that a nonsmoking person inhales without choice, particularly inside a closed area like an office building or house.

Researchers at the University of Utah found that women exposed to passive smoke for more than three hours a day were three times more likely to develop cancer of the cervix. Women whose husbands or other household members smoked a lot ran the greatest risk of cancer from passive smoke.

The Utah study — reported in *The Journal of the American Medical Association* (261,11:1593) — ran for three years and involved 270 white women ages 20 through 59, all of whom had developed cancer of the cervix. The researchers compared the cancer patients' smoking exposure to that of a control group of 408 women without cancer.

Although the report in *JAMA* was careful not to blame smoking for causing cervical cancer, it did suggest that smoking played a major role in the disease's development.

The Utah study is the first to link passive smoking directly with cancer of the cervix, although some scientists have speculated about it for a decade. Passive smoke has already been linked to lung cancer.

A second statistical study says indoor tobacco smoke is a major risk factor in developing breast cancer. Although the female hormone estrogen is believed to play the leading role in breast cancers, passive smoking might be as high as second on the list of causes, according to researcher A. Wesley Horton.

"Estrogen may be the principal promoter of human breast cancer," says Horton in a report in *Cancer* (62:6), "but evidence is mounting that indoor tobacco smoke can play a critical role."

One out of every 10 American women will develop breast cancer, Horton reports.

Breast cancer is the second leading cause of death among women in the United States. That puts a high priority on learning the causes of breast cancer and learning how to minimize the risk factors.

Horton, a professor at Oregon Health Sciences University, found that countries with high rates of lung cancer in men also have high rates of breast cancer in women, even when the women were not smokers. Countries with low rates of lung cancer in men also had low rates of breast cancer in women.

Although women can be exposed to sidestream smoke at home or at work, smoke from their husbands' cigarettes was the largest factor in breast cancer patients, Horton reports.

"The increased cancer risk from the passive inhalation of sidestream smoke is not limited to nonsmokers, but is significantly increased in smokers, too," a fact Horton attributes to D.P. Sandler in the *American Journal of Epidemiology* (121:37 and 123:370).

Horton believes that inhaling passive smoke may be more dangerous than actually smoking a cigarette. "Some of the chemical initiators [that cause cancer] are much more concentrated in sidestream than in mainstream tobacco smoke," Horton says. Mainstream smoke is smoke inhaled directly by the smoker.

Horton's report says it usually takes more than 20 years of inhaling passive tobacco smoke before a nonsmoking woman develops breast cancer.

According to the report, the current high rates of breast cancer could have been influenced by indoor, passive smoke inhalation during the late 1960s and early 1970s.

If you have never smoked and you have always lived and worked in a smoke-free environment, you're lucky: Horton suggests that you probably have a much lower risk of breast cancer than the one in 10 cited previously.

As for smokers, Horton urges them to "practice" their habit outdoors. "Designated smoking areas" and air conditioning with "recirculation of smoke-contaminated air more than doubles ... exposure to sidestream smoke," he concludes.

If your spouse smokes, beware of heart disease

You're a nonsmoker, so you think you're safe from cardiovascular problems that are caused by smoking. But you could be mistaken, especially if your spouse smokes.

A recent study compared the number of cases of cardiovascular disease among nonsmoking women who were married to smokers with the number of cases among nonsmoking women whose husbands did not smoke.

The study revealed that women whose husbands smoked were 1.5 times more likely to die of cardiovascular disease than the women married to nonsmokers, says the *American Family Physician* (42,4:1080).

The passive smoke from your spouse's cigarette is dangerous to both of you. That is a good reason to encourage your spouse to quit smoking — it will help both of you avoid cardiovascular disease.

Vitamin E works against damage by cigarettes

Worried about secondary smoke in the workplace or at home? A new study in *Alive* suggests that taking more vitamin E may reduce chances of lung damage.

Cigarette smoke creates free radicals, which are tiny particles that can cause lung tissue damage. The free radicals make it difficult for your lungs to turn the air you breathe into usable oxygen for the blood system.

Free radical damage has been linked directly to the development of lung cancer, emphysema and chronic bronchitis.

Vitamin E helps trap these free radicals and prevents them from harming the delicate lung tissue. So, if you can't escape smoke from other people's cigarettes, vitamin E may be your best defense against lung disease. But be careful! Too much vitamin E in the body can cause other serious problems.

Be sure to check with your doctor before you start taking extra vitamin E.

Smoking hides anemia by producing false hemoglobin

Feeling tired and worn down? But your doctor can't seem to find anything wrong with you to explain your fatigue and weariness? It might be because your body has hidden the real problem.

Women who smoke may be suffering from anemia and not know it because the anemia is "masked," warns a report in *The Journal of the American Medical Association* (264,12:1556). Anemia is a lack of iron in the body.

Apparently, smoking creates an increased level of hemoglobin in the blood. Hemoglobin is the part of the blood that carries oxygen and iron to the cells in the body. However, the hemoglobin produced by smoking is a kind of "false" hemoglobin — it doesn't carry oxygen and iron as it should.

So, when your doctor measures the amount of hemoglobin in your body to test for anemia, he sees an increased level of hemoglobin and assumes that you aren't anemic. But it's the false hemoglobin that he sees. In other words, the false hemoglobin levels could be hiding the lack of good hemoglobin and therefore "mask" your anemia.

So, if you smoke and you feel worn down and tired, ask your doctor to consider anemia even though your hemoglobin test denies it.

Smoking deadens your sense of smell

The longer you smoke, the less you can smell, say scientists at the University of Pennsylvania's Smell and Taste Center. Since the sense of smell affects the taste of food, smokers may also be depriving themselves of many of the pleasures of eating.

The good news: Quit smoking, and your sense of smell will return — slowly. If you've smoked two packs a day for 10 years, it will take about 10 years for your sense of smell to return to the level of a nonsmoker, says the report in *The Journal of the American Medical Association* (263,9:1233).

Smokers need more C

Scientists warn that smokers need more vitamin C than anybody else, according to *Medical Tribune* (30,30:8). Tobacco users need 100 milligrams of vitamin C a day, nearly twice as much as nonsmokers. The RDA for vitamin C is currently 60 milligrams.

You can stop smoking with this 13-step system

Even if you are a "hard-core" smoker — someone over age 55 who has smoked for more than 30 years — you can stop. All it takes is motivation and a system that replaces old habits with new ones, say researchers in *Senior Patient* (1,5:36). In this report, they detail a system to help older smokers kick the habit.

The system works, the researchers report, and the rewards are great. A number of studies have shown that older Americans who quit smoking reduce their risk of developing heart disease and their risk of dying from it.

The disease rates "are significantly lower for ex-smokers than for current smokers," researchers say. "And quitting benefits general health and vitality."

Here's a 13-step system that will allow you to take control of your smoking habit:

1) **Set a target quitting date.** Choose a day you think that stress will be minimal and you won't be around other smokers.

2) Once you've set a target date, **keep a record of your smoking habits,** including when you smoke and where. Keeping a diary will

help you recognize how much you smoke and why you smoke. Did a confrontation with a co-worker, rush-hour traffic or an upsetting phone call make you reach for your cigarettes?

3) **Designate a smoking place** in your home and at work. Don't smoke anywhere else. Choose a place that is inconvenient and uncomfortable. One person chose the corner of his basement; another chose the front lawn. If it's raining or very cold, you might decide to stay indoors rather than smoke. And you will look silly standing there smoking on your front lawn.

4) **Keep ashtrays and lighters only in this designated** smoking place.

5) **Don't carry cigarettes with you.** Ask nonsmokers (spouse, co-workers) to hold your cigarettes. You will have to ask for a cigarette whenever you want one.

6) **Smoke alone** and do nothing else (no watching television, drinking coffee or talking on the phone) while smoking. Take the pleasure out of the habit. Make smoking a chore.

7) **Change smoking postures.** If you hold your cigarette in your right hand, switch to your left. If you draw from your cigarette on the left side of your mouth, switch to your right. These changes should make smoking more awkward and uncomfortable for you.

8) **Buy one pack at a time,** and buy lower-tar brands.

9) **Postpone your first smoke of the day** and the first one after a meal. Start with a half-hour delay and work up to an hour.

10) When you want a cigarette, **don't light it right away.** Hold it in your hand and tell yourself, 'I don't need to light this just yet.' Once you begin to take control of your habit, the urge for a cigarette might pass.

11) **Set up a support network.** Choose sympathetic friends (perhaps ex-smokers) whom you can call when you feel the urge for a cigarette.

12) **Start an exercise program** to help prevent weight gain. But remember: Quitting is the goal. You can worry about any extra pounds later.

13) **Reward yourself often** for accomplishing your goals.

If you cut down smoking before your target date arrives, quitting should be less stressful for you.

If you have cold feet about this, talk to your doctor about prescribing nicotine gum, which will help control the urge to smoke.

Experts stress that you should use nicotine gum to quit smoking — not to cut down — because inhaled nicotine is more potent than the nicotine in chewing gum, and the gum will not work for you.

Acidic foods and drinks reduce the effectiveness of nicotine gum

If you're chewing nicotine gum to help you kick the tobacco habit, think twice before you order that soft drink or put ketchup and mustard on your burger!

Foods and drinks with high acid content can actually prevent you from absorbing the nicotine from the gum, warns *The Journal of the American Medical Association* (264,12:1560).

Normally, your body easily absorbs nicotine by way of the saliva released in your mouth as you chew the gum. But when you eat acidic foods and drinks, the acidity of your saliva changes. Then you can't absorb the nicotine released from the gum.

The next problem is that the nicotine that is not absorbed in the mouth is swallowed and ends up in the stomach where it can cause some unpleasant side effects.

If you have an acidic drink or food, you can still use nicotine gum ... just wait about 20 minutes. The saliva in your mouth will return to normal then, and you can get the full benefit of the nicotine gum.

The acidity of foods and drinks is measured on a pH scale of 1 to 14. The value of 7.0 is neutral. Water has a pH of about 7.0 and is neutral. All values below 7.0 are acidic — the lower the number, the more acidic it is.

See the following chart of food and drink pH values for further information about which foods and drinks to avoid while chewing nicotine gum.

Foods and drinks to avoid while using nicotine gum

Substance	pH value
Chocolate milk	6.76
Whole milk	6.72
Skim milk	6.58
Chicken soup	6.54
2% low-fat milk	6.53
Distilled water	6.02 - 7.28
Coffee	4.86 - 5.45
Tomato juice	4.37
Beer	4.00 - 4.60
Soy sauce	3.92
Apple juice	3.88
Orange juice	3.81 - 3.89
Ketchup	3.66
Pineapple juice	3.64
Mustard	3.34 - 4.87
Diet cola	3.32 - 3.36
Lemon-lime soda	3.22 - 3.28
Grape juice	3.17
Cola	2.30 - 2.76

Secret revealed — an easier way to stop smoking

The tobacco withdrawal syndrome gives a lot of grief to people trying to kick the smoking habit. Recent research may be able to help you quit a little easier.

The secret is this — at the same time you're cutting down on smoking and nicotine, cut way back on caffeine, too, a report in the *British Medical Journal* (298,6680:1075) says.

Researchers in San Francisco discovered that when you stop smoking, the caffeine levels in your blood skyrocket. They found that the caffeine levels in the blood of recent quitters were two-and-a-half times their caffeine levels when they were smoking.

The nonsmoker's body doesn't burn off caffeine as quickly as that of a smoker, doctors think.

In fact, they believe, smokers have to drink a lot more caffeine than nonsmokers do to get the same effect. The researchers studied 95 people and found that caffeine levels stayed about the same for those who continued smoking.

But, "plasma caffeine concentrations increase after people give up smoking and remain increased for at least six months," the report says.

Studies show that smokers trying to kick the nicotine habit tend to load up on coffee and caffeine-containing drinks and foods. In effect, they increase their caffeine intake to compensate for the loss of nicotine.

Three or four days after a smoker kicks the smoking habit, her body metabolism slows down its caffeine-burning rate. Thus, the new non-smoker gets a much bigger jolt from her customary amount of caffeine than before she quit smoking — the equivalent of suddenly drinking two times as much coffee.

That's the problem. "Assuming that consumption of caffeine is unchanged, high caffeine concentrations could contribute to the tobacco withdrawal syndrome," the *BMJ* report says. So drinking more caffeine is like adding a few boulders to an already heavy backpack.

When you quit, cut your daily caffeine consumption by at least half. If you were used to drinking two cups of caffeinated coffee in the morning while you smoked, cut back to less than one full cup as your body adjusts to nonsmoking. Watch out for caffeine in colas and chocolate, too.

Trying to quit smoking is tough enough. Don't add to your woes — or even sabotage your new-found freedom from smoking — by getting too much caffeine at the same time, the report urges.

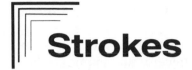

Strokes

Know the warning signs of stroke

If you had a sudden pain in your chest, you'd probably recognize it as a possible warning of a heart attack.

But what if one arm or leg suddenly becomes weak or numb? Or without warning, you get dizzy, have double vision or lose sight in one eye? You have difficulty speaking, standing or walking. Would you recognize these seemingly unrelated problems as warning signs for stroke, the third leading cause of death and a major source of disability?

About 10 percent of strokes are preceded by "transient ischemic attacks" or TIAs, the American Heart Association (AHA) reports. TIAs are sometimes called "little strokes" because the symptoms affect limbs, vision, balance or speech and last only for a few minutes.

TIAs should be considered a warning for a stroke, says the AHA. People who have experienced one of these temporary blockages of blood flow to some part of the brain are nearly 10 times more likely to suffer a paralyzing stroke than those who haven't had a TIA.

"It's important for the public to realize that the symptoms, or warning signs, for stroke are diverse," points out Dr. Louis R. Caplan of Boston, chairperson of the AHA Stroke Council. "They're not as clear-cut as heart attack symptoms."

The problem is that most people don't understand how the brain works, says Caplan. "So when these warning signs strike, they don't link it to the nervous system. Prompt medical or surgical attention to these warning signs can prevent a fatal or disabling stroke from occurring."

Since 38 percent of all stroke victims die within a month, the 30 days following a stroke are critical. Yet nearly half the people who survive the first month are still living seven years after their stroke, the AHA discovered. Quick medical attention can make an important difference in the effect of a stroke.

Most importantly, you should try to lower your risk of stroke. You can control many of the risk factors of stroke. High blood pressure, heart disease, high red blood cell count, transient ischemic attacks (TIAs), elevated blood cholesterol, cigarette smoking, excessive alcohol intake, physical inactivity and obesity are factors that increase the risk of stroke — but these factors can be treated or eliminated.

You can quit smoking, lower your blood pressure, increase your physical activity and lose weight to help lower your risk of stroke.

There are also several risk factors which cannot be changed — age, sex, race, diabetes mellitus, prior stroke, heredity and "asymptomatic carotid bruit" (a bruit indicates a blockage that may be reducing blood flow to the brain). People with several of stroke's risk factors should be especially careful to know stroke's warning signals and to watch for them.

In summary, here are the major warning signals of stroke:

> • **sudden weakness or numbness of the face, arm and leg on one side of the body**
>
> • **loss of speech, or trouble talking or understanding speech**
>
> • **dimness or loss of vision, particularly in only one eye**
>
> • **unexplained dizziness, especially when associated with other neurological symptoms**
>
> • **unusual and severe headaches**
>
> • **any paralysis on one side of the body.**

If you experience any of these symptoms, call your doctor and get medical help.

Early warning sign for impending strokes — the eyes have it

Permanent blindness is one of the most feared of all disabilities, according to several polls taken in the United States. As bad as blindness may be, a particular kind of temporary blindness may be a warning sign of something even worse — a stroke that might be fatal unless successful steps are taken to prevent it.

People over age 45 who experience a sudden loss of vision, lasting only a day or less, may be as much as 16 times more likely than the average person to suffer a massive, even fatal, stroke within a few weeks or months. That's the finding of British researchers reported in *The Lancet* (1,8631:185).

The medical term for such an attack of temporary blindness is lone bilateral blindness. The researchers are saying such attacks ought to be classified as telltale "preliminary" strokes. They are an advance signal of more life-threatening incidents soon to occur.

Here are the symptoms of this warning signal:

> - **A rapid dimming or complete loss of vision in both eyes at the same time**
>
> - **The blindness lasts 24 hours or less**
>
> - **More or less normal vision returns after no more than one day**

This particular temporary loss of vision occurs without any loss of consciousness, without any kind of seizure, and without any accompanying paralysis, dizziness or double vision. These symptoms distinguish this type of temporary blindness from some other types of vision problems.

Other kinds of temporary ("transient") blindness can occur during and after epileptic seizures, after childbirth, during heart attacks, after general anesthesia, as a result of brain tumors, and even during severe migraine headache attacks, the report says. However, these other kinds of temporary blindness are not advance signals of life-threatening strokes, according to the researchers.

For five years, the researchers kept track of 14 patients who had experienced all the symptoms of lone bilateral blindness. The tracking was part of a larger study that followed 512 patients who had experienced transient ischemic attacks (TIA).

A TIA generally is thought to be caused by high-blood-pressure-related problems, by blood clots in or near the brain, or by advanced diabetes.

Most of the 14 individuals said their loss of vision was either instantaneous or reached its maximum within seconds. Most said they experienced complete blindness very suddenly, but four patients "described their vision as dimming, frosting, or like looking through a haze or mist."

In all 14, the vision loss "was severe enough to make reading or recognition of faces impossible and most were unable to see well enough to get about." Five of the 14 also said a headache accompanied the attack of blindness. Several reported sweating, buzzing in the head and chest discomfort during the attack.

Of the 14 patients with lone bilateral blindness, five suffered their first-ever stroke within two-and-a-half years. Statistically, that's about 16 times the number of strokes that would normally be expected in that same age group (average age 67 years), the report says.

The researchers recommend that patients who have experienced attacks of lone bilateral blindness be considered at high risk for stroke. They should be treated just like patients with diagnosed TIA — "by control of vascular risk factors and ... prophylactic aspirin."

In nonmedical language, that means cutting down on cholesterol, losing weight, lowering blood pressure, quitting smoking and taking aspirin, the report indicates.

Daily aspirin dose could reduce your risk of stroke

If you suffer from an abnormal fluttering of the heart, you have a high risk of stroke; and a daily dose of aspirin might dramatically reduce your risk, according to a special report in *The New England Journal of Medicine* (322,12:863).

Researchers studied 1,244 men and women with atrial fibrillation, the medical term for heart flutter. They discovered that aspirin cut the risk of stroke by 50 to 80 percent. An anti-clotting drug, warfarin, which is available only by prescription, had the same effect as aspirin.

Researchers estimate that of the one million elderly people with atrial fibrillation, 75,000 will suffer a stroke this year.

In the study, heart-patient volunteers took aspirin, warfarin or a placebo (a harmless substance that only looks like a real drug). Among the people taking warfarin or aspirin, only 1.6 percent suffered strokes, compared with 8.3 percent of the people taking the placebo, the study reports. Those dramatic results prompted researchers to switch placebo patients to aspirin or warfarin. The people cut their stroke risk in half by taking one 325-milligram tablet of aspirin a day.

Many strokes happen when a blood clot blocks a blood vessel in the brain. Researchers believe aspirin and warfarin prevent strokes by making blood less "sticky," reducing its tendency to clot.

Aspirin and warfarin seem to work better at preventing minor, "minimally disabling" strokes than at stopping fatal ones.

Preliminary findings indicate that aspirin doesn't help people over age 75. Researchers don't know why, although previous studies have suggested that people over age 75 may have more diseases that increase their risk of stroke.

And the alternative treatment, warfarin, generally is not recommended for those elderly patients, researchers say.

They plan to follow up study patients every three months to determine the difference in benefits between aspirin and warfarin. They will also look at long-term effects of both drugs.

Before you start taking an aspirin a day, check with your doctor. Don't medicate yourself without getting good medical advice first.

Aspirin for stroke victims

An aspirin a day may be effective in preventing or reducing the effects of mental deterioration or dementia due to strokes.

Approximately 50 percent of dementia in elderly patients is related to Alzheimer's disease. However, the number two cause of dementia is multiple strokes. This dementia is known as MID (multi-infarct dementia). According to doctors at Baylor College of Medicine, Houston, about one-third of all dementia cases are caused by MID.

In a recent study, daily aspirin seemed to provide drastic improvements in MID patients. The researchers studied two groups of patients, whose average age was 67 years, with similar risk factors for stroke. They were treated identically, except that one group was given a single tablet of aspirin (325 milligrams) daily.

Blood flow in the brain and mental function improved significantly in the aspirin-treated patients, compared to the no-aspirin control group. The aspirin group also suffered fewer strokes or TIAs than the no-aspirin group.

"In the control group, 24 percent had subsequent strokes, while only 8.1 percent of the aspirin patients had strokes during the trial," the doctors reported. TIAs occurred in 39.4 percent of the control patients, compared to just 18.9 of the patients treated with aspirin.

"We haven't found a cure for Alzheimer's yet, but we've got something [aspirin therapy] that is helping MID," the researchers explained. "That's why it is important to identify the cause of the dementia and treat the two groups of patients separately."

Corn oil is latest weapon in war against strokes

Corn oil seems to be able to lower the level of plasma fibrinogen in the blood, reports *The Journal of the American College of Nutrition* (9,4:352).

Plasma fibrinogen is a kind of protein in the blood that helps make blood "sticky" and form clots. Too much fibrinogen causes the blood to "thicken" and clot abnormally.

Since some oils seem to lower the amount of fibrinogen, scientists wanted to find out which one does the best job: dietary fish oil, corn oil or olive oil. They fed the oils to three groups of volunteers for eight weeks and then tallied the results.

The fish oil group and the corn oil group were number one and two in lowering plasma fibrinogen. Olive oil was least effective and came in third.

Researchers already knew that fish oil lowers fibrinogen levels. But, what's new is the discovery that corn oil also does a good job in making blood more "slippery" and less liable to stick together in clots.

Corn oil might become the latest nutritional weapon against strokes and heart disease, the report suggests.

The nutrient that cuts the risk of fatal stroke by nearly half

There's an easy way to slash your risk of having a fatal stroke — eat one extra serving of fresh fruit or vegetables every day, declares a major new dietary study.

The super stroke preventer is the nutrient potassium, abundant in fresh fruits and vegetables, according to doctors Kay-Tee Khaw and Elizabeth Barrett-Connor and reported in *Medical World News* (30,11:30).

These researchers raised the possibility of potassium being a stroke fighter in a big study in 1987. Since then, three separate medical studies have demonstrated that increased potassium in the diet can dramatically lower your risk of death from stroke, the report says.

The studies found that groups of people who ate the most fruits and vegetables had 25 to 40 percent fewer fatal strokes than groups with lower potassium intakes. According to the report, women benefited from a high potassium diet even more than men. The people in the studies all were 59 or older.

"Americans could raise their potassium levels significantly by simply cutting down on junk food and substituting orange or grapefruit juice for soft drinks," the report says.

Fitness a key to lower stroke risk

"One way to reduce your risk of joining the half million Americans each year who suffer a stroke is to stay physically fit," says a report in *The Physician and Sportsmedicine* (17,9:37).

Researchers at the Dallas-based Institute for Aerobics Research studied the rates of stroke among 8,421 healthy people for an eight-year period.

They found that of those healthy people, the ones who were classified as "high fit" were almost three times less likely to suffer a stroke as those in the "low fit" category. They assigned the people to either high, low or medium fitness levels based on treadmill tests.

This is the first large study to suggest any link between fitness levels and risks of nonfatal stroke, the report says. This "preliminary" finding doesn't surprise Dr. Joseph C. Maroon, director of neurosurgery at a Pittsburg hospital. He notes that fit people usually have high levels of HDL ("good") cholesterol in their bloodstreams. That helps carry off the type of cholesterol that clogs blood vessels.

Several studies suggest that exercise lowers the risk of artery blockages that lead to heart attacks. Artery blockage is pretty much the same thing, whether in the heart or in the brain, Maroon reasons.

Artery blockages lead to tissue death, whether brain cells or heart muscle, Maroon says. Because of that, he sees exercise as beneficial for potential stroke victims as well as for people with heart attack risks.

Low cholesterol linked to strokes in some men

A man who has a combination of high blood pressure and low levels of total cholesterol may face an increased risk of death from a bleeding stroke, according to a new research report.

But the researchers warn that low cholesterol levels are still desirable for most people because the risk of death from heart and artery disease, or from a nonbleeding stroke, is much greater than the risk from a bleeding stroke.

For bleeding strokes, known as hemorrhagic strokes, "the death rate was highest in the lower cholesterol category (less than 160 milligrams of cholesterol per deciliter of blood volume) and decreased with increasing cholesterol levels," according to the report in *The New England Journal of Medicine* (320,14:904).

Very low serum cholesterol levels plus high blood pressure cause an increase in bleeding strokes because low cholesterol seems to weaken the walls of arteries in the brain.

Just as water under pressure seeks a weak spot in a hose to burst through, high blood pressure increases the strain on the weak walls of the arteries and increases the number of ruptures or bleeding strokes, they believe.

However, high levels of cholesterol are known to cause an increased risk of death due to heart or artery disease, and due to nonbleeding strokes.

"Within every cholesterol-level category, age-adjusted death rates for coronary heart disease were higher than for all strokes." In this study, 60.5 men out of 10,000 died of coronary heart disease compared to just 2.36 who died from a bleeding stroke.

According to the American Heart Association, only about 10 percent of all strokes result from cerebral hemorrhages, when a defective artery in the brain bursts, flooding the surrounding tissue with blood.

The loss of a constant supply of blood means that some brain cells no longer can function. The accumulated blood from the burst artery may put pressure on surrounding brain tissue and interfere with the way the brain operates.

The study seems to indicate that for a few men, high cholesterol levels are better.

For these men, the danger of having a bleeding stroke may be high enough to warrant an increased risk of other kinds of diseases caused by high cholesterol levels. That can be determined only after medical testing and talking with a doctor.

But for most people, lowering blood cholesterol is still a healthy target.

Stroke recovery hampered by some medications

Certain medications, if taken shortly after a stroke, can slow down your recovery, according to a report in *Medical World News* (31,6:11).

Dr. Larry B. Goldstein and his colleagues at Duke University Medical Center, Durham, N.C., studied the records of 58 stroke patients to determine the effects of different drugs on recovery.

Of the 58 patients, 24 took clonidine (a drug used to lower high blood pressure) at the time of their stroke or during their treatment. Patients who did not take clonidine improved more quickly than those who did.

Dr. Goldstein said he does not give stroke patients haloperidol (an antipsychotic drug) or diazepam (a tranquilizer), stating, "We're just starting to learn which drugs can be harmful under what circumstances."

Thyroid Problems

Is your thyroid too active or not active enough?

If you suffer from constipation, brittle nails and dry skin, ask your doctor to check your thyroid gland, advises Dr. David Cooper in *Medical World News* (30,19:54).

These three symptoms might be indications of an underactive thyroid gland, otherwise known as hypothyroidism. Other markers include fatigue, depression and coarse hair.

People over 60 are twice as likely to have an underactive thyroid gland as younger people, according to the report. Hypothyroidism affects about two of every 10 women and one of every 10 men past middle age. The condition is commonly misdiagnosed in elderly people, Dr. Cooper adds.

The thyroid gland is about the size of a walnut and is located at the base of the neck near the windpipe. It produces hormones that, when released into the bloodstream, help the body convert oxygen and nutrients into energy. An underactive thyroid gland doesn't produce enough hormones to keep your energy levels high.

On the other hand, an overactive thyroid gland produces too many hormones, resulting in nervousness and diarrhea. That condition is known as hyperthyroidism.

Think of it this way — "hypo" is too little and "hyper" is too much.

One reason for misdiagnosis, Dr. Cooper says, is disagreement on the normal hormone levels for elderly people.

As you age, your thyroid gland naturally may produce more hormones. However, this increased production of hormones still may not meet your body's needs, the report indicates. But the increased production may fool your doctor, who may say that your thyroid is functioning normally.

Hypothyroidism is easily treated with hormone-replacement therapy, Dr. Cooper says.

Two cautions: This therapy may cause mineral loss from bones. For those with osteoporosis, the "brittle-bone" disease, such therapy could make a bad condition worse. And second, taking extra thyroid hormone could tip you over into hyperthyroidism — too much thyroid hormone.

The treatment must be closely monitored by your doctor.

Symptoms of hypothyroidism resemble menopause

Feeling unusually tired and fatigued? Suffering from dry skin and thinning hair? Tired of that puffiness around your eyes?

Yes, you say, I am tired of all those things, but my doctor told me to expect these things during menopause.

Well, menopause might not be the problem. You could be suffering from hypothyroidism. Hypothyroidism is often misdiagnosed or underdiagnosed, especially among menopausal women, because its symptoms resemble other common disorders, warns a recent report in the *Medical Tribune* (31,21:2).

Menopausal women often mistake the symptoms of hypothyroidism for the symptoms of menopause. These symptoms include fatigue, impaired memory, dry skin, thinning hair, puffy eyes and depression.

Even if the doctor suspects and tests for hypothyroidism, the true results of the thyroxine tests are often "hidden" by estrogen therapy. Apparently, estrogen therapy can cause an abnormal thyroid test to look normal.

Researchers suggest that doctors should test for levels of thyroid stimulating hormone (TSH). This hormone level can accurately tell if the thyroid is functioning properly without the result being masked by estrogen therapy.

Avoid thyroid 'health foods,' doctors say

There's one "natural" product widely sold in health food stores and by mail that could turn out to be very unhealthy for you, say doctors at Tufts University School of Medicine and the VA Hospital in Boston, Mass. The product to avoid is desiccated thyroid, usually sold in freeze-dried, tablet form, they say.

One man with thyroid imbalances tried several times to treat himself with the health-store tablets, the doctors reported in *Archives of Internal Medicine* (149,9:2117).

He took two different "natural" thyroid preparations while he was under treatment for problems caused by Graves' disease (old-fashioned goiter, now known as hyperthyroidism). He had had his thyroid gland partially removed years before.

When he finally told his doctors that he was treating himself with the health store tablets at the same time they were trying to treat him with a thyroid hormone, he had a high heart rate, weight loss and unbalanced hormone levels. Those are symptoms of too much thyroid hormones in the blood.

Doctors analyzed the store product that had advertised itself to be free of thyroxine, a thyroid hormone that's used by doctors to treat thyroid problems.

"Despite the disclaimer, the preparation we studied does indeed contain thyroxine and can cause hyperthyroidism if taken in excess," doctors C.T. Sawin and Maria H. London write. Too much thyroid hormone can poison you, leading to seizures, heart attack or death, the doctors warn.

Many things sold as "health food products" are OK, the doctors say. "Except for the thyroid preparations, none are likely to cause harm, except for their cost. The thyroid products are another matter."

They recommend that you steer clear of such products, usually made from ground-up cows' glands.

Some health-store thyroid tablets include tissue from cow ovaries, bull testes, pancreas, prostate, liver, heart and intestines, says the *Archives* report.

Since such tablets are neither drug nor food, there are no government regulations that require minimum standards for content or purity.

Ironically, most such health-food-store thyroid tablets cost more per tablet than prescription doses of thyroid hormones bought at your pharmacy, the report says.

Ulcers

Treatment helps heal 9 out of 10 peptic ulcers

You know the symptoms. The burning, gnawing and aching feeling in your stomach means your peptic ulcer has flared up — again. The antacids relieve the pain and discomfort for a while, but you can't seem to find any long-term relief. And your doctor can't seem to find a cure.

Until now, that is.

Scientists may have found a way to prevent ulcers from flaring up in people who have histories of recurring peptic ulcers, reports *Medical World News* (31,16:17).

Scientists think that peptic ulcers might be linked to a kind of bacteria known as *Helicobacter pylori* (formerly known as *Campylobacter pylori*). The scientists' theory is that if they can eliminate the bacteria, they can eliminate the ulcers. And their research seems to support this theory.

The treatment — using an over-the-counter antacid and diarrhea fighter — seems to deliver a knockout punch to painful, sometimes life-threatening stomach ulcers.

In a recent clinical test, new "triple therapy" — bismuth subsalicylate (Pepto-Bismol) in combination with antibiotics and the ulcer drug ranitidine (brand name Zantac) — eliminated both the bacteria and the internal stomach sores in ulcer sufferers. This study indicates that healing ulcers and preventing the formation of new ulcers is linked to eliminating the bacteria. Spicy foods and stress levels apparently play much less important roles in ulcer formation than previously thought.

At a recent conference on digestive disorders, Dr. David Graham of the Houston Veterans Administration Medical Center reported that the group taking "triple therapy" only had one ulcer recurrence. But eight of every 10 people in the control group had new ulcers flare up again within six months. Everybody in the control group took only the prescription ulcer drug and nothing else.

"Accelerated healing was observed in the triple therapy group, with nearly twice as many healed at four weeks and 100 percent healed at 12 weeks, compared with 16 weeks needed for total ulcer resolution in the group given only ranitidine," Dr. Graham says in *Medical World News*

(30,12:9). Dr. Graham once was vigorously skeptical about a germ-ulcer link. Now he's a believer.

A study by Dr. Thomas Borody, director of the Centre for Digestive Diseases in Sydney, showed that patients who were cleared of *Helicobacter pylori* remained free of ulcers for 16 months. Take away the bacteria, and you take away the ulcers, the study indicates. When the *Helicobacter pylori* recurs, the duodenal ulcers recur.

Until recently, doctors have enjoyed only temporary success in the treatment of ulcers. More than 80 percent of all ulcers that were treated reappeared after the treatment ended. As a result, those with ulcers had to take continuous doses of medicine to prevent the ulcers from reappearing.

However, scientists now believe that the *H. pylori* bacterium is the key to ending this frustrating cycle. The researchers in the Sydney study found that killing the bacteria resulted in zero cases of peptic ulcer relapse at the end of one year. In other words, killing and removing the bacteria "cured" the ulcer and prevented it from recurring.

Studies show that nine out of 10 people who suffer from ulcer flare-ups have *H. pylori* bacteria present in their digestive tract. So researchers think that killing the bacteria would eliminate ulcer flare-ups in nine out of 10 people suffering from ulcer disease.

Just how someone "catches" the bacteria is not known. However, when four members of the same family developed ulcers in The Netherlands, doctors found that they all were infected with *H. pylori*. So were four other family members without ulcers living in the same home.

Since all eight people were infected with the identical strain of the bacteria, researchers believe that either they were all infected at the same time or that the bacteria can be transmitted from person to person.

Not all ulcers are associated with the bacteria, according to Dr. Lawrence Laine of the University of Southern California. For instance, he says that people with ulcers caused by nonsteroidal anti-inflammatory drugs (NSAIDs) generally aren't infected with the *H. pylori* bacteria.

Is a natural treatment for ulcers on the way?

Years ago, doctors usually had only general advice and one main treatment besides surgery for patients with ulcers. The advice was "watch what you eat." The customary treatment was "a bland diet," meaning lots of milk, little fiber and no spices.

That's changed considerably in recent years. Doctors now have whole arsenals of drug treatments for ulcer victims. And while doctors still advise us to avoid those foods that irritate the digestive system, bland diets for ulcers seem to have gone the way of cod liver oil.

But the future for ulcer sufferers may contain something of the past. Diet may again take a leading role in managing ulcer disease, according to a report in *FDA Consumer* (23,5:14). During the past two decades, the rates and severity of ulcer attacks have gone down.

Many researchers think that's because of changes in our diet, mainly a switch from animal fats and tropical oils in cooking to use of plant protein and vegetable fats. Many doctors and nutritionists have urged such changes to lower our blood cholesterol levels and reduce our risks of heart disease. The side benefit of that switch may have been fewer ulcers along the way. As a result, researchers are looking into the possibilities of natural ulcer fighters.

Vegetable oils provide polyunsaturated fats, including one essential fatty acid — linoleic acid — that the body requires for processing certain nutrients. Linoleic acid and another polyunsaturated fat, arachidonic acid, help the stomach produce hormone-like substances called prostaglandins. These prostaglandins help protect the stomach's lining and speed up healing.

Researchers hope to learn more about linoleic acid and how it contributes to this natural healing mechanism for ulcers. Your body can make linoleic acid if it's forced to. But nutritionists recommend that you take in about 2 percent of your daily calories in the form of linoleic acid. Good sources include oils made from corn, safflowers and soybeans (but not olive oil or coconut oil). Even if you are on a strict, low-fat diet, you should take about a tablespoon of such polyunsaturated oil every day, according to *Jane Brody's Nutrition Book*.

Special advice for seniors: Sometimes ulcers can strike people over 55 without the usual accompanying symptom of pain. These painless ulcers can stay hidden for a long time and do a lot of damage.

Check with your doctor about your ulcer risk and potential natural ways to manage an ulcer problem.

Common ulcer drug triggers life-threatening case of diarrhea

A 56-year-old woman almost died recently trying to avoid a stomach ulcer. Her doctor had prescribed an anti-ulcer drug, and two days later, she found herself in the hospital in a life-threatening situation.

A common side effect of some NSAIDs is ulcer disease, and many doctors try to avoid those ulcers by prescribing anti-ulcer medications, such as misoprostol.

However, for this woman, that was almost a deadly action, reports *Annals of Internal Medicine* (113,6:474).

The woman began taking misoprostol to treat the bleeding ulcers that had been caused by her NSAID therapy. Two days after she started taking misoprostol, she developed a life-threatening case of diarrhea.

She was admitted to the hospital for treatment. The misoprostol treatment was stopped immediately, and the adverse symptoms disappeared over the next five or six days.

Apparently, the woman had a mild case of inflammatory bowel disease that had gone unnoticed for several years, and she forgot to tell her doctor about it. So, the doctor prescribed misoprostol, which aggravated the bowel disease and caused the dangerous diarrhea.

Researchers suggest that people with any form of bowel disorder should avoid misoprostol treatment. You should also make sure your doctor knows about all illnesses or health conditions you have before he prescribes your medications. A complete health history will help him prescribe the safest and most effective medications for your needs.

Urinary Problems

Don't be embarrassed to discuss UTI with your doctor

Discussing a urinary tract infection (UTI) with your doctor may be embarrassing, but it's necessary. If left untreated, a UTI could damage your kidneys, according to *Lifetime Health Letter* (2,3:3) and the *Annals of Internal Medicine* (111,11:906).

UTIs affect 20 percent of the female population. They are responsible for five million doctor visits a year. Although they occur in both men and women, they are most common in women after menopause.

The entire urinary tract can become infected by invading bacteria, but the bladder is most often pinpointed, especially in women. Unhappily, one infection seems to spawn others, so your first infection probably won't be your last.

Women are the primary target of recurring urinary tract infections due in large part to sexual intercourse. This makes some women feel awkward talking to their doctor about the frequency of their infections.

The type of contraceptive used can also increase UTI risk. "Women who use diaphragms have considerably more UTIs than women who use oral contraceptives," according to the *Health Letter* report. Contraceptive foams and condoms also increase the risk slightly.

Pain and discomfort from UTIs can appear quickly. Some women report symptoms as early as the day following sexual activity.

Symptoms often vary, depending on the location of the infection, but two common complaints are a frequent need to urinate and pain during intercourse. Most often the pain is described as a burning sensation, although some women complain of a "stomach ache" right below the navel area, where the bladder is located.

Women past the age of menopause are especially prone to infections. This seems to be attributable to the thinning of vaginal and urethral tissues brought about by menopause. Fortunately, estrogen in the form of hormone-replacement therapy helps prevent thinning tissues and infections.

UTIs can be treated effectively with antibiotics, but you must see your doctor right away, especially if you've had UTIs before. Often, your doctor can do a simple test in the office rather than sending a urine sample to a laboratory. Many women who are prone to UTIs take small, regular amounts of antibiotics to ward off infections.

Drinking lots of water after intercourse will help prevent UTIs. "In effect, you're washing away the bacteria before they have a chance to cause an infection," according to the report. You should also urinate frequently throughout the day, rather than "hold it."

Since UTIs can mimic other medical problems, such as vaginal inflammation, it is important to see a doctor for an accurate diagnosis. When left untreated, the urinary tract infection can spread to the kidneys, where the potential for kidney damage can then turn the UTI into a serious health problem.

So far, studies have failed to show that bubble baths, hot tubs and swimming pools contribute to urinary tract infections.

Cranberry juice may be a weapon against urinary infections

Does cranberry juice prevent or fight urinary tract infections? Several clinical studies suggest that drinking the sweetened juice of the otherwise bitter berry may cause two changes in the body. The two beneficial changes help fight infections in the pipeline from the kidneys through the bladder.

Researchers think the juice raises the acid level of urine, causing it to become hostile to germs. They also think the fructose (a kind of sugar) used to sweeten the juice somehow makes mucous tissue inside the urinary system "slippery" to bacteria — the germs can't grab onto body tissue and multiply.

In one study reported in *U.S. Pharmacist* (14,5:35), 60 people with urinary infections drank a pint of cranberry juice each day for 21 days. Otherwise, they took no special medications.

More than half showed a significant improvement. Two out of 10 were slightly better, and about three out of 10 showed no improvement. In addition, six weeks after they all stopped drinking the juice, more than half those who showed improvement came down with another urinary infection.

Two other studies reported in the journal also showed improvements in people after they drank the juice.

Urinary incontinence in the elderly

It's troublesome, aggravating and, most of all, embarrassing. And it affects at least 10 million adults in the United States today — urinary incontinence.

It is defined as "the involuntary loss of urine so severe as to have social and/or hygienic consequences." It is a problem that should not be taken lightly or ignored. The complications of urinary incontinence include rashes, sores and skin and urinary tract infections. People who suffer from urinary incontinence also experience limitations in social activities, which can lead to isolation and depression.

According to a report in *U.S. Pharmacist* (15,3:58), there are several different kinds of urinary incontinence.

❏ **Stress incontinence** is the leakage of small amounts of urine that occurs when laughing, coughing or sneezing.

❏ **Urge incontinence** is the most common form of incontinence in the elderly. Those who suffer from this type experience a sudden need to urinate, but cannot hold the urine long enough to reach a toilet. Usually only a small amount of urine is lost, but this may occur every few hours.

❏ **Overflow incontinence** consists of a fairly continuous flow of urine — also known as "dribbling."

❏ **Functional incontinence** involves losing a large amount of urine all at once. The problem here lies in physical or mental handicaps — the person either cannot physically get to the bathroom in time, or he doesn't mentally recognize the need to urinate until it is too late.

❏ **Mixed incontinence** usually involves a combination of stress and urge incontinence. This form is common in the elderly.

Although some cases of incontinence must be treated with drugs or surgery, there are some simple at-home remedies that may help in the management of incontinence.

❏ **Pelvic muscle exercises** (Kegel exercises) strengthen the muscles that help control urine flow. To perform these exercises, contract the muscles that will stop the flow of urine. Do this ten times, relax, then do ten more. Gradually increase the number you do each day. Do this several times a day for several minutes at a time. Do not do many of these on the first day — you'll be sore the next day. Kegel exercises are successful in helping with incontinence in 30 to 90 percent of all women.

❑ **Biofeedback** is useful for management of stress and urge incontinence. People are trained to have better control over the storage of urine (check with your doctor for more information on this training).

❑ **Bladder training** helps you control incontinence voiding at regular, short intervals. Gradually, you lengthen the intervals to a maximum point that you can maintain. This remedy is especially helpful in urge and stress incontinence, and most people experience some relief using this method.

❑ **Palliative treatment** doesn't actually "treat" the incontinence, but it helps you feel less socially isolated. This treatment means using absorbent products (Depends, Serenity), external collecting devices for men (Texas or condom catheters) and bed pads.

These simple remedies may be helpful in the management of urinary incontinence. However, they are not a substitute for a medical evaluation.

If you have any trouble with urinary incontinence, check with your doctor immediately to determine the cause and discuss possible treatments.

Urinary incontinence is a nuisance, but it doesn't have to be a permanent handicap. The combination of your doctor's advice and simple at-home remedies can help you manage the problem and resume your normal daily activities.

Vaginal Infections

A cup of yogurt a day keeps the gynecologist away

Eating a cup of yogurt a day dramatically reduced recurring vaginitis in 11 women participating in a year-long study at the Long Island Jewish Medical Center in New York, according to a report in *Medical World News* (30,20:41).

Women suffering five or more episodes of vaginitis a year were eligible for the study. Simply eating yogurt was so beneficial that two dozen women refused to participate in the "no treatment" portion of the study.

"The number of infections fell from a mean of three to less than one during six months of daily yogurt consumption," according to the report. Vaginitis is an infection of the female vagina, resulting in pain, burning and uncomfortable secretions.

Not all brands of yogurt will work, however, researchers point out. Only yogurt containing the bacteria Lactobacillus acidophilus is effective.

When good hygiene's a bad idea

Douching regularly may bring on painful infections, reports *The Journal of the American Medical Association* (263,14:1936).

Researchers studied a group of women who routinely douche once a week. This group was nearly four times as likely to come down with pelvic inflammatory disease (PID) as women who douche less than once a month.

Many women rinse out the vaginal canal following sexual relations or as part of ordinary hygiene. That might be medically unsafe for some, suggests the Seattle study of 1,000 women.

Why? Because douching might flush out protective bacteria and introduce harmful germs, the scientists speculate.

Curiously, women had more problems with PID when they used disposable bottles of commercially prepared douching solutions. Women had fewer infections when they used plain water or homemade water-plus-vinegar solutions, the report says.

PID is a severe infection of the reproductive tract. It sometimes causes sterility or abscesses. Infected abscesses may rupture and require immediate surgery.

Vascular and Circulatory Problems

How to stop phlebitis and blood clots

If you sit much of the time, or spend hours on your feet without other exercise, you may be at high risk for phlebitis. That's a painful condition in which a vein becomes inflamed, and a blood clot forms.

Clots, especially in the large leg veins, are dangerous. Sometimes clots break up and travel to the lungs or heart, causing serious damage or death.

Phlebitis most often affects the legs, although it can occur anywhere in the body, says Dr. Thomas Riles, a surgeon at New York University Medical Center.

Leg injuries sometimes trigger phlebitis, but clots usually develop when people don't get enough exercise to keep blood circulating in their legs.

Police officers, teachers and bedridden patients are commonly affected. Phlebitis is more common in older people, and women get it more often than men.

Phlebitis can occur in veins close to the skin — superficial veins — or in veins deeper in the body. The deeper ones cause the most trouble.

Blood clots in superficial veins look like knots or cords and are easily seen. The vein is painful and tender. Deep-vein phlebitis causes severe pain and may involve the entire leg, not just the vein. The calf or thigh may swell and turn blue.

The good news is that phlebitis is preventable. Here are some tips from Dr. Riles:

- ❏ If you stand for long hours while on the job or have varicose veins, wear support hosiery.

- ❏ While traveling, be sure to stretch every half hour. A short walk will help keep blood circulating in your legs.

- ❏ Consider losing weight. Overweight people are more likely to suffer from phlebitis.

You can ease the pain by elevating your legs and taking aspirin. Warm compresses will also help. If infection sets in, your doctor will prescribe antibiotics.

In all cases of suspected phlebitis, see your doctor immediately. This can be a very serious condition.

Polycythemia vera — not a sign of good health

The deep red skin color in Uncle Jake that you always attributed to good health and extra sunshine possibly could be the hallmark sign of a serious blood disorder known as polycythemia vera.

This blood disorder causes the body to produce too many red blood cells, and the disorder could be life-threatening if not recognized and treated immediately.

Here's the catch — polycythemia is treatable, but it is very hard to recognize and diagnose. The most obvious symptoms of the disease are often confused with other less-dangerous conditions.

The most obvious symptom is a gradual change in skin color from the normal flesh color to various shades of red. According to *The Journal of the American Medical Association* (263,18:2481), the change in skin color is so gradual that it is often overlooked. The high red color is usually thought to be from robust health or exposure to the elements. Bloodshot eyes are another symptom of polycythemia vera. However, people often mistake them for conjunctivitis, allergies or overindulgence in alcohol.

A symptom that is unique to this disorder is pruritus (severe itching), which is occasionally aggravated by bathing. Other symptoms may include mental sluggishness, lethargy, weakness and fatigue.

The dangers of polycythemia vera, if left untreated, are the risks of thrombosis (blood clots, which could lead to strokes and heart attacks), ulcers and intestinal hemorrhages. The longer the disorder is untreated, the greater the risk of these conditions.

The good news is that polycythemia vera can be treated and managed effectively to ensure a normal lifestyle. Check with your doctor for answers to questions about the diagnosis and treatment of polycythemia vera.

Relief from Raynaud's

Raynaud's disease is associated with a decreased blood flow to the fingers and toes. The fingers or toes turn blue or white, with some degree of numbness, and they rewarm very slowly.

Raynaud's sufferers have always been advised to wear warm socks and gloves in the wintertime, but now scientists have devised a new at-home treatment plan to help manage the symptoms, says a recent report in *The Physician and Sportsmedicine* (18,3:129).

The steps for this procedure are as follows:

1) Fill two bowls with water of about 120 degrees. Place one bowl in a cold area (either a room or outdoors), and place the other in a warm room.

2) Dress lightly, as you would for room temperature. In the warm room, put both hands in the 120-degree water for two to five minutes.

3) Wrap the hands in a towel and go to the cold room. Again put both hands in the 120-degree water for two to five minutes.

4) Repeat step 2 — put hands in warm water in the warm room for two to five minutes.

5) Repeat this procedure three to six times a day for a total of about 50 trials.

Following these simple steps can give relief from the problems of Raynaud's disease.

Exercise decreases risk of blood clots

A walk in the park may be just what your body needs to help protect you from dangerous blood clots. According to a recent report in *The Physician and Sportsmedicine* (18,3:43), regular exercise increases your body's ability to dissolve blood clots.

A study at the University of Washington in Seattle shows that exercising regularly increases the activity of TPA (tissue plasminogen activator) in the body. TPA is a protein substance in the body that dissolves blood clots and reduces your chances of developing blood clots.

Dr. John Stratton from the University of Washington studied 16 healthy men from ages 25 to 74 for six months. The subjects were placed on walking, jogging or bicycling programs for the six months to observe the effects of regular exercise.

At the end of the six months, the researchers measured the amount of TPA in the blood, and they found a significant increase of TPA in the blood, especially in the older men. In fact, some of the older men experienced as much as a 39 percent increase in the amount of TPA in their blood. The greater amount of TPA in the blood reduces the risk of forming blood clots.

Dr. Stratton's study also showed that fibrin, a protein which causes blood clots, decreased by about 14 percent with regular exercise.

Since the protein fibrin actually promotes blood clots, the researchers noted that fibrin is "a clear-cut risk factor [for blood clots] in the same order of magnitude as cholesterol." And scientists say that high levels of fibrin have been connected to deaths from heart disease.

Since regular exercise reduced the amount of fibrin in the blood, the exercisers obviously had a decreased chance of developing blood clots.

The combined effects of more TPA and less fibrin in the blood work together to help protect people from blood clots and heart disease or strokes. Therefore, people who formulate an exercise program with their doctor have a great chance of preventing blood clots and avoiding heart attacks and strokes.

Researchers also have found that regular exercise can help regulate the levels of TPA and fibrin in the blood after a heart attack and help reduce the risk of a second heart attack.

Check with your doctor to develop an exercise program that is best for you.

Blood vessel disease — 'B'-ware!

If your doctor has warned you about your risk of strokes or blood vessel diseases, but you're not suffering from high cholesterol levels, vitamin B may be just what you need.

The American Heart Association reports that a metabolic defect that can lead to blood vessel disease and increase the risk of stroke may be corrected with vitamin B supplements.

The defect is known as "mild hyperhomocysteinemia." This condition results in slight to moderate elevations of homocysteine, an amino acid that circulates in the blood. At normal levels, this amino acid is harmless. But research indicates that mildly elevated levels may damage blood vessels and possibly lead to atherosclerosis (hardening of the arteries).

The American Heart Association reports that excess homocysteine seems to damage blood vessels. Homocysteine, much like cholesterol, causes sores and scars to form on blood vessel walls. If a blood clot forms on the lesions and blocks blood flow to the heart or brain, it can trigger a heart attack or stroke.

The good news is that vitamin B can help break down extra homocysteine in the blood and prevent dangerous buildups of the amino acid.

B vitamins (biotin, B6, B12) convert the homocysteine to a harmless kind of amino acid called methionine. Eliminating the extra homocysteine from the blood greatly reduces risk of blood vessel diseases.

People who have suffered from hardening of the arteries that could not be explained by high cholesterol levels are the most likely suspects for mild hyperhomocysteinemia.

But don't try to treat yourself without your doctor's advice! If you're concerned about your risk of blood vessel disease, talk to your doctor about the best type of therapy for you.

Vitamin E helps protect arteries from hardening

Vitamin E may be helpful in protecting you from atherosclerosis (hardening of the arteries), according to reports in *Medical Tribune* (31,19:11) and *Nutrition Today* (25,5:5).

Based on recent studies, vitamin E seems to help prevent the development of atherosclerosis, and it also seems to help reduce the damage if atherosclerosis has already begun.

The study in *Nutrition Today* reports that lab animals that were fed diets without vitamin E had about 79 percent more artery blockage than those animals fed the same diet but containing vitamin E.

Researchers also fed vitamin E enriched diets to lab animals that had been suffering from atherosclerosis for at least one year. After two years on a diet rich in vitamin E, the animals went from having 35 percent artery blockage to 15 percent.

Vitamin E works as an "antioxidant" in the cells of your body. This means that it prevents oxygen molecules from combining with parts of the cell that would result in dangerous products.

For example, LDL cholesterol molecules occasionally combine with oxygen molecules to create "oxidized LDLs." These oxidized LDLs seem to damage cells, and scientists suspect that they may be one of the root causes of atherosclerosis.

Researchers suggest that dietary antioxidants such as vitamin E could be a vital part of the treatment strategies for people with atherosclerosis as well as a good protection device for people seeking to avoid the disease.

Large amounts of vitamin E can be harmful, so never take vitamin E supplements without first talking to your doctor.

Salt causes brain damage?

Too much salt in your diet may be harmful to more than just your blood pressure. According to *Science News* (137,15:238), researchers think that salt may cause brain tissue damage.

Apparently, too much salt in the diet damages and narrows artery walls. These narrow arteries cut off blood supplies to the brain, which results in brain tissue damage and could lead to a stroke. Maintaining a low-salt diet can decrease the risk of brain tissue damage.

Vitamins and Minerals

Can vitamin and mineral supplements make you smarter?

We've often been told that we "are what we eat," but a new study takes that a step further. It suggests that our intelligence level may be linked to adequate amounts of vitamins and minerals.

In just one school year, tests on 90 high school students in Britain showed an increase in IQ scores in children taking nutritional supplements. Children taking a placebo (a harmless pill) and children not taking anything were used for comparison. The children receiving the supplements had a marked difference in their nonverbal IQ scores, according to *The Lancet*, a British medical journal.

Nutritionists know which vitamins and minerals aid development in different parts of our brain and body. Yet most believed that people in Western countries received adequate amounts of the necessary vitamins and minerals through their everyday diet. This is the first study that has been able to document changes in intelligence based on vitamin and mineral supplementation in people who were not technically deficient. David Benton, who conducted the study, considers the results preliminary.

If you want to start taking more vitamins and minerals, you should use supplements that contain them in the ratios set by the U.S. government and known as the Recommended Dietary Allowance (RDA).

Vegetarians need vitamins

People on strict vegetarian diets may run a greater risk of developing vitamin B12 and vitamin D deficiencies than nonvegetarians.

According to a report in *The American Journal of Clinical Nutrition* (50,4:718), a recent French study indicates that vegetarians and non-vegetarians had equal amounts of thiamin, riboflavin, folates and vitamins B6, A and E. However, the vegetarians had lower amounts of vitamin B12 and vitamin D than the nonvegetarians.

To prevent vitamin deficiencies, vegetarians should eat more foods rich in vitamin B12 and vitamin D or consider taking vitamin supplements to complement their diet.

Pills' crumbling and dissolving times are important

Have your calcium supplements passed the vinegar test?

If not, your body might not be getting the benefit of what you're feeding it, suggests a report in *Nutrition Action Health Letter* (17,5:1).

The vinegar test can show how quickly and completely your calcium tablet crumbles and dissolves. If your tablet flunks the test in vinegar, it probably won't dissolve in your body either, says the report.

Here's how to find out whether you're getting the nutrients you're paying for:

Put one tablet in a glass of plain apple-cider vinegar. That's to simulate the acid environment of your stomach, the first stop for anything you take by mouth. Time how long it takes the tablet to completely disintegrate (crumble apart). In addition, measure how long it takes for the crumbled tablet to dissolve in the liquid and become part of the liquid solution.

Crumbling time of an hour or more might indicate a problem. If the tablet hasn't crumbled by the time it leaves your stomach, the calcium carbonate probably won't get absorbed into your bloodstream, says the *Nutrition Action* report. Dissolving time of more than a half-day should be a warning sign that your body isn't absorbing the calcium, whether it's regular calcium or timed-release.

Try a similar test with your other vitamin-mineral supplements. Drop a tablet into a glass of plain water. Again, if it takes more than four or five hours to dissolve, much, if not most, of the nutrients will just pass on through your system without getting absorbed.

"Tablets that do disintegrate may not get into the bloodstream," the report quotes University of Maryland researcher Ralph Shangraw. "But if it doesn't disintegrate, that's a pretty good indication that it won't get absorbed." Shangraw calls for much quicker crumbling times — under 30 minutes.

Some brands do better than others. Supplements with potentially poor dissolving rates include generic-brand multi-vitamins and multi-minerals, timed- or slow-release tablets and big, solid pills like calcium-magnesium-zinc combinations. Some slow-release tablets may not dissolve at all.

The report tells of one supplement user who opened his septic tank for repair and discovered a layer of undissolved vitamin pills.

Generally, capsules out-perform solid tablets or pills, usually because capsules have a gelatin outer-skin that dissolves quickly in the stomach. Liquid forms, of course, are the most quickly absorbed.

Severe form of leukemia halted with vitamin A drug

French researchers report promising results in treating a severe kind of blood cancer with a concentrated form of vitamin A.

Using retinoic acid, a derivative of vitamin A, three out of four people with acute myeloid leukemia were disease-free up to nine months after treatment stopped, according to a report in *The Lancet* (2,8665:746).

Confusion may mean a nutritional deficiency

It's considered a medical emergency. Doctors see signs of mental confusion, verbal nonsense, wobbly walk, uncoordinated movements and eyesight disturbances in people with a severe deficiency of vitamin B1, also called thiamine.

"The age-old and potentially fatal nutritional deficiency ... requires immediate thiamine [B1] replacement to ensure the best long-term outcome," says an article in *Emergency Medicine* (21,7:13). "Withholding treatment for only a few hours from patients you think may have the disease may worsen the prognosis."

The condition, known medically as Wernicke's encephalopathy, can strike not only alcoholics but also people with kidney disease, patients with thyroid gland problems and compulsive dieters suffering from self-induced starvation, a condition called anorexia nervosa.

While its symptoms are serious, the disease itself "is probably totally reversible if treated early," the report said. Even a previously healthy person can drain her body's entire supply of thiamine within three weeks, the report warns. That's especially true if the person is for any reason receiving an intravenous infusion of glucose over a period of several days.

Thiamine is a water-soluble vitamin, the first of the B vitamins to be isolated in its pure form (that's why it's known as B1). Normal levels of thiamine are necessary for converting carbohydrates in food into energy, for the proper operation of the nervous system and for growth and repair of body tissues.

Thiamine is found naturally in yeast, liver, whole-grain products, wheat, eggs, milk, nuts, potatoes, kidney beans, seeds and leafy, green vegetables.

"The need for thiamine is increased when carbohydrate consumption is high," according to *Vitamin and Mineral Encyclopedia* (FC&A Publishing).

Exercise or emotional stress may increase the energy needs of the body and the body's need for thiamine. More thiamine is needed in pregnancy, during breast-feeding, when fever is present, during and after surgery and in cases of hyperthyroidism.

Other things that deplete thiamine include sulfa drugs, oral contraceptives and estrogen hormone treatments, air pollution and certain food additives like nitrates and sulfates.

Adult men normally need about 1.5 milligrams of thiamine each day. Adult women need somewhat less, about 1.1 milligrams. However, if special conditions, like those listed above, warrant, your regular thiamine intake may need to be supplemented.

Always be sure to ask your doctor or health-care provider about supplements, however, because certain people should not take thiamine. For diabetics, for example, thiamine supplements can interfere with insulin levels in the blood.

An internal insect repellent?

Taking vitamin B1 supplements, known as thiamine, may provide a natural repellent against insects.

In a small study at Michigan's Lake Superior State College, thiamine supplements seemed to protect volunteers from mosquito bites. Students took the supplement or a placebo (a fake supplement) immediately before they went out into the woods and then kept track of the number of mosquito bites they received.

There were fewer mosquito bites on people who took the thiamine. Researchers are now trying to duplicate the study with more people to confirm the results.

Some niacin cautions

High-dose niacin, in whatever form it's taken, is no longer a vitamin, but a drug, warns Denise Arthurs of the Tufts University Nutrition Center in Boston.

"At the levels recommended by popular [nutrition] books and by people in the lay public — 1,500, 2,000, 3,000 milligrams — niacin ceases to be a vitamin and is, in fact, a drug," Arthurs says. "It has side effects like most drugs do."

She urges that such high doses be taken only under the direction and constant monitoring of a doctor, reports *Medical Tribune* (31,16:14).

Niacin in high doses should be avoided by some diabetics, warns a recent report in *The Journal of the American Medical Association* (264,6:723).

Megadose niacin dramatically lowers cholesterol levels, including LDL ("bad") cholesterol. But, people with non-insulin-dependent diabetes may suffer from a niacin side effect, the report says. High-dose niacin treatment causes diabetics to lose control of blood sugar levels.

The researchers recommended caution in using nicotinic acid for these diabetics.

Vitamins and nerve damage

If you've been experiencing weakness, loss of sensory abilities, confusion and a tendency to stumble and fall, you may be short on vitamin B12.

Researchers in *U.S. Pharmacist* (15,3:78) report that these symptoms may be caused by a vitamin B12 deficiency and could result in damage to the nervous system.

However, nervous system damage can easily be avoided by eating more foods rich in vitamin B12 or with vitamin supplements to complement the diet.

Check with your doctor before you begin eating larger amounts of vitamin B12. Too much can be as dangerous as too little!

Women's vitamin deficiencies masquerade as deadly leukemia

Under the doctor's microscope, the abnormal blood cells seemed to shout one dreaded diagnosis — cancer of the blood, leukemia!

But in two cases, looks were deceiving, even to trained scientists, reports the *British Medical Journal* (300,6734:1263).

After a bone biopsy in one case showed additional leukemia-like cells, doctors at Hammersmith Hospital in London even ordered an intravenous (IV) needle inserted to start chemotherapy.

The 43-year-old woman escaped unnecessary medication when late-arriving blood tests showed she had a severe shortage of vitamin B12 (also known as cobalamin).

That shortage apparently caused pernicious anemia (a lack of nutrient-carrying red blood cells), which was successfully treated with shots of vitamin B12.

Another woman, 52, also had abnormal blood and bone-marrow cells, similar to leukemia. It turned out that she had a shortage of another B-complex vitamin, folate (known to a few people as vitamin B9; another form is folic acid or folacin). Her anemia was cured by taking extra folate.

In both cases, after the women got the needed vitamins, their blood tests returned to normal, and the leukemia-like cells disappeared. Both women had lung or airway infections when they took the blood tests. Doctors speculate that the combination of respiratory infection and anemia might have affected the test results. Such cases might not happen often, but they do point out the need for extra care in making medical judgments.

The Recommended Dietary Allowance for folate (folacin) is 200 micrograms for men over 50, and 180 micrograms daily for women past age 50. According to the National Research Council publication *Diet and Health* (1989), women tend to take in less folacin daily than men do.

Natural sources of folate include dark-green, leafy vegetables; liver; dry beans, peanuts; wheat germ and whole grains. Heat destroys the vitamin, so cooking and canning can cause very high folate losses, the report says. As much as 5- to 15-milligram supplements of folic acid daily appear safe for healthy people, according to a report in *The American Journal of Clinical Nutrition* (50,2:353). Folic acid overdose may mask symptoms of severe anemia and interfere with zinc absorption.

Vitamin B12 comes naturally only in foods of animal origin. Liver, muscle meats, fish, eggs, milk and milk products supply B12. The RDA for vitamin B12 is two micrograms for men and women over age 50. Check with your doctor before taking either vitamin B12 or folate supplements.

Boost immune response with more vitamin C

Taking a 1,000-milligram tablet of vitamin C increases body temperature, quickly floods the bloodstream with the nutrient and seems to boost the immune system's resistance to infections. So indicates an Arizona State University study in *The Journal of the American College of Nutrition* (9,2:150).

Turning up the heat is one way the body fights invading disease germs. That rise in temperature triggered by the big dose of C might be why the vitamin seems to protect some people from the common cold, suggests researcher Carol S. Johnston. In the study, healthy men and women took the equivalent of 17 times the RDA every day. They took by mouth one tablet of the sodium ascorbate form of vitamin C.

Besides raising their body temperatures, the big dose also lowered the concentration of iron in their blood. While that sounds bad, it's actually not, since germs multiply more slowly with lowered iron levels.

The raised temperatures and lowered iron levels happened only when the people took that single large daily dose of vitamin C. The same beneficial effects probably wouldn't happen if they simply took regular vitamin-mineral supplements every day, the report suggests.

That implies that you might be better off avoiding vitamin C in supplement form until you feel a cold or other infection coming on. In any event, don't take supplements or megadoses of any nutrient without checking with your doctor first.

You can get vitamin C in its natural form by eating at least two servings a day of citrus fruits, broccoli, brussels sprouts, strawberries, cantaloupe and dark-green, leafy vegetables.

How vitamin C fights heart disease and stroke

A newly discovered role for vitamin C might be fighting cholesterol plaque buildup in arteries, suggest two studies reported in *Medical Tribune* (31,16:14) and *Science News* (136,9:133).

Vitamin C stays on the job far longer than vitamin E in fighting oxidation of low-density lipoprotein (the "bad" LDL form of cholesterol). University of Texas researchers believe oxidized LDL triggers atherosclerosis, or hardening of the arteries.

Because vitamin C does such a good job of battling this cholesterol, Dr. Ishwarlal Jialal suggests that the RDA should be doubled, from 60 milligrams to 120, the article says.

Scientists at the University of California at Berkeley are also calling for an increase in the recommended daily allowance of vitamin C. Studies there also showed that vitamin C neutralizes free radicals in the blood that band with LDL cholesterol and initiate clogged and hardened arteries. Vitamin C "disarms" free radicals, these researchers say.

"I was quite surprised at how much better a scavenger of free radicals [vitamin C] was, especially when compared to vitamin E," says biochemist Balz Frei. Vitamin C performed even better than naturally occurring substances in the blood that fight toxic intruders, the *SN* report says.

Hardening of the arteries causes heart disease and some strokes.

Vitamin E helps restore muscles to healthy state after exercise

If you exercise regularly, you probably need to eat more green, leafy vegetables and more apples and apricots. These foods contain large amounts of vitamin E, and studies suggest that people who exercise regularly need more vitamin E than those who do not exercise with any regularity, reports *Nutrition Today* (25,5:5).

Due to the muscular stress that accompanies many types of exercise, most people experience slight muscle damage during exercise.

Based on recent studies, researchers report that vitamin E helps minimize tissue damage that could be caused by exercise and then helps restore muscles to a healthy state after exercise.

If you exercise regularly, talk to your doctor about your daily intake of vitamin E. He can advise you on how much vitamin E you should be taking in daily to minimize muscular damage and maximize the benefits of your exercise.

Vitamin E: who, what, where, why and how much?

- ❏ **Sources:** Green leafy vegetables, shrimp and other seafood, margarine, nuts, vegetable oils, apples, apricots, peaches, wheat germ and whole-wheat flour.

- ❏ **Function:** Promotes normal growth and development; helps reduce tissue damage after exercise; helps prevent atherosclerosis; acts as an anti-clotting agent in the blood; helps protect blood cells from oxidation (cell damage).

- ❏ **Who needs more of it:** People over the age of 55; those who exercise regularly; people with hyperthyroidism; those with alcohol or other drug abuse.

- ❏ **Effects of deficiency:** Anemia, inability to concentrate, muscle weakness or damage, irritability, lack of energy and vitality, decreased sexual performance.

- ❏ **Effects of too much:** Possible increase in level of cholesterol in the blood; increased chance of blood clots; impaired sexual function; changes in immune system responses, higher death rates.

- ❏ **Recommended daily allowance:** Men over age 50 need 10 milligrams daily; women over age 50 need 8 milligrams daily.

Source: *FDA Consumer* (24,9:31)

Magnesium: an overlooked 'miracle' mineral?

You are probably one of the eight of every ten Americans with a significant deficiency in the mineral magnesium. As an average American, you consume only about 40 percent of the daily amount of magnesium you need.

You may be subjecting yourself to higher risks of high blood pressure, diabetes, pregnancy problems in women and cardiovascular disease, including abnormal heart rhythms, according to *Science News* (133:356).

Other studies link magnesium deficiency with increased cancer risks, especially esophageal cancer, reports *Maximum Immunity*.

Recent research showed abnormally low levels of magnesium in the heart muscles of victims of sudden death from heart attacks, indicating that magnesium plays a hitherto unsuspected role in preventing or lessening the effects of heart disease, says *Popular Nutritional Practices*.

The further good news about this "miracle" mineral is that recent studies involving humans and animals demonstrated that magnesium-spiked diets decreased the bad effects of pulmonary [lung] high blood pressure, lowered blood cholesterol levels by more than one-third, dramatically reduced migraines and high blood pressure associated with pregnancies, and even prevented the formation of high blood pressure in rats that had been specially treated to make their blood pressure rise.

In another study, researchers found that intravenous solutions of magnesium given to victims immediately after severe heart attacks cut their death rate in half in the critical four weeks following the attacks, when compared to victims who received only IVs without the added magnesium.

The studies strongly suggest that all of us need to take another look at this little-known element. While it's been heralded in recent years as an anti-stress mineral, it may be much more important than we realized for maintaining cardiovascular health and for preventing other serious problems, including cancer and high blood pressure.

Because most people don't get even half as much magnesium as they need daily, according to studies presented at the 22nd annual Conference on Trace Substances in Environmental Health and reported in *SN*, "many people face serious consequences — including death — from preventable magnesium deficiency ... and contributing to the problem is that this deficiency is likely to be silent until it is severe," according to Mildred S. Seelig, executive director of the American College of Nutrition in Scarsdale, N.Y.

The studies show that higher levels of dietary magnesium not only prevent development of several serious health problems, but also play a definite role in fighting the bad effects of high blood pressure and fat-rich diets. For example, in animal tests, results showed that salt-induced hypertension was actually prevented by adding magnesium to drinking water at four to eight times the recommended daily allowances of the mineral.

In another test, rats getting increased magnesium showed few of the ill effects of high blood pressure, induced chemically in their lungs, while rats without the added mineral tripled their lung pressures, doubled their heart sizes, and suffered three to seven-fold thickening of artery walls with corresponding shrinkages of arterial diameters.

In still another test, this time with rabbits on "normal" cholesterol diets, the researchers showed that increasing magnesium levels to about five times recommended daily allowances resulted in 30 to 40 percent reductions in blood levels of cholesterols and other lipids, when compared to low-magnesium diets.

Equally significant, rabbits on high cholesterol diets got megadose magnesium and cut their blood lipid levels by more than half, the study showed. (Lipids are fats or fat-like materials.)

Migraine headaches and high blood pressure, both problems for many pregnant women, are directly linked to inadequate magnesium levels, according to an East Tennessee State University researcher.

Low magnesium levels also may contribute to stillbirths, miscarriages and low-birth-weight babies, studies with both humans and animals showed. Magnesium supplements greatly reduced such problems, the report said.

While experts believe more than eight of every ten Americans don't get enough magnesium, the highest risk people are alcoholics and those taking "water pills" (diuretics), digitalis and other heart drugs, and some antibiotics and anti-cancer drugs, according to Seelig. These substances "bind" with magnesium, prevent its absorption into the body and speed it through the body without letting it have its good effects. Such high-risk people need to check with their doctors about getting a special higher daily supplement of magnesium, the studies suggested.

Soft drink fans also may not absorb enough magnesium because of the "binding" effect of the phosphates contained in most sodas. For example, a regular 12-ounce soft drink may bind up to 30 milligrams of magnesium and flush it out of the body before it can do its good work.

The recommended dietary allowance (RDA) of magnesium is 350 milligrams for males over 18 and 280 milligrams for females. The RDA for pregnant women and lactating (milk-producing) mothers is even higher — 355 milligrams, according to the RDA published by the National Research Council.

Three or four soft drinks a day could cause significant deficiencies in magnesium absorption, even in those few people who take enough of the mineral every day.

Good dietary sources of magnesium are leafy, dark-green vegetables, whole-grain cereals, figs, lemons, grapefruit, yellow corn, almonds and other nuts and seeds, apples and seafoods.

However, experts say it's hard to get enough of the mineral just by eating the right foods. They suggest that everyone consider taking a daily supplement in tablet form. One researcher said magnesium would be the one supplement he would recommend for everyone.

You should take magnesium in equal amounts with calcium, several studies said. It can also be bought as magnesium oxide (you get 150 milligrams of magnesium from one 250 milligram tablet of magnesium oxide).

It's commonly available in tablets of 133.3 milligrams and may be taken four times a day. Take between meals because magnesium neutralizes stomach acid (remember milk of magnesia?) and acts like an antacid.

Few studies show any poisonous effects of higher-than-RDA doses of magnesium. Experts suggest no more than 3,000 milligrams per day for patients who suffer kidney dysfunctions.

One study suggested huge doses of the mineral could be linked to excessively low blood pressure and depressed breathing in a few cases. Any long-term use of magnesium in megadoses should, of course, be done only with your doctor's knowledge and permission. Strong indications are that you will be seeing much more in the near future about this overlooked "miracle" mineral.

In summary, magnesium has been shown in recent studies to do the following:

- **Prevent formation of salt-induced high blood pressure.**

- **Cut blood cholesterol levels by more than one-third.**

- **Stop migraines in pregnant women.**

- **Cut death rates in half for post-heart-attack patients.**

- **Prevent formation of several forms of cancer.**

- **Increase oxygen use by muscles, leading to better fitness.**

- **Regulate body's blood sugar metabolism, raising energy level.**

- **Fight depression and act with calcium as a natural tranquilizer.**

- **Help prevent heart attacks.**

- **Aid in stopping calcium deposits, kidney stones, and gallstones.**

- **Keep teeth healthier.**

Needed: more of that other 'M' mineral

Most of us need more of another "trace" mineral: manganese. It's an important fighter against osteoporosis (dangerous bone loss among older persons, especially women over 50). It also acts like a traffic cop to insulin, signaling how much to produce and when to release it into the bloodstream, and helps heal tissue damage caused by ozone and other environmental pollutants.

Studies reported in *Science News* (130:199) indicate the body has trouble absorbing manganese even when we eat enough of the right foods. Further, even the recommended dietary allowance (RDA) of 2 to 5 milligrams per day may be too low.

A University of Texas research project showed that you must eat at least 3.8 milligrams each day to keep from running low on the mineral.

The problem is that other ingredients in manganese-rich foods — like spinach, wheat bran and tea — cause the mineral to slip through the digestive tract without much of it being absorbed. The manganese present in meats, milk and eggs, though in smaller amounts than in other foods, is more easily absorbed, which makes these "bio-available" sources of the mineral more important in a nutritious diet. A better approach may be to take manganese supplements in the form of daily tablets, but watch when you take it and with what other minerals.

Studies show that mineral supplements containing iron, calcium, and magnesium cut down on the body's absorption of manganese. So if you take a manganese supplement, wait several hours before taking other kinds of mineral tablets.

The tip-off to the link between bone problems and manganese deficiency occurred to biologist Paul Saltman after he studied the chronic bone fractures suffered by basketball superstar Bill Walton. X-rays showed Walton had a form of osteoporosis, resulting in continuous bone loss and breakage. Blood tests showed the athlete had no manganese and half the normal levels of zinc and copper. The researcher took Walton off his macrobiotic diet and put him on mineral supplements, and within six weeks Walton resumed his career playing basketball. The mineral plays an important role in helping specialized cells break down old bone tissue and replace it with new bone cells. A manganese deficiency weakens the bone-building cells, resulting in increasingly porous bones and symptoms of osteoporosis, the report says.

Another study of Belgian women with severe osteoporosis showed the women had one-fourth the manganese levels in their blood as women of the same age without the bone disease.

The moral of the story is clear: Supplement your diet with manganese, being careful not to take it with blocking agents like magnesium, iron and calcium, phytate and fiber in bran, oxalic acid in things like spinach, and tannins in tea.

Eat fresh fruits and veggies for proper balance

Some scientists have suspected that higher levels of the mineral potassium might help protect you against intestinal cancers. Now an animal study suggests that it's the ratio of potassium to sodium in the body that gives you protection. The higher the potassium-to-sodium ratio, the better, indicates a study in *Nutrition and Cancer* (14,2:95).

Researchers found that rats with four times as much potassium as sodium in their supplemented diets had one-eighth the number of intestinal tumors as rats fed a diet containing only twice as much potassium as sodium. Taking in much more potassium than sodium also helps keep your blood pressure under control.

Nutritionists recommend that you get at least 1,600 to 2,000 milligrams per day of potassium in your diet. That's not hard if you eat a lot of unprocessed fruits and vegetables and fresh meat.

Getting too much potassium can be as bad as getting too little. A daily intake of around 18 grams (that's 18,000 milligrams) can cause serious heart disturbances, even cardiac arrest. Check with your doctor before taking potassium or any kind of dietary supplements.

Low selenium levels linked to cancers, digestive ills, asthma

Men seem to be more sensitive than women to a deficiency of the mineral selenium. Men with low levels of selenium in their blood were more likely to develop cancers of the lung, stomach and pancreas, reports the *Journal of the National Cancer Institute* (82,10:864).

That finding comes from a big, 10-year Finnish study of nearly 40,000 men and women. Women had a marginally higher risk of cancer because of low selenium, but not nearly so much as men, according to researcher Paul Knekt. Men who averaged 59.1 micrograms of selenium per liter of blood had the highest risk of cancer. Men with an average of 62.5 micrograms had the lowest risk, the report says. People in Finland, a Scandinavian country bordering the Soviet Union, don't get much selenium in their diets, the report says.

The U.S. Recommended Dietary Allowance (RDA) for selenium is 70 micrograms daily for men over 50, and 55 micrograms for women 51 and above.

Low selenium levels also seem to be linked in some way to bladder cancer. Thirty-five people developed bladder cancer out of a group of 25,802 people that researchers were keeping tabs on. Those with bladder cancer had significantly lower blood levels of selenium than people who were cancer-free, according to a study reported in *Cancer Research* (49,21:6144).

In another Scandinavian country, Sweden, researchers measured blood levels of selenium in people who were being treated for diseases of the heart and digestive system. The biggest shortages were found among people with digestive diseases. People with stomach and intestinal diseases might have selenium deficiency, the report indicates. A selenium shortage could further harm their immune systems and delay their recovery.

Two studies suggest that low selenium levels might contribute to the development of asthma. People with symptoms of asthma have low levels of selenium in their blood and blood plasma, says a British study reported in *Clinical Science* (77,5:495).

In New Zealand, people with the lowest levels of selenium are twice as likely to develop asthma as those with the highest levels. Also, those with low levels of glutathione peroxidase had five times the asthma risk as those with high levels, says a study in the British scientific journal *Thorax* (45:95). Glutathione peroxidase is a natural anti-inflammatory enzyme produced by the body. Selenium forms part of the chemical makeup of this enzyme, which battles the inflammation of lung tissues caused by asthma. A New Zealander typically gets less than 30 micrograms a day of selenium.

Selenium apparently works closely with vitamin E, a powerful antioxidant, to neutralize harmful free radicals circulating in the blood.

Natural sources of selenium include salmon, tuna, swordfish, shrimp, lobster, oysters, whole grains and sunflower seeds. Brazil nuts are an especially rich source, mainly because they are grown in soil high in selenium. In fact, a quarter-ounce of Brazil nut meat — about the size of one nut — provides 76.8 micrograms of selenium, well above the RDA. But, be aware that one Brazil nut is about 85 percent fat, and one-third of that is saturated fat.

Check with your doctor before taking a selenium supplement. Even small amounts of selenium above the RDA can cause side effects like nail damage, hair loss, nausea, diarrhea, skin odor, fatigue, irritability and even damage to the nervous system, says *Recommended Dietary Allowances, 10th Edition* (National Research Council).

Zinc can help you live longer

Low levels of zinc can reduce your body's immune response and increase your risk of infections. But too much zinc can reduce the effectiveness of copper, iron and other minerals in your system.

A recent study in *Journal of Nutrition for the Elderly* (8,1:3) indicates that the RDA provides enough zinc to keep a normal person's immune system responding well without harming the needed absorption of other minerals. Adults should get 15 milligrams of zinc daily, the RDA according to the federal government. Liver, seafood (especially herring and shell-fish), dairy products, meat, whole grains and eggs are good sources of zinc, while vegetables are poor sources of zinc.

Adequate zinc consumption may actually help to lower death rates. That's because a less healthy immune system results in more infections among elderly people. And more infections result in higher death rates for seniors.

In tests in hospital patients, people with healing problems like leg ulcers or pressure sores also had the lowest levels of zinc in their bodies, reports the *British Journal of Nutrition* (59,2:181).

Zinc also may help prevent "macular degeneration," a deterioration of the nerves in the eyes. In a study at the Louisiana State University Eye Center, older adults who took zinc supplements for up to two years had less eye deterioration than people who didn't receive the supplements.

In addition, zinc also has been reported to help fight cancer and skin disease, to improve the sense of taste, and to shorten the length of the common cold, says the *Journal of Nutrition for the Elderly* (8,2:49).

Aging alone does not cause low levels of zinc, according to *The American Journal of Clinical Nutrition* (48,2:343). Older people, especially those in institutions, aren't getting enough zinc because they don't eat as much food as they used to. A study at Bowling Green State University found that "dietary zinc intakes were inadequate in 67 percent" of the elderly.

The journal *Human Nutrition and Applied Nutrition* (40,6:440) reports that in one acute medical care ward studied, the meals served by the institution provided only about one-half the RDA of zinc — even if the patient ate everything on the plate!

Phytic acid, found in grains and other dietary fiber, interferes with the absorption of zinc, so people on high fiber or vegetarian diets may not get adequate amounts of zinc. Normal cooking "decreases the phytic acid content and improves zinc absorption," says the *Journal of Nutrition* (117,11:1898).

Zinc supplements above the RDA interfere with the body's metabolism of copper and iron. "Many women might be at risk for iron deficiency" even with supplements of less than four times the RDA of zinc, says *The American Journal of Clinical Nutrition* (49,1:145). Decreased levels of copper, which helps in the formation of bone, hair and skin and is important in the formation of hemoglobin and red blood cells, are also caused by excessive doses of zinc supplements.

While the proper amount of zinc greatly helps the body's immune system, too much zinc has the opposite effect. Excessive intake of zinc is suspected to impair the immune system's response, says *The Journal of the American Medical Association* (252,11:1443).

Too much zinc also lowers the level of "good" cholesterol known as HDL, according to *Metabolism* (34:519).

Consuming the RDA of zinc is essential for good health. But high doses should be avoided because of its effects on other minerals and because of possible negative effects on cholesterol levels and the immune system.

Older Americans need more vitamins D and B6

Elderly Americans, especially those who are bedridden, may need higher amounts of vitamin D to prevent rickets-like disease, according to a report in *Drug Therapy* (19,8:63).

Studies suggest that the older you get, the less efficient the skin is at producing vitamin D. In addition, the intestines cannot effectively absorb supplements, the report says.

Sun exposure increases vitamin D production in the body, but in one study, even people living in sunny climates had lower vitamin D levels.

Older Americans need to eat more vitamin D-rich foods — milk, cod liver oil, egg yolk, butter fat, and salmon and cod livers.

If you are over 50, you may be short-changing yourself on vitamin B6, suggests a report in *The American Journal of Clinical Nutrition* (50,2:391).

Recommended daily allowances (RDAs) of vitamins and minerals are based on the needs of young, healthy adults, say Danish researchers. The current RDA for B6 is 2.0 milligrams for men and 1.6 milligrams for women.

The researchers suggest that RDAs for the elderly be based on the older person's individual needs. Those needs likely are different from those of a young person.

The scientists are particularly concerned about vitamin B6, the levels of which decrease in the body with increasing age, sometimes leading to a deficiency. Vitamin B6 promotes healthy skin, red blood cells and teeth and gums.

Researchers encourage older people to eat more fruits, vegetables and potatoes. A carefully balanced, healthful diet usually ensures the right amount of B6 and other vitamins. But people who don't get enough nutrition from their regular diets may need vitamin B6 supplements, the report says.

Weight Loss

Being overweight can hurt your chances for a long and healthy life

In addition to detracting from your appearance, being more than 15 percent overweight can lead to many health problems including joint disease, coronary artery disease, stroke, high blood pressure, high cholesterol levels, diabetes, gallstones, gouty arthritis, osteoarthritis, cancer, skin problems, breathing difficulties, sleep apnea, kidney disease, increased risk during surgery, increased risk of complications during pregnancy and a delay in the discovery of abdominal diseases.

Obesity also leads to — believe it or not — traffic accidents, according to a report in *The American Journal of Clinical Nutrition* (49,5:993).

Being overweight is just one more risk factor that raises your chances of becoming ill. For example, high blood pressure increases your stroke and heart-disease risk; smoking increases your heart-disease risk even more. If you're overweight, you can raise the odds on stroke and heart disease and add diabetes to the list.

"On the whole, diet plays a very important part in the development of [heart disease], cancer and diabetes," the report says. One last reminder: "[Diet] becomes even more meaningful if the harmful effects of heavy alcohol drinking are taken into account."

More to lose than weight

Scientists have found a new weight-loss incentive for all those would-be dieters who haven't gotten serious about their diets yet.

The results of a recent study reported in *The New England Journal of Medicine* (322,13:882) suggest that all women who are mildly to moderately overweight have a risk of heart disease 80 percent higher than women who maintain their ideal body weight.

Weight gain during adulthood increases the risk of coronary disease. And the older you get, the greater your risk becomes. These results indicate that being overweight is a major cause of death from heart disease among women in the United States.

Weight loss: Your sex and age are a factor

Weight loss is guilty of both age and sex discrimination. That's the finding announced by the Centers for Disease Control in Atlanta, a federal health agency. Young women gain more weight than young men, but older women lose more weight than older men, according to the new CDC study.

Due to reduced physical activity and other lifestyle changes beginning in early adulthood, men and women between ages 25 and 34 are likely to gain an average of seven pounds over their next 10 years.

But the CDC research shows that just over six percent of adults in that age group will gain nearly 30 pounds over a 10-year period — putting them at a substantially greater risk of high cholesterol, high blood pressure and heart disease.

Younger women are more likely than men of the same age bracket to add extra weight. The average American male can expect to pick up an additional 6 pounds between his 25th and 35th birthdays.

The average woman will gain about 7.75 pounds during that same decade. And while about 4 percent of the younger men will gain more than 30 pounds in 10 years, women of the same age are nearly twice as likely to gain this much excess weight, the CDC reports.

In the first nationwide study of its kind, investigators from the CDC analyzed data on 9,897 adults aged 25 to 74. Each person's weight was recorded twice over a 10-year period. Nearly 13 percent of the 25- to 34-year-old adults in the study who had started with normal weights had become overweight 10 years later.

Researchers found that the average adult tends to gain weight until about age 55, regardless of the sex of the individual — but the incidence of major weight gain is roughly twice as high for women as it is for men. Interestingly, it was the skinny guys who were most likely to put on added pounds. "The men in the study who were underweight during their first weighing had the highest risk of major weight gain," according to the report.

However, among women, the ones who were fat just got fatter. Women who were overweight at the first weighing had the highest risk of major weight gain over the next decade.

In the study, a 20 percent increase in body weight was considered a major weight gain. In other words, a man who weighed 175 pounds in the first weighing period and then put on 35 pounds over the next 10 years would qualify as a "major" weight gainer in the study.

"After age 55, however, both men and women tend to lose weight," said CDC study director David Williamson. "We found that individuals lose an average of two to 10 pounds between the ages of 55 and 64, but in this age group, women actually lose more weight than men. For some reason, women seem to be more extreme in both trends."

The CDC researchers believe that the weight gain experienced by most younger adults is potentially hazardous to health, even if it doesn't lead to obesity. "Most of the weight being gained by younger adults is in the form of fat, not muscle," Williamson warned. "We want to emphasize that the process of gaining weight can increase the likelihood of high cholesterol levels or high blood pressure, even if you aren't classed as obese."

Physical activity needs to be a bigger part of weight control — diet alone is seldom enough, the investigators say. "The weight gain that begins in early adulthood may be a direct result of changes in the average person's exercise habits," Williamson said. "Teenagers typically are very active, but physical activity often tapers off in adulthood."

The best time to deal with the problems of body fat and being overweight is before they occur, Williamson stressed, "because, as anyone knows who's ever tried it, it's very difficult to lose weight once you've gained it. It may be easier to keep it off in the first place."

The danger of yo-yo dieting

The more often you diet, the harder it is for you to lose weight, a new study reports. Not only that, but there's a danger to on-again-off-again dieting. Losing weight quickly, then gaining it right back, may increase your risk of sudden death from heart disease, according to a new study by researchers at Northwestern University.

"Men who showed the greatest up-and-down weight swings also had the highest risk of sudden death from coronary heart disease," says weight loss expert Dr. Kelly Brownell of the University of Pennsylvania School of Medicine.

Weight loss and weight gain, known as weight cycles or yo-yo dieting, is a way of life for many people. However, researchers are discovering that yo-yo dieting may be more harmful than not losing weight at all.

Here are some of the pitfalls of yo-yo dieting:

❏   It may slow your body's metabolism and make it more difficult for you to lose the weight again. Studies on animals by Dr. Per Bjorntorp of Sweden found that losing and regaining weight greatly increases "food efficiency."

The report in *The American Journal of Clinical Nutrition* (36,3:444) defines food efficiency as how much weight is gained compared to the amount of calories that are consumed.

Only if someone was facing starvation would this natural defense mechanism be helpful. Under normal circumstances, "increased food efficiency" simply makes dieting more difficult.

In *Physiological Behavior* (38,4:459), Brownell explains, "frequent dieting may make subsequent weight loss more difficult." In his study, animals that went through two cycles of weight loss and weight gain, "showed significant increases in food efficiency" in the second weight loss/weight gain period.

"Weight loss occurred at half the rate and regain at three times the rate in the second cycle. ... At the end of the experiment, cycled animals had a four-fold increase in food efficiency compared to obese animals of the same weight who had not cycled." The tests show, in other words, for every new weight-loss diet you try, it's likely you'll lose weight more slowly and regain it more quickly.

If your diet is successful and you do lose weight, you'll have to eat a lot less from now on than you're used to eating. Tests by Dr. Jules Hirsch of Rockefeller University in New York reported in *Metabolism* (33,2:164) also show that obese people who have lost weight on a diet require less energy (or calories) to maintain their body weight.

"In order to maintain a reduced weight, some reduced-obese ... patients must restrict their food intake to approximately 25 percent less than" what would be expected for their new, lighter body size, Hirsch says.

❒ Yo-yo dieting usually shifts weight from your hips and thighs to your stomach, where it is more dangerous to your health. A fat stomach or waist is linked to an increased risk of stroke in men and higher rates of heart failure in both sexes, according to researchers from Boston University, reports *Natural Healing News* (1,2:1).

❒ Yo-yo dieting actually may increase your desire for fatty foods. Studies by Reed and Rodin reported in *Physiological Behavior* (42,4:389) found that animals on a severely restricted diet chose more fatty foods once they were taken off the diet. Since fatty foods are less healthy for us, an increased desire for fats "may have negative health consequences."

❒ Yo-yo dieting may increase your body's proportion of fat to lean tissue. According to Brownell's Weight Cycling Project, when people lose a lot of weight by dieting — especially on crash diets or low-protein diets — they lose muscle tissue along with the fat. However, when they regain the weight, the addition usually comes back as fat, not as muscle, Brownell says.

This is a good reason to combine diet with exercise — exercise will help you to lose fat and not muscle so you'll be less likely to gain the weight back. "The addition of exercise in the diet treatment did show an effect in weight and fat loss," reports *The American Journal of Clinical Nutrition* (49,3:409).

Yo-yo dieting strains your body and increases your risk of sudden death from heart disease. But for many people, a permanent weight reduction is a good thing. The point is to keep the weight off once you lose it. That may mean eating about one-fourth less calories from now on — a permanent diet, instead of a yo-yo diet.

Before going on any diet, check with your physician first. And be sure to work with your doctor or health-care provider to discover a safe weight-loss and weight maintenance program that you can follow — from now on.

Learn to suppress your appetite naturally

If overeating is your problem, learn these tricks to suppress your appetite and control your weight.

Drink a glass of grapefruit juice, tomato juice or unsweetened lemonade as an appetizer about 20 minutes before you eat. The acid in the juice and the volume of fluid that you drink will help you feel full, and you will be able to eat less.

Throughout the day, you can drink lemon-water as a natural appetite suppressant. Just add the freshly-squeezed juice from a lemon to a glass of water. Slowly sip on this drink throughout the day. Drinking just two glasses of lemon-water a day will help you control your appetite.

Place a bottle of mouthwash in front of your refrigerator door, suggests the Good Wellness Program for Weight Management. If you stray into the kitchen looking for "something to eat," you will have to move the mouthwash first.

Use the mouthwash before taking anything out of the fridge. Rinsing with the mouthwash may help satisfy the cravings without consuming any calories.

Try squeezing your earlobe for 60 seconds before you eat. This is an ancient technique of acupressure that may help curb your appetite.

Also, be sure to eat slowly. Put your utensils down after each bite. It takes several minutes for the stomach to tell the brain that it is full. Eating slowly will help you realize you're full before you overeat.

Easy 'OJ diet' might help you lose weight

You don't need to send off for it if you see an ad for an "orange juice diet." That's because you've got the whole diet right in your supermarket produce section or chilled juice case.

It's simple: Scientists have discovered that water mixed with fructose suppresses your appetite better than glucose with water or even diet drinks. Fructose is the kind of sugar found in fruits.

Drink a glass of fructose-rich orange juice a half hour to one hour before a meal, the results suggest. You'll eat fewer calories during the next meal and still feel comfortably full, indicates a Yale University researcher in *The American Journal of Clinical Nutrition* (51,3:428).

The diet drink, glucose-water and fructose-rich fruit juice all seem to work as appetite suppressants. It's just that fructose works better than sugar-water, and the glucose-water works better than drinks flavored with the low-calorie sweetener aspartame (brand names NutraSweet and Equal). Plain water was least effective of the four.

In the Yale study, overweight men who drank fructose-rich orange juice ate nearly 300 fewer calories at lunch. Overweight women consumed an average of 431 fewer mid-day calories. Their intakes were compared with similarly overweight men and women who drank plain water before lunch.

Even when the participants switched fruit drinks, the results were the same. The people drinking the fructose-sweetened lemonade mixture ate fewer calories than those drinking the other lemonade-flavored mixtures.

But what about the calories in the fructose drink itself? You might well ask. Since the fructose drink was about 200 calories, the net calorie suppression was about 100 to 230 calories per meal. That still puts the orange juice diet ahead of its glucose, aspartame and plain water competition.

If only for one meal a day, that still adds up to a savings of 700 calories a week or 36,400 calories a year, certainly enough to make a difference over the long run. Long-term, slow weight loss is the healthiest form of weight loss for most people.

The diet benefit, however, doesn't carry over to soft drinks sweetened with high-fructose corn syrup. People who drank a lot of aspartame-sweetened diet drinks reduced their intake of calories from sugar more than those who gulped regular, high-fructose soda pop, says a report three months later in the same journal (51,6:963).

Caution on the 'grapefruit diet'

It took three months of vitamin and mineral treatment to pull a 47-year-old New York woman out of a diet-caused nose dive into anemia, fatigue, leg swelling and abdominal pains and bloating.

She had used the so-called grapefruit diet for two years and had lost about 50 pounds, but her health had faded during the process, according to a doctor's report in *The Journal of the American Board of Family Practice* (2,2:130). She had been eating unrestricted breakfasts, dinners and snacks but nothing at lunch but a grapefruit.

Her doctor found that she suffered from an iron deficiency, causing anemia, and a severe case of vitamin B12 shortage. The doctor put the woman in the hospital and gave her a red cell transfusion to beef up her blood.

For the next three months, the doctor put the woman on a regular nutritional diet with the addition of a multivitamin supplement, one milligram of folic acid by mouth daily, iron sulfate by mouth twice a day, and monthly injections of B12.

A year later, the woman was still eating balanced normal nutritious meals, had regained her energy and had kept her weight to within five pounds of what she weighed when she first saw the doctor, the report said. What she discarded, the doctor said, was the grapefruit diet.

Raise resting metabolism rate with exercise

You've argued with your conscience about it before. You know you need to lose some weight, but you're afraid to diet because dieting is supposed to lower your metabolism so much that you gain all the weight back. It's a legitimate fear. But now that fear appears to be unfounded.

Until now, scientists have thought that people who lose weight through low-calorie diets ended up in a catch-22 situation: Losing weight slows down the body's resting metabolic rate. Your resting metabolic rate is the amount of energy needed to maintain basic body functions, such as breathing and heart beat.

A slower metabolic rate is your body's way of coping with less food. It helps the body function normally with a smaller amount of food. The problem is that a slower metabolism makes it easier to gain weight and harder to keep off those unwanted pounds.

However, studies now are showing that exercise can help restore a healthy metabolism, says *The Journal of the American Medical Association* (264,6:707).

Apparently, people who lose weight by combining a low-calorie diet and exercise will experience a drop in their metabolism at first. In fact, the exercise may even increase the initial drop. However, after a few weeks of this routine, the metabolism springs back to a level that is normal for their new, lower body weight.

The new metabolism will be slightly slower than the original metabolism. However, the new metabolic rate is perfect for the new body weight.

So, dieters should not be concerned about a plunging metabolic rate. As long as you exercise, your metabolic rate will spring back up to a healthy level that will suit your new, thinner body.

Thirty minutes of daily exercise can burn off 150 to 200 extra calories a day according to *Stay Healthy* (3,12:46).

And here's more good news from *Good Health Bulletin* (2,3:2): Regular exercise also keeps your heart healthy by producing an enzyme that breaks down fats in the bloodstream.

Exercise helps you maintain, not lose, weight

You've just started a new exercise program and are excited because the exercise is going to help you lose weight, right?

Well, researchers have added a new twist to that theory. According to a report in *The Physician and Sportsmedicine* (18,7:113), exercise is not a big help in losing weight — you would have to walk about 22 miles to lose one pound. However, exercise is extremely helpful in helping you keep the weight off once you've lost it through eating less. Exercise also helps you lose fat, not muscle, so you'll be less likely to gain the weight back. Exercise should be viewed as a "weight-maintenance tool" rather than as a weight-loss tool.

It is fairly common for people who have lost some weight to gain it back simply because they didn't begin an exercise maintenance program. On the other hand, those who commit themselves to an exercise program after their weight-loss program are usually successful in keeping the old pounds off.

Lose weight by changing when you eat

How about a weight-loss diet that lets you eat everything you're eating now? Would you try it?

Most people can shed unwanted pounds by changing the time of day they eat, according to *Postgraduate Medicine* (79:4,352). Eating earlier in the day could let you lose as much as 10 pounds in a month.

More than 600 volunteers lost between five and 10 pounds each in one month in a study done by Tulane University researchers. The participants didn't change what they ate, just the time of day it was eaten. Breakfast and lunch became the main meals of the day, with only a light snack in the afternoon. People in the study could not go to bed at night within eight hours of their last meal. The researchers speculate that eating the major part of our daily calories early in the day allows the food to be used to produce energy; therefore, fewer calories are left over to change into fat.

Dieting is more effective when the calories are consumed earlier in the day, a study by Dr. Frank Halberg at the University of Minnesota confirmed. People on 2,000-calories-per-day diets lost 2.2 pounds per week if they ate all 2,000 calories at breakfast. But people who ate the 2,000 calories at dinner gained weight or lost very little.

How you sleep can affect your weight

Sleeping in a cold room can increase weight loss, reports *Harper's Bazaar*. Just as exercise helps burn off calories, having your body work to maintain its normal temperature will help you lose weight while you're sleeping. Helping your body to "exercise" during a comfortable sleep cannot be considered a rapid diet technique, but in the long run, it can help burn off unwanted calories.

A cool room at night with fresh air circulating is also thought to contribute to a good night's sleep.

Dieters' blues

If you're tempted to eat everything in sight each time you open the refrigerator, try a blue bulb. The color blue often helps curb an overactive appetite, says a digest in *Vitality* (4,3:N6). Installing a blue light bulb in your refrigerator may help curb your appetite and prevent you from eating yourself out of house and home.

Help reverse drug-induced impotence by losing weight

Many men who take diuretics or "water pills" to help control their hypertension suffer from a physically and psychologically unpleasant side effect — sexual impotence.

But scientists may have discovered a way to reverse this aggravating side effect. Moderate weight loss may help reverse the drug-induced sexual problem, suggests a report in *Science News* (138,12:189).

In a recent study, 35 men who suffered from drug-induced impotence went on diets and lost an average of about 10 pounds each. All but three of the men who lost the weight reported obvious improvement in erectile ability. In other words, 90 percent of the men in the study who lost weight experienced relief from the drug-induced sexual impotence.

Researchers suggest that men who suffer from drug-induced impotence should talk with their physicians.

The doctor can prescribe a safe diet that will help the men control their hypertension as well as lose weight to reverse the drug side effects.

Being too thin may shorten your life span

Being thin is not as in vogue as it used to be, especially if you are between the ages of 55 and 74, says the *Archives of Internal Medicine* (150,5:1065). Apparently, it's better for elderly people to carry a few extra pounds rather than be underweight.

Researchers are finding that older skinny people are up to 1.6 times more likely to die than medium-weight or overweight people. Being overweight caused more problems than being too thin only when the extra weight complicated high blood pressure or diabetes (two weight-related conditions).

When are you too thin? Researchers from this study defined the average height for men to be 5 feet 9 inches and the average height for women to be 5 feet 4 inches. Average-height "thin" men weighed under 149 pounds, and "thin" women of the average height weighed under 126 pounds.

Ask your doctor to help you determine your ideal and healthiest weight.

9 D's of dieting

If you aren't trying to lose weight, but the pounds are dropping off nonetheless, should you be concerned? Yes, doctors say, if you've lost 5 percent of your normal body weight over the last year.

You should check with your doctor, for example, if you are a 170-pound man who's lost 10 pounds, or a 125-pound woman who's lost 6.5 pounds unexpectedly.

But before you see your doctor, you can help him by taking a look at the major causes of weight loss in the elderly, according to a recent outline in *Geriatrics* (44,4:31). If you are having any of these problems — called the nine D's of elderly weight loss — tell your doctor.

The more information you can provide, the less time and money you will spend on unnecessary tests to find the cause of your weight loss.

❑ **Dentition**. This is a fancy word for dentures and teeth. Poorly fitting dentures may make chewing painful and eating a less pleasurable activity. Always clean your dentures well; "dirty dentures" may affect taste. Gum disease also affects taste, so regular dental checkups are in order, even if you wear dentures.

❑ **Disease.** Some diseases, such as heart disease and cancer, sap the body's strength and may lead to weight loss. If you have such an illness, talk to your doctor about what you can do to keep up your appetite.

❑ **Dysgeusia.** Another fancy term, this means that as you age, your abilities to taste and smell diminish, which in turn takes the pleasure out of eating. Certain drugs, such as theophylline, may add to the problem. Try adding more herbs and spices to your food.

❑ **Depression.** This is one of the most common causes of elderly weight loss and affects one in 10 older Americans. Lifestyle changes, such as retirement, loss of a spouse and health or financial problems, may trigger depression. Once you recognize depression, however, it can be treated.

❑ **Diarrhea.** People who suffer from diarrhea usually eat less to avoid it. Diarrhea is always a symptom of another condition, and once it's treated, your appetite should return.

❑ **Dysphagia.** This means difficulty in swallowing, coughing or sneezing. People with nervous disorders such as Parkinson's disease often have dysphagia. Some may have the sensation of food sticking in their throat. The condition is treatable.

❑ **Dementia.** People suffering from dementia, such as Alzheimer's patients, are not able to watch their food and beverage intake and may let themselves get hungry and thirsty. They may not enjoy eating and have trouble swallowing. These people need assistance when dining.

❑ **Dysfunction.** Dysfunction means the social causes of weight loss: An elderly widower who never learned to cook for himself; a widow trying to save money; or elderly people who have no transportation to the grocery store or who fear walking on icy sidewalks or in dangerous neighborhoods.

❑ **Drugs.** Antidepressants and diuretics, among others, may cause dry mouth, which interferes with taste and swallowing. Other drugs, such as theophylline, may cause stomach upset. Still others affect taste and smell. If you are taking medication, ask your doctor about its side effects.

Concluding Remarks

The power of prayer

The secrets in this book are based on medical reports of natural healing, but don't overlook the *supernatural* healing power of God. God is our Creator and Master Physician.

If you put your faith and trust in God, by following Jesus Christ, we believe that your prayers for healing will be answered according to God's will.

Although God may not answer "yes" to every request, there is ample evidence of the power of prayer that is submissive to God's will.

Not only are there many anecdotal reports of unexplained miracles, but one scientific study reported in the *Southern Medical Journal* (81,7:826) has shown that prayers to "the Judeo-Christian God" were effective in treating seriously ill hospital patients.

Researchers studied 393 people admitted over a ten-month period to a hospital's coronary care unit. After the patients agreed to participate in the study, the doctors randomly assigned 192 of them to an "intercessory prayer group." This was a group of Christians praying outside the hospital for the sick people.

The group of patients who was prayed for had fewer health problems than the other group even though there was no significant difference in the two groups before they entered the hospital. The people who weren't prayed for required ventilatory assistance, diuretics and antibiotics more often than the "prayed-over" people.

The data seem to show that prayer has a beneficial effect on people admitted to a coronary care unit.

If you would like to know more about how to know God and have eternal life through a personal relationship with Jesus Christ, please write to FC&A, Dept. JC 99, 103 Clover Green, Peachtree City, Georgia 30269. We believe getting to know God better will change your life!

INDEX